Media Environments
and Mental Disorder

Media Environments and Mental Disorder

The Psychology of Information Immersion

WILLIAM INDICK

McFarland & Company, Inc., Publishers
Jefferson, North Carolina

The research presented in this book was supported (in part)
by funds from a Summer Research Stipend from the Research Center
for the Humanities and Social Sciences at William Paterson University,
as well as from William Paterson University's Assigned
Released Time for Research Program.

LIBRARY OF CONGRESS CATALOGUING-IN-PUBLICATION DATA

Names: Indick, William, 1971– author.
Title: Media environments and mental disorder : the psychology
of information immersion / William Indick.
Description: Jefferson, North Carolina : McFarland & Company,
Inc., Publishers, 2021 | Includes bibliographical references and index.
Identifiers: LCCN 2021017440 |
ISBN 9781476678825 (paperback : acid free paper) ∞
ISBN 9781476642512 (ebook)
Subjects: LCSH: Mental illness—Psychological aspects. | Mass media. |
BISAC: PSYCHOLOGY / Mental Health | COMPUTERS /
Design, Graphics & Media / General
Classification: LCC RC455.4.B5 I53 2021 | DDC 616.89—dc23
LC record available at https://lccn.loc.gov/2021017440

BRITISH LIBRARY CATALOGUING DATA ARE AVAILABLE

ISBN (print) 978-1-4766-7882-5
ISBN (ebook) 978-1-4766-4251-2

Front cover image © 2021 Metamorworks/Shutterstock

Printed in the United States of America

McFarland & Company, Inc., Publishers
Box 611, Jefferson, North Carolina 28640
www.mcfarlandpub.com

For Sophie Drake

Table of Contents

Preface

Victims of Sight, Victims of Sound

A medium creates an environment.
An environment is a process; it is not a wrapper.
It's an action, and it goes to work on our nervous system
and on our sensory lives, completely altering them.

—Marshall McLuhan (1966)

Media—the means of communication among people—make victims of us all. The media are invasive. They invade our senses. We have little control. Advertisements surround us. We cannot avoid or un-see them. The sounds of radio and public address systems envelop us; we have no "earlids" to shut them out.[1] One can attempt to "tune out" the media, but it's difficult, as media are contrived and constructed to capture and hold our attention. When my children are at a restaurant with a television on, they cannot *not* watch it ... nor can I.

Most people can only tune out media by tuning in to another form of media. Thus, the phones and gadgets come out, even in places that are permeated with media, such as nightclubs and theaters, and even in the company of others with whom we're *supposed* to be socially engaged. This afternoon, as I ate lunch in the campus cafeteria, I spied a college student sitting across from me. This student was sitting with a group of peers, but he was not speaking or looking at them. There were television monitors scattered across the cafeteria, an "MTV University" program on the screen, with pop music emanating from the speakers. He occasionally glanced at the TV screen, but he wasn't really watching or listening to the broadcast. He was mostly staring at his iPhone, visually engaged. Simultaneously, he had earbuds in, aurally engaged. I saw that he was tapping his feet in rhythm to the music that he was listening to, but he also had a textbook open, and seemed to be splitting his visual attention between his book, the TV, and his phone. He was engaged in at

1

least four different media simultaneously: three visual and one auditory. I also noticed that his cap and t-shirt were covered with logos advertising sports teams, and that both of his arms were covered with tattoos displaying symbols of various forms. In short, this young person was completely saturated with media: over the surface of his body, on the actual skin of his body, in his sense perceptions, and inside his mind. There was literally no place in which to stuff more media. His body itself, covered with tattoo images and logoed clothing, seemed to be a medium in-and-of-itself for various companies, organizations, and designs. The invasion, in this sense, was complete. Media, the environmental imperialist, came, invaded, and conquered the young man: body, mind, and soul. He was a victim of sight and sound ... but a *willing* victim?

Marshall McLuhan wrote that a fish has absolutely no concept of water, because the fish is entirely saturated and immersed within a water environment, and has never experienced the "anti-environment" of water ... dry air.[2] So too, we're all saturated and immersed in media environments, to the extent that we're largely unaware of the media that surround us, and how they influence our minds and behaviors. The danger of ignorance towards our media environments is very real, and quite severe. If we understand the brain as a sophisticated electro-organic network molded by millions of years of evolution to help us adapt to our ever-changing environments, then we can understand "mental disorder" as a pathology of adaptation. The "mentally disordered" person is someone who is maladapted to his environment, making him sad, angry, or anxious; and causing maladaptive, self-destructive, and often antisocial behaviors. Furthermore, if the modern environment is defined not so much by physical obstacles and goals, as in ancient times—such as a deer to hunt or a field to plow—but by media obstacles and goals—such as an email to write or a lecture to present—then the media we consume and utilize must have critical effects on our mental health, up to and including the point at which media become the cause of some, or even most, of our so-called "mental disorders." Given that nearly half of all people in the U.S. meet the criterion for a diagnosis of mental disorder at some point in their lives,[3] there is clearly something gravely wrong in the way that we as a species are interacting with our environment. In this book, I explore the effects of media on "mental disorder." My purpose is to reveal the invisible environments that surround our bodies and infiltrate our minds. I explore the notion that much of what we consider to be "mental disorder" may in fact be interpreted as adverse reactions and maladaptations to our media environments.

I'm in no way a Luddite or a proponent of banning any form of media. Not only do I think those stances to be impractical and largely impossible on a population level, I also think that they simply won't work; just as prohibiting alcohol didn't work to solve the problem of drunkenness; just as the "War on Drugs" didn't solve the problem of substance abuse; and just as censorship can never solve the problem of "obscenity." I also don't think it's feasible or advisable to require media corporations such as Facebook, Twitter, Instagram, Google, or the corporations that provide media software and hardware, such as Apple, Microsoft, and Samsung, or the corporations that provide internet service, such as Verizon and AT&T, to limit or self-censor either the content of the media they disperse, or the extent or nature of the media themselves. Corporations are and always will be primarily concerned with profits, and to expect a corporation to adopt and perpetuate a primary concern for the mental health of its customers is naïve—it would be like expecting a lion to self-impose limits on its own prey—or expecting a leopard to change its spots. Corporations provide us with our media environments, but we live in them, and we must accept the responsibility of learning to adapt to them even as the modern media environment constantly changes at breakneck speed.

I believe that understanding the nature of our media environments and how they affect our mind and behaviors is the next frontier in the field of psychology, and that this new approach to psychopathology may allow us to reduce and eventually eliminate our dependence on psychopharmaceuticals for the treatment of mental disorders—a dependence that even the most script-happy psychiatrist must admit has spun out of control—especially for the tens of millions of children who take powerful psychoactive substances every day just to adapt to a specific media environment that they have difficulty adapting to (school). My hope for the future is that we as a species will understand how our media mold our thoughts and behaviors, so that we can adapt our media environments to the unique and infinitely diverse minds of our children, rather than chemically altering their brains with potentially toxic and dangerous drugs in order to force their minds to conform and adapt to media that are inhospitable to their ways of perceiving and understanding the world. My wish is for us to cease allowing ourselves and our children to be victims of sight and of sound, first by understanding the media environments that envelop us, and then by controlling these media so that they adapt to us, rather than the other way around.

Our entire species as a population are the subjects of an unprecedented mass experiment. The independent variable is that of digital media, a new stimulus abruptly introduced to the whole population over the past few decades. The method of experimentation is the complete revolution in which we communicate and use information, a revolution that has dramatically changed nearly every aspect of our lives. There are no controls. The experimenters are not psychologists or scientists, they're global corporations such as Apple, Samsung, and Microsoft, whose only interest in the experiment is financial profit. The dependent variable is our own sanity. The results of the experiment are not being comprehensively measured by anyone, though we're all rather curious about the outcome. If the results are ever measured and an outcome concluded, it will not happen in time to affect us adults, but we may have time to figure out better outcomes for our children. Children are the real subjects of the experiment. They were born into it, having never been exposed to a media environment other that the digital one we live in now. Children are at once the least aware of the media surrounding them, and the most affected by them. We owe it to them to begin analyzing this grand experiment, and to start administering some controls. We need to figure out better ways for them to grow up in a world saturated with media that they didn't create, and which they don't understand, even though they'll be forced to immerse themselves in this media in order to survive.

Introduction

The Hall of Mirrors

Environments are not just containers, but are processes that change the content totally.

—Marshall McLuhan (1965)[1]

No environment is perceptible, simply because it saturates the whole field of attention.

—Marshall McLuhan (1966)[2]

The most basic form of media, and also the most invasive, is the human voice. Modern parents never cease to complain about their "media addicted" children. Their complaints transcend their physical voices digitally, flowing out in a never-ending stream of emails, texts, tweets, blogs, posts, and chats. However, there's very little wonder why a child would prefer a TV show or videogame to a person. People's voices can be intrusive, obnoxious, and annoying. Unlike a TV show, they cannot be paused, muted, rewound, fast-forwarded, stopped, restarted, or turned off. People, such as parents, speak when speech is unwanted, say messages that children don't want to hear, and make demands that children don't want to meet. The media of the TV show, on the other hand, is completely controllable. The medium itself is amusing, non-judgmental, patient, and undemanding. While the TV invites attention, it doesn't demand it, as the parent does—nor does the TV request that other rival media be turned off—while the parent tiresomely does so. No wonder a child prefers TV to Mom or Dad. We parents get annoyed with our children when they refuse to disengage from various media— but we provided them with these distractions, knowing full well that they elicit deep immersion engagement, and that splitting attention among rival media causes distractedness, aggravation, and hostility. When users are pulled out of their preferred medium (e.g., television), there may be aggravation and hostility toward the new medium, the parent.

We adults express the same preference for nonhuman media, every time we choose to go to an ATM rather than a bank teller, every time we purchase something online rather than in person, every time we send a text message instead of speaking to someone face-to-face, and every time we spend the evening networking on Facebook or Instagram, rather than spending time with actual people. Nonhuman media are in so many ways less stressful, more efficient, and even more pleasurable than interactions with actual people. In the modern media environment, humans are perpetually fighting nonhuman media for the attention of other humans, such as our children, spouses, students, and friends. Humans are at a distinct disadvantage, and are losing ground by the minute, as new media increasingly become more adaptive, more pleasing, more interactive, more instantaneous, more powerful, and more engaging. And while adults can remember life before digital media, children cannot. The next generation of the human species will not even be able to conceive of an environment that isn't saturated with infinite and instantly accessible information. Like McLuhan's fish, children are the least aware of their media environment, and they are the most affected by it. Like the fish, they're entirely dependent on the invisible environment they're immersed in, and their minds are molded by that environment.

In this book, I will trace the development of media from the most basic forms—the sights and sounds expressed by the human body—to the most technologically complex media created to date, the digital media that shoot through the atmosphere into space, bounce off satellites, and rain down to saturate the Earth. As each medium of communication is explored, I will suggest how it is related to specific "mental disorders," using the categories and nomenclature designated in the current edition of the *Diagnostic and Statistical Manual of Mental Disorders* (the DSM-5), as a standard reference point. I'll propose how each form of media actually *creates* certain mental disorders. The reasoning behind this paradigm is quite simple. The media we use create our information environments. New media create new environments. Our brains must immediately adapt to these new environments in order to harmonize our behaviors with our surroundings. Since our environment, to a large extent, is shaped by the way we perceive, understand, and communicate information, then we can think of mental disorders as symptoms of maladaptation to our media environments.

In Chapter One, the rationale for a new model of mental disorder is provided, by pointing out the deficiencies of prior models, and the benefits of a "media ecology" model.³ In Chapter Two, an underlying neurological model for the way that media influence the structure and connectivity of the brain is revealed. The model is based on the premise that certain functions related to media—such as language—are lateralized in the left hemisphere of the brain. As our media environments increased in sophistication over the course of evolution, the brain adapted to them by shifting language functions increasingly towards the left hemisphere of the brain. This "leftward shift" hypothesis underlies the theory that media in their different forms are both indirectly and directly causing many mental disorders, by engendering a functional imbalance between the hemispheres of the brain. Each subsequent chapter studies specific disorders in relation to the various media affecting them, within the framework of the leftward shift hypothesis. The development of the disorders in relation to the historical changes in media that have influenced them, up to and including the influence of digital media in the present day, are also traced.

Beginning with Gutenberg's revolutionary invention, print technology extended the influence of literacy around the globe, changing the media environments that almost all humans are obliged to adapt to, and in turn, changing the human mind. Without print, mass literacy would not have been possible. Without mass literacy, the progress of human learning and ingenuity would not have proceeded past the intuitive wisdom of the ancients. The Enlightenment, the Industrial Revolution, and the modern Information Age were generated and propelled by the ability of people to learn, understand, and disseminate mass amounts of standardized information quickly and expediently over vast distances. Over the past five centuries, the effects of print technology have molded the shape of the modern world, and also the way that we understand and express ourselves. These revolutions in culture and society are mirrored by neurological changes within the human mind—epigenetic adaptations to the new media environments that have enveloped us. Chapters Three and Four explore the provocative theory that the neurological adaptations human brains have undergone in order to foster the revolutions in our media environments that have made the modern world possible, have—as unwanted and unforeseen side effects—created maladaptions to these media environments, in the form of autistic and schizophrenic minds.

Chapter Three explores the notion that in order to accommodate the neurological functioning required for abstract intellectual analytic thought, the brain has become so left-hemispheric dominant in some people that vital right hemispheric input is inhibited to the point of pathology. The pathology, in this case, is referred to as "autism." The leftward shift hypothesis will be applied to the growing epidemic of autism spectrum disorder, a pathology that currently affects 1 in 68 children,[4] with numbers continuing to rise. If the influence of such media as language, literacy, and print have been driving higher order cognitive processing leftward for over a million years, then autism would represent the endpoint of this process: a mind that is dominated by left hemispheric thought, to the over-exclusion of right hemispheric input.

Though the steep increase in the diagnosis of autism is largely attributable to changes in the awareness and diagnostic criteria of the disorder, the sheer vastness of the increase suggests that something causative may be going on in the environment. Diagnoses of autism rose from 1-in-5,000 in 1975 to 1-in-68 in 2014.[5] My son, right now, is 74 times more likely to be diagnosed with autism than I was when I was a boy his age. The leftward shift hypothesis suggests a spectrum of variation in the expressions of the genes that control for lateralization of language in the brain. Some people's brains will be lateralized more strongly to the left than others. Autism, I suggest, represents the far end of the spectrum, a brain that is lateralized so far to the left that the critical input from the right hemisphere, especially in relation to social cognition and behavior, is inhibited to a pathological degree.

Nevertheless, though there is clearly a neurological and almost certainly a genetic root to autism, the underlying environmental factors—media—are still at play, both at the broad level of the entire species over the course of a million years of evolution, and also at the narrow level of the individual child living in today's media environment. The brain of the infant and small child is very "plastic" and moldable, with most of its higher order connections for language and thought un-configured until late in childhood. If the child's media environments, including the current electronic and digital media, really do influence the process of hemispheric lateralization (the neurological "wiring" of the brain and the balance of processing between the hemispheres), then an understanding of how these environments affect thinking, combined with a knowledge of the child's genetic neurological predisposition, could help us to design more adaptive media environments for these children. This could reduce or even eliminate the neurodevelopmental causes of autism in millions of children.

Chapter Four explores the theory that in order to accommodate the neurological functioning required for language, the mind had to "split" itself in two, by inhibiting some forms of communication between the left and right hemispheres of the brain. The "split mind" that has emerged as a result of this neurological adaptation gave birth to a growing number of individuals whose "split" is incomplete, resulting in the maladaptive overlapping of two separate simultaneous streams of verbal thought emanating from the twin hemispheres of the brain. The product of this unwanted and dissonant "cerebral feedback" are the hallucinations, delusions, and thought disorders that are symptomatic of schizophrenia.

Chapter Five focuses on the disorders created by oral language—or more specifically—disorders created by the function of internalized language, otherwise known as private verbal thought, or more simply, as the "voice of consciousness." Anxiety and depression are disorders that are made possible by the ability of humans to dwell and ruminate upon their own existences as figures in an ongoing narrative that has a long past, an uncontrollable future, and an inevitable but unpredictable end. Language, the intellectual tool that empowered humans to conquer the world, inflicts upon its bearers the unfortunate "consequences of consciousness," experienced as "hyperconscious" ruminations upon our own depressing shortcomings, and anxiety-inducing predictions of future failures and pitfalls. In short—without language there would be no consciousness—and without consciousness there would be no anxiety or depressive disorders.

Chapter Six explores the consequences of literacy, the medium that extends oral language via reading and writing. When a culture adopts a medium such as literacy so completely and so unconditionally that every individual who cannot completely master the medium is considered mentally disordered, then we must consider that culture to be intolerant towards individuals with those neurological dispositions. Our culture requires that all children must go to school. The media environment of schools is dominated by the medium of literacy. Children whose minds are not neurologically disposed towards mastering literacy are diagnosed with "intellectual disabilities" and "learning disorders" such as dyslexia. Behavioral disorders such as ADHD could also, to a very large extent, be considered syndromes consisting of behaviors that are elicited as reactions to a media environment that forces children to master a medium that they are simply not neurologically predisposed towards mastering. Simply put, there would be no such thing as learning disorders, intellectual disability, and ADHD, if children weren't forced to go to school, and forced to master literacy in schools.

Electronic media is generally unidirectional. We listen to the radio or a CD. We watch TV or a movie. The information streams in one direction—towards us—and we are the passive consumers of the media content. Literacy is also, generally, a unidirectional experience. We read a book or an article, but few of us actually write books and articles. When we do write, our writing is almost always a one-to-one correspondence such as a letter, text, or email to a colleague or friend. Digital media, however, allow all of us to actively engage in bidirectional and one-to-many correspondence. When we use a digital social media site such as Facebook, for instance, we not only see pictures posted by others, we post our own pictures that are seen by others. Such media are bidirectional, as the user is both the consumer and the generator of the media content. The media also transcend the limits of one-to-one correspondence by providing a many-to-many dialogic transmission system, in which many users can interface with each other simultaneously. So, unlike a letter sent from one person to another, a Facebook post can be seen by an enormous number of users, who can then reply to the user who generated the post, initiating dialogues of postings that can host almost endless readers and responders. In short, digital media in general and social media in particular are true revolutions in the history of communication, forever changing the way we interact with each other and exchange information. The psychological impact is vast. The effects of digital media and social media are explored in Chapter Seven, which focuses on the ways that these new media extend our senses of self into the ether, drastically reshaping our perceptions of our own identities.

Images of our person, once a private matter, are now public. Images and videos of ourselves that exist on the internet are accessible to countless other persons on the planet. We also have unprecedented access not only to images of other people, but to endless amounts of both public and private information about other people. The internet has unlocked the closets of our personal lives to the world, baring to everyone the skeletons within. Privacy is an obsolete concept. The sense of self that was once an inner world of self-conscious experience is being extended outwardly into the ether, where it comingles in virtual space with the extended selves of so many others in our digitalized species. The effect on our psyches of the new media can be seen in the burgeoning of various mental disorders of the self.

In an age when humans interact more with machines and computers than with other humans, when information takes precedence over communication, we experience a sense of depersonalization that, in extreme cases, leads to disorders of dissociation. A dissociated state is when someone experiences a period of time in which they are cut off and separated from their own identity. As a reaction to the modern state of communication and interaction, when real and meaningful social connections are being abandoned in favor of anonymous digital interfaces between distant strangers, it's no wonder that some people are becoming strangers to themselves. And in a time when people's identities are deconstructed, digitized, and projected into the ether as objects of desire, adulation, spectacle, scorn, and ridicule, we should not be surprised when our children begin to view their own bodies as alien objects, and when they treat these unhuman objects callously by mutilating, starving, exposing, exploiting, and otherwise objectifying their own bodies. The primary focus of Chapter Seven is the connection between social media use and the phenomenon of narcissistic personality disorder, as well as other issues related to a sense of disconnection with the self and with others, issues that I argue are directly linked to social media use.

To borrow yet another metaphor from McLuhan, if we imagine the mythical Narcissus gazing spellbound into the reflective media of the still water, his response is numbed and desensitized, as the water has a "narcotic" effect on him. (McLuhan pointed out that the name "Narcissus" comes from the same Greek root as the word "narcosis.") The narcotic numbness is sustained by the fact that Narcissus is unaware of the medium he's engaged in (his reflection in the water). He's therefore unaware of the allure of the content of the medium (himself). Narcissus is under the false impression that he's gazing at someone else, and it's the uncanny but unconscious recognition of his own self in the mirror that fixates and hypnotizes him.[6] Narcissism, in this sense, is not just about self-adoration, it's about *obliviousness* towards one's own self-adoration. However, if Narcissus were to be temporarily pulled away from the water and made aware that the water itself is a medium, and that the content of the medium is himself; Narcissus would be disabused of his illusion, disenchanted from his trance, relieved of his narcosis, and freed of his addiction to the reflective medium. The illusion that media present us with—*the central metaphor in this book*—is the illusion that media connect us with others. In truth, all media merely reflect our own thoughts and feelings about ourselves...

Every Medium Is a Mirror

When we gaze at a screen, the initial image we see before we turn on the device is the true content. That shiny black screen is a mirror, reflecting our selves. Once the device is turned on, the magic ether conjures alluring images of what we believe are others, and the illusion begins, as does our narcotic fixation on the illusion. In this media-saturated environment, drowning in our own illusions, we could either sink or swim. We can learn to float, stroke, swim, and even sail. We can find balance and harmony in this all-encompassing saturating environment, or we can drown in it. Fully adrift in the Digital Age, we spend entire days and entire lives staring at screens ... gazing into the mirror. We find ourselves in Narcissus's predicament, unwittingly addicted to our own reflections, desperately lost in a hall of mirrors.

Returning once again to McLuhan's fish metaphor, if we assume a problem in the fish's environment is causing maladaptation, the most obvious solution—taking the fish out of the water—is, unfortunately, not viable. Just as total water deprivation is impossible for the fish, total media deprivation is impossible for the human being. Like it or not, we created the media environment we live in, and we're going to have to adapt to it. That realization doesn't make us helpless. In fact ... it empowers us. The all-important questions are:

> 1. *How can our awareness of the effects of our media environments help us adjust to their influences?*
> 2. *How can we adjust our media environments to make them more adaptive to us?*

This book focuses on the first question. It's an inquiry into the psychological effects of our media environments, as well as an attempt to raise awareness about this issue. The next question—*What can we actually do about it?*—is addressed briefly in the Conclusion to this book, but that subject is too vast and important to leave as an afterthought, which is why I'm doing research for a follow-up book, on media mindfulness.

• ONE •

A Media Ecology Model of Mental Illness

> *The divided nature of our reality has been a consistent observation since humanity has been sufficiently self-conscious to reflect on it. That most classical representative of the modern self-conscious spirit, Goethe's Faust, famously declared that "two souls, alas! dwell in my breast…" it seems like a metaphor that might have some literal truth. But if turns out to be "just" a metaphor, I will be content. I have a high regard for metaphor.*
> *It is how we come to understand the world.*
>
> —Iain McGilchrist (2009)[1]

Before a problem could be dealt with, a model for how the problem came about and how it could be solved is necessary. The model isn't "real" in any way … it's a metaphor that helps us see the problem from a certain perspective. If something is unknown to us, the only way to make it known to us is by comparing it to something we do know, hence the need for the metaphor. The metaphoric model is indispensable. There is literally no other way we could understand the problem. However, the specific model in use must change as our understanding of the problem changes; otherwise, the model becomes outdated and must be abandoned in favor of a newer, more pertinent model.

That moment when an individual, a group, or even an entire society realizes that the old model is no longer working and abandons it in favor of a newer model is known as a "paradigm shift," which often fosters "revolutions" in thinking or behavior. The moment in history several hundred years ago when Western societies such as England, France, and America realized that the old model of monarchic rule should be abandoned for a new model of democratic rule sparked various revolutions in governance, some bloody and tumultuous, others more smooth and peaceful.

Resistance to a paradigm shift comes from individuals who are so heavily invested in the old paradigm that they cannot imagine letting it go. King George III, for example, was resistant to the independence and self-rule of the English colonies. Generally, these individuals believe that the old model is the only model that could work, and that no other viable model could ever replace it. That kind of resistance to change is dangerous, as it will halt the progress towards the creation and adoption of newer and better models, in favor of the comfort and security of the status quo. Nevertheless, when enough people realize that a new model is more suitable than an old model, the paradigm shift will inevitably happen, regardless of the resistance to it. I believe that the time has come for a new model of mental disorder; a model that focuses on the effects that media have on our mind and behavior. Before presenting this model, I would like to review the other models of mental illness that preceded it, in order to explain why a new model is needed.

The Demonology Model

The oldest, most universal and—in some parts of the world—still the most prevalent model of mental disorder is "Demonology," the idea that maladaptive behavior has at its source the influence of demons or malicious spirits, either within us or around us. Evidence of the practice of trepanation, the intentional drilling of holes into the skull in order to release the malicious spirits within, is revealed by the archaeological discovery of early Neolithic skulls across multiple continents that have precisely round holes bored into them. (These head-holes could not have occurred naturally, accidentally, or as the result of random violence.) The holes offer physical evidence of the belief in demonology that goes back at least 7,000 years. Written records and illustrations of the practice trace the belief in demons through the Neolithic and the various metallic ages into the Dark and Middle Ages right through to the modern day, where it's still practiced in certain remote corners of the world. However, the most common (and least invasive) demonological procedure for the correction of misbehavior was cure through a spiritual or religious ritual, such as an ordeal or exorcism (oftentimes being one and the same).

Though we think in metaphors, we don't necessarily recognize the fact that our models for the world, and our models for ourselves in the world, are metaphorical. It may be easy for us to recognize that a person from a primitive culture who thinks about mental disorder as an affliction in which an individual's soul is possessed by demons, is using a model for mental disorder that is outdated and unhelpful. We can see that because we recognize the basic elements of his model—the soul and demons—as metaphors or symbols for our own psyches. Yet, at the same time, we ourselves may not be able to recognize the fact that our own understanding of mental disorder is also purely metaphorical—an abstract model of thought—which is also outdated.

There's a tendency for people to think of mental disorders in the same way that we think of physical injuries, like a broken arm or a burst appendix. This conceptualization is flawed, because the names we apply to mental disorders such as "Depression" and "Anxiety" and "ADHD" are really just metaphors for all sorts of thoughts, feelings, and behaviors that psychologists have decided to group together under specific categories as a means towards developing treatment models. The categorization is necessary, but when we begin to think of the categories as real physical ailments, like broken arms and burst appendixes, we lose sight of the true nature of mental disorder, and thus devise and cling to models of mental disorder that are not apt, outdated, and unhelpful. We must remember that mental disorders are not physical ailments; they are metaphors that we devised out of thin air to reflect upon our own minds and behaviors.

Somatogenesis

Following demonology, the next metaphorical model for mental disorder is somatogenesis, the belief that mental illness is caused by an imbalance of bodily fluids, or a bodily malfunction. This metaphor is epitomized by the model developed by the ancient Greek physician, Hippocrates, who claimed that both mental and physical health are dependent on the proper balance of the four fluid "humours" in the body: yellow bile, black bile, blood, and phlegm. Hippocrates' model was forgotten in the Dark Ages, but revived in the Renaissance, and then forgotten again. Ironically, this now-ancient metaphor for mental health and mental disorder has some remarkable similarities with the current neurochemical model that now dominates the field of clinical psychology and psychiatry. In particular, the modern belief that mental health is dependent upon a proper balance of neurotransmitters—in particular the four cardinal neurotransmitters, serotonin, dopamine, norepinephrine, and acetylcholine—is eerily similar to Hippocrates' model of the four humours.

Also, and possibly more significantly, Hippocrates' model predates the notion of a Cartesian split between body and mind, which assumes that the body and mind are quite disparate parties, that function and exist on different planes. Hippocrates' model assumes that the mind (our thoughts and feelings), is simply a product of the brain (the physical organ inside our skull). Since the brain is merely another part of the physical body, the same principles that govern the functioning of the body also apply to the functioning of the brain, and therefore the mind. The modern neurochemical model is based on a similar metaphor, that is: the mind is a function of the brain, which is a function or part of the body no different in principle from the rest of the body. Just as the body is governed by physical entities such as blood, organs, and neurochemicals; so exactly is the brain. There is no Cartesian split; the brain and body are one.

Though I admit that, obviously, the physical brain is part of the physical body, I must insist that there is indeed a body/mind split, though not strictly Cartesian. The brain is quite unlike the body in that it's constantly adapting itself to its environment in real time. The brain at any given moment is evolving and changing via the process of adapting (or "rewiring") its neural connections. The physical body is incapable of real time evolution, or nearly instantaneous adaptation to its environment. For instance, it's thought that it took millions of years for our hominid ancestors to evolve thumbs with the precision grip adaptive for the creation and use of stone hand tools. The process of physical adaptive evolution of the body is excessively slow. However, a human brain can adapt itself to the use of a new tool at a remarkably fast pace. Just see how long it takes a toddler to master the use of a relatively sophisticated tool, such as the iPad or iPhone.

Similarly, if I lose my arm in an accident and it's not immediately reattached by a surgeon, I'll never be able to use that arm again. However, if I lose a part of my brain due to a stroke or aneurism, the brain will immediately begin the process of rewiring its own neural circuitry in order to process the same function done by the damaged part of the brain, using a different part of the brain. Thus, while the brain is admittedly a physical property like the body that contains it, in function—specifically in its ability to evolve, adapt, and change itself, i.e., its "plasticity"—it's remarkably *dissimilar* to its physical host. Hence, the product of the brain, the metaphysical functioning of the mind, is really much different from the product of the body, the physical functioning of somatic body parts. The Hippocratic model of somatogenesis is therefore an outdated model.

Psychogenesis

By the late 19th century, the dominant view of mental illness was psychogenetic, the view that mental illness was caused by a combination of genetic and psychological factors. Though this model was indeed enlightened, it was too broad, and desperately in need of more precise models to fill in the spaces. How do genetics actually predispose someone to mental disorder? What psychological factors are in play?

As psychological factors are influenced by the individual's environment, how does the environment come into play?

These questions were addressed by a myriad of models, most of them fascinating, all of them wrong. There was the popular theory of "Degeneration," based on the premise that the process of evolution had reversed itself and that human beings were devolving into baser, less sophisticated beings. There was Mesmer's theory of "Animal Magnetism" or "Mesmerism," the belief that the body and mind were controlled by invisible magnetic forces, and that mental disorder could be cured via the adjustment of such forces. There was also "Phrenology," the belief that mental and moral character could be assessed by measuring the shape, size, and topography of different areas of the skull. There was no shortage of theories for how and why mental disorder exists, and how it could be dispelled, but all of them seriously fell short of explaining anything comprehensively.

Psychoanalysis

It was Sigmund Freud, at the turn of the 20th century, who offered a modern attempt at a comprehensive psychogenetic theory of mental illness. Specifically, Freud argued that mental activity was split into dual regions, the conscious and the unconscious. In order to live respectable lives as members of society, humans must constantly repress their unacceptable sexual and aggressive drives. Forbidden incestuous urges, murderous oedipal fantasies, and repugnant lecherous cravings must not be granted conscious awareness, but instead must be perpetually walled off in the penal antechamber of the mind—the unconscious storehouse of inhibited desires, unremembered dreams, forgotten fantasies, and repressed memories. Severe anxiety (referred to as "hysteria" in Freud's day), as well as depression and other forms of neurosis, were all the result of unconscious drives offending or assaulting an under-defended ego.

Freud's model was breathtaking in originality, astounding in scope, miraculous in insight. It was a true paradigm shift, pushing forward the field's thinking about mental disorder such as no other single model had ever done before, or since. Freud, as no one else has done, revealed ourself to ourselves. He pointed out that the human psyche is, indeed, a metaphor for the self. Consciousness and unconsciousness, id and ego, conscience and libido—these are all metaphors for our own sense of duality, our own sense of unknowingness, our own attempt to understand ourselves, to control our own thoughts and desires, to know who it is that speaks our thoughts to us, and to subdue them, in order to banish forever those unwanted ideas and feelings from the kingdoms of our minds, and to capture and keep prisoner in perpetuity that one feeling we all desire but find the most elusive—happiness.

In demonstrating that the human mind is pure metaphor, Freud revealed a deeper truth to our existence, but didn't necessarily solve the problem of mental disorder. Indeed, while a generation of well-off neurotics who were able to afford psychoanalysis did reap its benefits, the vast majority of people who suffered from mental disorder either suffered in silence or found solace in a bottle. Those who suffered serious mental disorders in the first half of the 20th century simply wasted away in asylums, hidden far from view of "normal" society, oftentimes kept in dilapidated conditions and abusive situations. Asylum treatments for the severely mental ill recalled the barbaric demonological rituals of early times, with trepanation recast as surgical lobotomy, and physical ordeal recast as electroconvulsive (shock) therapy.

Freud once said, "When you think of me, think of Rembrandt, a little light and a great deal of darkness."[2] Indeed, Freud's greatest insight is that we have precious little insight into the greatest mystery of all, the mystery of our own mind. He framed the problem as no one else had done before, but there's still the problem. He pointed out quite clearly that the ego, the conscious self, is "not the master of its own house"— but then who is the master—and is he even at home? The solution Freud himself offered, psychoanalysis, now, in perfect hindsight, seems too reductionist, too focused on the sexual to the exclusion of all else, too solipsistic, as the answer to each question keeps pointing back to the bottomless unknowable void of the unconscious.

In a way, his model also seems to recapitulate demonology, with the dark unknowable parallel dimension of the supernatural replaced with the "dark continent" of the unconscious psyche, the demons and spirits recast as repressed memories and unexpressed fantasies and desires, and psychoanalysis as the new inscrutable and elaborate ritual of exorcism. It all seems so metaphysical ... but there must be something knowable and tangible about the brain, that can help us solve the mysteries to the ailments of the mind.

The Medical Model

Freud himself was a neurologist and a psychiatrist, a medical doctor. He began each new patient's assessment with a thorough physical on the examination table, the artifact of which has become the infamous "psychiatric couch." Only after concluding that there were no physical or neural causes to the patient's psychiatric problems did Dr. Freud proceed to psychoanalysis. In founding and propounding the "talking cure," Freud pushed the field of psychiatry forward by leaps and bounds. Psychoanalysis offered the possibility for patients to cure themselves by understanding their own minds and their psychological issues as metaphors for themselves—metaphors that, once interpreted, could be reinterpreted into more adaptive metaphors for themselves and their environments.

Prior to Freud, most of psychiatry was involved in the institutional care of the "incurably mentally ill" in asylums. For the potentially curable mentally ill who had money, there were experimental treatments such as hypnosis and electrotherapy that offered little hope for sustained improvement. Though the field of clinical psychology existed since the end of the 19th century, clinical psychologists were primarily researchers and academics. The actual treatment of the mentally ill was considered a branch of medicine to be practiced only by psychiatrists, medical doctors trained in the field of mental illness. Thus, the approach towards mental disorder for the past few centuries has been dominated by the medical model, a model that is not well suited for the understanding of mental disorder.

What's wrong with the medical model? In presuming that mental disorders have a biological cause, the medical model approaches mental disorders as physical things—not as metaphors for the human experience. If I go to a medical doctor complaining of a hurt arm, the doctor can make a physical examination and provide objective physical proof of a damaged arm, via an ex-ray or physical observation. But if I go to a doctor complaining of a depressed mental state, the doctor cannot physically examine my internal mental state, the doctor can only listen to my explanations and interpretations of my behaviors, thoughts, and feelings, which are, in essence, metaphors of myself.

There's a real danger in presuming to tell people that their metaphors for themselves are physically flawed, just like a broken arm is physically flawed. Essentially, the doctor would be asserting that my thoughts about myself are not metaphors at all, but real things, like bones and muscles, that can be quantified and pointed to in the pages of a book. However, that's simply not the case. Thoughts and feelings are not similar to bones and muscles. Feeling sad or depressed could be understood as a metaphor for how one may be thinking about oneself right now—a metaphor that can be interpreted in manifold ways—because it is, in truth, a figment of one's own consciousness. Understanding oneself as a "depressive" because one was told by a doctor that their brain is inherently flawed due to a real disease called "Major Depressive Disorder" is transforming a metaphysical issue into a physical issue, which could be helpful for some people, but could also be harmful for others.

Other assumptions of the medical model include the notions that all patients are "ill," that all illnesses have a biological basis, and that all illnesses can be treated or cured. If I walk into a doctor's office and say that I'm feeling sick and I think I may have the flu, I would want my doctor to make all of the assumptions mentioned above: That I'm a patient there because I have a real illness, that there's a biological basis—such as the flu virus—to my illness, and that the doctor can provide a cure or corrective treatment for my illness. Such is not necessarily the case with mental disorders. If I walk into a psychiatrist's office and say that I'm feeling depressed, that doesn't necessarily constitute "illness," because depression is a normative human experience. Furthermore, the symptoms of depression are self-described as subjective metaphors, or reflections on myself, not objective physical symptoms, like a runny nose or red eyes. The doctor-patient relationship presumes real sickness on the part of the patient, but real sickness for mental health patients is not so clear-cut.

Furthermore, the medical doctor's presumption that there is a biological basis to my illness is not necessarily true in the case of mental disorder. For instance, even if real disorder is established, the primary cause could be almost exclusively environmental, with hardly any biological basis at all. I could be depressed because my cat died, or because my girlfriend broke up with me. However, the medical doctor, by practice, will treat the patient, not the environment. The medical doctor will usually presume that he can treat or cure his patient's illness, but mental disorders aren't necessarily curable. The aim of most psychotherapy and psychoanalysis is for the patient to help himself, by interpreting his maladaptive internal metaphors and then reinterpreting them to be more adaptive. Therefore, the medical model is in many ways unfit for the treatment of mental problems.

Humanistic psychologists such as Carl Rogers rejected the medical model and revamped their approach to treatment. Patients are called "clients" rather than "patients," to clarify that there isn't necessarily anything sick or disordered about them, even though they're receiving mental health treatment. The word treatment was replaced with nonmedical terms such as "counseling." Doctors, likewise, are referred to as "therapists" or "counselors," to remove the presumption of illness or disorder. The entire process is referred to as "client centered therapy," or more recently, "person centered therapy," indicating that all progress comes from the client himself, and that the therapist is merely a guide and facilitator in this self-helping process.

These strides were important, but the fact is that in the past few decades, in large part due to the advent of psychopharmacological drugs, the entire field of psychology has moved dramatically back towards the medical model, while humanistic and psychoanalytic approaches are becoming increasingly marginalized.

The medical model could be considered a binary model, in which people are categorized into two distinct groups: the healthy and the sick—or, in the parlance of psychology, the normal and the abnormal. In the medical model, a mental health patient is, by default, sick or abnormal, and the doctor, by default, must cure this sickness or abnormality as efficiently as possible. In today's reality, to "cure" means to prescribe medication that will "balance" an inherent neurochemical "imbalance" in the patient's brain, that is presumed to be the root of the problem. In short, the function of the medical practitioner is to prescribe the correct medicine, and it's the medicine that will achieve the cure. There are many, many, *many* problems with this approach. They all arise when we mistake metaphors for objective realities. When the mind is perceived as an objective reality, rather than a metaphor for the processes that take place in the physical brain, we wind up with a medical model of psychiatry in which no distinction is made between the metaphorical mind and the physical brain. The mind/brain are envisaged as one physical machine. The medical model is, in essence, a mechanical model of the brain ... but the mechanical model is completely unfit as a metaphor for both the mind and the brain.

The Mechanical Model

The model of mental disorder that we've been working with for centuries is a mechanical model. It was borne out of the Industrial Age, the time when people realized that machines could perform manual labor better than people could, and so machines, little by little, were engineered to apply to virtually every form of physical labor. The mechanical model assumes that the brain, like the body and all other human devices, functions like a machine. That is, it's a self-enclosed mechanism that functions in a specific way and continues to function in the same way in perpetuity. This is a very appropriate model for a world in which mechanisms such as the printing press, the railroad engine, and the pocket watch dominated the landscape of the human psyche. It's a static model. These mechanisms function the same way every day. They do the same jobs over and over and over again. They're essentially similar to each other, and aren't capable of changing their own function, just as they're incapable of changing their own cogs and gears.

A simple machine, like a lawnmower, is a closed system. It has set functions and operations that can only be changed by its manufacturer or operator, and though it can be adapted to operate in different environments by its operator, it does not adapt itself automatically. (Please note, I'm referring to a simple machine here, not a digitalized machine with a computer, which would give it artificial intelligence, making it more than a simple machine.) The simple machine is completely unlike the brain, which is an open interactive system, constantly adapting itself to its environment, perpetually adjusting itself to find and maintain a state of homeostasis between the internal and external planes of existence. A simple machine is relatively indifferent to its environment and is often used to master its environment. The lawnmower masters the grass. The automobile masters the road. The tractor masters the field. The forklift masters the pallet. The brain, on the other hand, must always be completely engaged with its environment, and its purpose is not necessarily to master the environment, but to live harmoniously within it.

A machine works in a sequential order of mechanical actions. In a car, the spark plugs fire, causing cylinders to combust, thrusting the pistons that turn the crankshaft that rotate the gearbox that channels the circular motion to the driveshaft and into the spinning of the wheels. One mechanism drives the functioning of another mechanism in sequential order until all mechanisms are functioning together. It's very tempting to think of the brain as such a mechanism, but it isn't. The brain is an organism. It's born, it lives, it grows, it adapts, changes, degenerates, and dies. It is not a machine. When a machine malfunctions, it breaks down and needs repair to its original pristine state. When the brain's processes are maladaptive, it re-adapts and corrects itself into a new, different, more adaptive state.

The brain communicates with itself via electric signals that travel at the speed of light within relatively tiny distances, making its processes synchronous and instantaneous, not sequential, like a machine's. The state of homeostasis the brain is perpetually trying to find and maintain between itself and its environment depends on synchronous processing of stimuli and constant adaptation to the changes within the environment. To put it simply: A machine functions, the brain adapts. Though we're tempted to make the machine/brain analogy, the analogy is *not* apt. In order to understand ourselves, we must imagine metaphors that better represent the actual processing of the brain, so we can then imagine metaphors that better represent our minds.

Another issue with the mechanical/medical model of clinical psychology is that it assumes a binary stance towards any psychological condition—it's either normal or abnormal—healthy or pathological. Psychological conditions are of course more complex, because the brain is always rewiring itself in adaptation to its environment. Therefore, any deficiency in mind and behavior will be compensated for by the brain by strengthening its response to the environment in other ways. For example, it's often said that dyslexics "compensate" for their reading deficits with superior memories. This statement is both true and untrue. It's true that dyslexics often have superior memories in comparison with "neurotypicals," and it's true that an excellent memory can compensate in some ways for a reading deficit. However, it's untrue that dyslexics consciously develop better memories as a mechanism of compensation.

The truth is that all humans are born with the capacity for excellent memory; some children even display "eidetic" or "photographic" memory for images and events with extraordinary vividness and detail. However, when children learn to read and write, the brain must "assign" significant quantities of neural capacity to the cognitive functions of literacy, and since literacy makes extraordinary memory somewhat of an obsolete ability—(why remember something if you can write it down or look it up?)—the brain co-opts neural capacity otherwise used for memory and applies it towards neurological processes that are more highly in demand by the environment, such as the processes that enable language and literacy. Hence, photographic memory generally fades away in children once they start school, with the exception of some people, like dyslexics, who never lose the ability, because they never stop using it.[3] (Extraordinary visual memories are also common in preliterate cultures, for the same reason.)

Similarly, autistic savants and autistics in general display extraordinary talents and abilities in specific areas, despite gross deficits in other areas, as Isabelle Rapin explained: "Extraordinary proficiencies of some autistic children for putting together puzzles, taking apart mechanical toys, or decoding written texts may reflect the consequences of attention and learning being inordinately focused on nonverbal visual-spatial tasks to the exclusion of, or perhaps because of, the lack of demand for learning verbal skills."[4] My point here is that the mechanical/medical model perceives psychological conditions such as autism and dyslexia only in terms of their deficits, rather than understanding the conditions as varieties of neurodiversity, with both deficits *and* their corollary advantages. Oliver Sacks expressed the problem better than I can:

> "Deficit," we have said, is neurology's favourite word—its only word, indeed, for any disturbance of function. Either the function (like a capacitor or fuse) is normal—or it is defective or faulty: what other possibility *is* there for a mechanistic neurology, which is essentially a system of capacities and connections? What then of the opposite—an excess or superabundance of function? Neurology has no word for this—because it has no concept. A function, or functional system, works—or it does not: these are the only possibilities it allows.... And this alone

suggests that our basic concept or vision of the nervous system—as a sort of machine or computer—is radically inadequate, and needs to be supplemented by concepts more dynamic, more alive.[5]

The Clinical Model

In the post–World War II era, clinical psychologists became more involved in the direct assessment and treatment of mentally ill patients, due to the overwhelming demand for mental healthcare for the millions of returning veterans from the European and Pacific theaters of war. The old method of shipping the mentally disordered off to asylums seemed unfit for these "shell shocked" boys, and the medical doctors, including psychiatrists, were already over-extended treating all of the physical injuries. The infusion of clinical psychologists into the field of treatment for the mentally ill brought a more research-based, academic approach to the fold. Clinical psychologists treated patients primarily with psychotherapy, i.e., the "talking cure," though Freudian psychoanalysis eventually waned in popularity in favor of other paradigms, such as Humanism and Cognitive-Behaviorism. The primary element of the clinical model is the application of a research-based "categorical" approach, based on the presumption that mental disorders could be deconstructed according to groupings of symptoms, and then categorized according to these groupings.

The "bible" of clinical psychology in America became the DSM—the *Diagnostic and Statistical Manual of Mental Disorders*—published by the American Psychological Association. The DSM is now in its fifth revision. The key presumption presented in the DSM, which is thereby assumed by all clinical psychologists and psychiatrists using the DSM, is that the distinction between normal and pathological behavior is one of *kind* rather than *degree*. That is, people can be categorized according to their behavior (or their thoughts about their behavior), into one of two categories—normal or abnormal—and beyond that, there are a myriad of other subcategories that could be applied to the abnormal person based on specific disorder, i.e., Major Depressive Disorder, Generalized Anxiety Disorder, Attention Deficit Hyperactivity Disorder, etc. Every sort of abnormal behavior has a category, and every abnormal person can be assigned to a category.

What's wrong with the clinical model? The categorical approach of the clinical model assumes qualitative differences among people based on distinctions that assume issues like depression and anxiety are "real" illnesses, as opposed to metaphors for internal mental states. As such, it's making a mistake very similar to that of the medical model. In making a diagnosis of me as someone with clinical depression, the clinical psychologist is stating authoritatively that the thoughts and feelings that I may dictate on one day of assessment justifies the decree that I am in a category of person different from other people.

I am not a normal person; I am a depressive. I have a disorder, and this disorder reflects something inherently flawed in my mind and my brain, not just a maladaptation to my environment. The disorder in a very significant way defines me as a person. In a binary system in which there is normal and abnormal, I am abnormal, even though we all admit that sometimes we feel one way and sometimes we feel another. In a world where everyone feels and thinks differently every day of the week, who's to say what's normal or abnormal? Who's to say that your moody Monday is "normal" depression, but that my sad Tuesday is "clinical depression?" The clinical psychologist, that's who.

Clinical psychologists, when presuming that mental disorders are physically real illnesses in the way that medical conditions like cancer or pregnancy are physically real, categorize disorders based on groupings of symptoms that overlap to a great extent. For example, many of the symptoms of anxiety overlap with the symptoms of depression. So, if an individual is complaining of disturbances in sleep, irritable mood, difficulty concentrating, feelings of self-loathing, and lethargy—does this individual suffer from anxiety or from depression? The fact is, these symptoms are listed in the DSM for both disorders. The psychologist, if making a diagnosis, is forced to make a judgment call that's oftentimes rather arbitrary. There's a notoriously low degree of inter-assessor reliability among different psychologists assessing the same person. In the same person being assessed, one psychologist is likely to call "depression" what another psychologist is likely to call "anxiety." To play it safe, many psychologists make a "comorbid" diagnosis of both anxiety and depression.

Ok, but as long as people who are suffering get treatment, what does it matter? It actually matters a lot! With the advent of psychopharmacology, and especially with the advent of providing licensure to clinical psychologists and physician's assistants to prescribe psychiatric medication, the clinical model of treatment has become essentially the same as the medical model of treatment. If most mental disorders are presumed to have a biological basis in the neurochemistry of the brain, then most mental disorders can be treated with psychotropic medication that changes the neurochemistry of the brain, in which case distinctions between a diagnosis of "anxiety" and a diagnosis of "depression" are anything but arbitrary, because the medication prescribed for one disorder is chemically different than the medication prescribed for the other disorder. By presuming that mental disorders are physically real, biologically based, and categorically distinct from each other, we go way beyond the risk of mixing metaphors for different mental states. We run the very real risk of prescribing medication that is contra-indicated (i.e., incorrect), with negative effects as well as side effects and interaction effects that could be catastrophic for the patient.

One common example is when a child who has manic behaviors (a symptom of Bipolar Disorder), is misdiagnosed with ADHD (the most commonly diagnosed behavioral disorder in children). To a diagnostician, the symptoms of ADHD and the symptoms of mania can seem almost identical, especially in a child who's unable to verbalize his internal mental states and explain his thoughts and feelings. However, when the manic child is given the most common form of medication prescribed for children with ADHD, a powerful psychostimulant such as Ritalin, the drug is likely to intensify the child's manic behaviors to the point of full-blown psychosis, which could destroy the child's entire mental life. Clearly, there's a problem not just with the medication in some particular cases, but with the entire way that the field is conceptualizing the origin and treatment of mental disorders.

The Neurochemical Model

The neurochemical model adopted by almost all modern mental health practitioners as the core dynamic of their clinical model is really just a more refined version of the medical model, which in principle is a mechanical model. Ironically, all of these roads lead to the same place: psycho-pharmaceutical medication. The brain, in the mechanical model, is conceived of as a mechanism, a machine. Psychiatric medication prescribed to treat the disordered patient is conceptually similar to the oil administered by a mechanic to facilitate the functioning of the machine. But here's where the machine/mind metaphor breaks down. Let's say your car is acting clunky and the "check engine" light comes on, so you go to a mechanic. The mechanic checks the car and tells you that the problem with your car is that it needs more oil, which he adds. Everything works fine, but a couple of days later, the car is clunky again and the "check engine" light reappears. The same mechanic tells you that the problem is that the car is low on oil, and so he adds some and everything is fine, until the same problem recurs a day later. At your third visit, the mechanic explains that your car suffers from a perpetual deficit of oil, and his recommended fix is to perpetually add more oil every day.

Though this fix may address the day-to-day problem of clunkiness and "check engine" light illumination, you intuitively know that the mechanic is clearly missing a deeper and more integral problem. In the same way, if your psychiatrist tells you that your depression is caused by a perpetual deficit of serotonin, and that the treatment is to perpetually take a drug that increases the presence of serotonin in your brain, and that it's quite likely that you'll have to take this drug every day for the rest of your life, you should intuitively know that the psychiatrist is clearly missing a deeper and more integral problem.

Let's say you go to your doctor complaining of a runny nose, sore throat, stuffed head, etc. The doctor would be likely to diagnose you with a cold, and prescribe medication. When asked if the medication will cure the cold, the doctor, of course, would say: "No. There's no cure for the common cold; but the medication will treat the symptoms." Similarly, any psychiatrist would admit that psychotropic medication does not cure mental illness, it merely treats the symptoms. If the medication cured the illness, you wouldn't have to take it every day in perpetuity, because at a certain point, you'd be cured. Any medication that needs to be taken indefinitely is not curing an illness; it's treating symptoms, just as adding oil to your car is not really fixing the car. The metaphors of both the car and the cold break down when we try to equate them with mental disorder. The car is a physical machine, so therefore the problem with the car is unequivocally a physical problem, such as a leaky engine. Similarly, the cold is caused by a physical virus that runs its course and then goes away. The mind, however, is not a machine.

Unlike the closed system of a machine, the open system of the mind functions by interacting with the environment and adapting itself to its environment, creating a homeostasis, a balance between the internal functioning of the mind and the external functioning of the body in the environment. The mind adapts itself by providing feedback to the brain, which is constantly refining and retuning its neural connections by adjusting the balances of various neurotransmitters that manage the connections. The principal assumption of the neurochemical model is that mental illness is caused by chemical imbalances of neurotransmitters. The corollary that follows this assumption is that adding chemicals to the brain to readjust the imbalances will treat the illness. The all-important question that's not addressed by this model is, *Why do the chemical imbalances exist in the first place?*

If we return to the principal function of the mind/brain—the maintenance of homeostasis between an individual and their environment—we must conclude that the cause is either some inherent structural neurological flaw in the brains of mentally disordered people, causing perpetual imbalances, or something in the environment that makes it difficult or even impossible for the brain to adapt itself, so that balance is rarely if ever achieved. I admit wholeheartedly that there are probably some cases in which inherent structural neurological flaws exist, although for most mental illnesses, despite decades of searching by countless researchers with the most sophisticated equipment, almost none have been found. The theory I'm suggesting in this book is that there's also an environmental cause to the imbalance—stimuli in the environment that the mind/brain of many people cannot adapt to—and that these stimuli are the media of information that, in many cases, are very new arrivals to our environment.

The chemical imbalances, if they exist, are *symptoms* of the problem, not the problem themselves—just as the oil deficit in the car is a symptom of a leaky engine—not the problem in-and-of-itself. In administering medication to readjust these imbalances, we're tampering with the symptoms of the problem (the imbalance), which in turn influence the behavioral symptoms that indicate the existence of the problem (the disorder). Medication, far from addressing the problem, is merely treating the symptom of the symptoms. The fact that most psycho-pharmaceutical medications must be taken perpetually without causing any cure whatsoever, and oftentimes with minimal effect on the symptoms themselves, is a pretty good indicator that the treatment model itself is inherently flawed.

The further fact that the toxicity of psycho-pharmaceutical medications causes serious side effects and interaction effects, not to mention critical issues such as addiction, tolerance, dependency, and misuse, all add to the point that the neurochemical model of mental illness is not only ineffective, it's dangerous. In this sense, practitioners of the model are unwittingly violating the prime directive of all healers: "First do no harm."

The current clinical model, which incorporates the neurochemical model, which in turn incorporates the medical and mechanical models, is outdated. In stationing the cause of all disorder inside the brain, it ignores the more likely causes existing outside of the brain. In doing so, it treats its subjects in the most invasive way (altering the brain), rather than taking the least invasive approach (altering the environment). Perhaps the biggest problem with the clinical model is that it disempowers the mentally ill, convincing them that the root of their problems is in their own flawed brains, despite the lack of any evidence to support this hypothesis. Rather than being empowered to proactively change their environments or their role in their environments, they're put in the passive role of disabled people, who must rely on medication for the rest of their lives in order to function, despite the great deal of evidence that the majority of psycho-pharmaceutical medications are only marginally effective beyond the placebo effect. In short, the current clinical model is probably causing more harm than good.

The Spectrum Model

A specific model of a machine—a '57 Chevy Bel Air, for example—functions in a specific way. All of the same models of that specific machine, therefore—all '57 Chevy Bel Airs—function in exactly the same way. There's no functional diversity within a model of a machine. If a machine of that specific model functions differently from the other machines, then that machine is a broken machine. The primary problem with the neurochemical model is that it reduces brains to the status of machines, and then assumes that all brains are designed to function exactly the same way—the "normal" way. Any brain that doesn't function in the normal way is "abnormal," requiring it to be normalized by adding drugs to balance the chemical imbalance that's presumed to be causing the abnormal functioning. This model is conceptually flawed.

Brains, of course, aren't "designed" by anyone. The hardware of the brain has evolved over millions of years to perform one function: To adapt to the individual's environment. While we're born with all the neurons we're ever going to have, most of our neurons are unconnected at birth. Maturation at the neuronal level is a process of creating and re-creating neural connections. So, while the structure of the brain between individuals is remarkably similar, the processing of the brain—a product of the way that the neurons have connected to each other as a function of adapting to its environment—is entirely dissimilar among individuals. The brain's remarkable "plasticity" dictates that no two brains will ever be exactly the same, because each brain is individually molded by each individual's unique experiences and interactions with his particular environment. The brain is therefore completely *unlike* a machine.

From an evolutionary perspective, it certainly makes sense for the brain to be capable of a very broad spectrum of functioning for every possible behavior, so that there's a maximum amount of flexibility in the way that each brain can adapt to its environment. Diversity, in evolutionary terms, is always adaptive. Unfortunately, as renowned biologist Milton Diamond is fond of saying: "Biology loves diversity, society hates it!"

"Neurological Diversity" is a relatively new movement in the field of psychology. This perspective accepts the individuality of each brain as a product of its own plasticity. The spectrum model of mental illness incorporates neurological diversity as a basic principle. In its broadest conception, the spectrum model holds that the binary categorization of people's behaviors into "normal" and "abnormal" categories is at best too simplistic and at worst harmful to the people labeled as "abnormal." According to the spectrum model, every behavior can be assessed along a broad spectrum, and every person's behavior falls somewhere along the continuum of that respective spectrum. There is no "normal" and "abnormal," just infinite diversity across an indefinite number of spectrums.

The field of psychology has already begun to implement the spectrum model, as seen in the reconceptualization of "Autistic Disorder" in the DSM-IV, into "Autism Spectrum Disorder" in the DSM-V, and the reframing of "Schizophrenia" and a variety of other psychotic disorders into the category of "Schizophrenia Spectrum Disorder." We can assume that future revisions of the DSM will re-conceptualize other disorders such as Depression, Anxiety, and ADHD as spectrum disorders. After all, just as it's conceptually problematic to label a child as either "normal" or "abnormal"—"normal" or "autistic"—it makes even less sense to label someone as either "normal" or "depressed," "normal" or "anxious," etc.

Surely, all of these psychological issues fall along a broad spectrum of behavior, rather than a binary one-or-the-other distinction. Nevertheless, the entire mental health industry has been built upon the clinical model that assumes a binary distinction. The folks who actually pay the bills, the insurance companies, will not reimburse a clinician for fees unless his client is diagnosed with a specific disorder. At the end of the day, in order to get mental health treatment, an individual needs to be diagnosed as "disordered" in some way. The same distinction applies to children getting treatment for autistic symptoms. Spectrum or no spectrum, at the end of the day, the child is still being labeled "autistic."

Parents, teachers, and clinicians may use the more politically correct term, "on the spectrum," in reference to the child, rather than calling the child "autistic," but this wordplay confuses rather than clarifies the issue. If we assume that every behavior, including autistic behaviors, falls along a broad spectrum of behaviors that exist for everyone, then saying that someone is "on the spectrum" makes no sense at all, because *everyone* is on *every* spectrum. Saying "on the spectrum" is just a more sensitive way of saying "autistic," just like saying "intellectually disabled" as per the new DSM-V nomenclature is just a more sensitive way of saying "mentally retarded."

Though the new terms are certainly more sensitive, they still engender the same old binary distinctions that in essence express the most basic categorizations: "normal" or "abnormal." Though the spectrum model is an improvement upon the traditional clinical model, it doesn't really change our approach to mental disorder. If we really want to embrace the ideals of true neurological diversity, an actual paradigm shift is required, not just nominal changes in terminology.

Neurological Diversity

The cochlear implant is an ingenious device that bypasses the function (or dysfunction) of the ear in people with hearing problems, such as partial or complete deafness. The hearing aid works by receiving sound waves from the environment, digitizing the waves, and then resending them as electric signals directly into the cochlear nerve in the brain. The cochlear nerve then transmits the same electric signals towards the neurons in the auditory processing centers of the brain, where they're interpreted and perceived as sound.

The mind-blowing thing about this procedure is that it's that simple. Digitized sound transmitted as electric signals are immediately recognized and decoded by the neurons in the brain and translated into sound—no other hardware or software is needed to complete this interface. The brain, amazingly, can take any pattern of electric signal, decode it, and perceive it as sensory information. The implications of this simple fact are staggering! The brain is an electro-animate organism that can format itself to virtually any kind of electronic stimulation in its environment. We can use even the most simple electronic device to digitalize stimuli such as sound into electric signals, or to stimulate specific neurons in order to enhance or inhibit the release of specific neurotransmitters (as in the case of Deep Brain Stimulation implants for Parkinson's patients), or to directly interface with the brain, bypassing the senses altogether. The use of electroshock therapy was the blunt hammer version of this tool, which is now reaching the age of the precision needle. But there's room to be wary...

The protests of the deaf community against the implantation of cochlear transmitters in deaf babies revolves around the controversial assumption that hearing is "normal" and deafness, "abnormal," an assumption that they reject. From the perspective of neurological diversity, there is no "normal" and "abnormal," just diversity. Therefore, a world in which the brains of deaf infants are immediately implanted with cochlear transmitters is a world in which deafness as an identity and as a culture is not tolerated and, in effect, wiped out. This, according to some in the deaf community, is tantamount to cultural genocide.

The controversy over the cochlear implant is clearly the canary in the coal mine for future issues regarding neural implants, especially in the case of mental disorder. Would an implant that could inhibit all of the symptoms of schizophrenia be another case of cultural genocide? How about an implant that would inhibit all symptoms of ADHD, or anxiety, depression, or autism? How far are we willing to go in our assumptions of abnormality in behavior, in our denial of neurological diversity, in our desire to mold each individual's behavior to conform to the narrow specifications of the norm? Will we proceed until the plastic adaptivity of the brain is molded and proscribed by drugs and implants to such an extent that there's no such thing as mental disorder anymore?

Will we proceed until there's no such thing as an "individual" anymore? If so, what would be left in its place? A species with a brain that is electronically preset to function within such strict limitations of behavioral norms that true individuality of mind and behavior are restricted to the point of elimination in favor of absolute and universal normality … the absolute tyranny of the "normal?"

Diversion from the norm at a species level is not just important, it's essential for survival. Evolutionary adaptivity requires diversity. Ridding the species of neurological diversity would therefore be dangerous to the survival of the species. What may be considered abnormal in one environment could be considered beneficial, superior, or even essential in a different environment. Is it possible that behavior patterns that we now categorize as "ADHD," "Autism," or "Schizophrenia" were actually adaptively beneficial in past environments, or would become adaptively beneficial in a future environment? If so, then ridding ourselves of these behavior patterns would be maladaptive to the species as a whole.

Another danger that would arise in a dystopian world of universal normality is the subjugation of the mind of the artist. Artists are individuals in society whose perceptions and expressions are sufficiently divergent to the norm as to give the rest of us pause. They provide divergent perspectives that we've never encountered before, thereby expanding the consciousness of society as a whole. Divergence is why the creative artist is often considered mentally ill, and why they suffer for their art. To be divergent in a world of convergence, to be square in a world of round holes, is to be different, estranged. Marshall McLuhan explained it this way:

One of the functions of the artist that is understood in recent decades is that it is, above all, to prevent us from becoming adjusted to our environments. There's always a danger of becoming a robot, of becoming well-adjusted or conditioned like a man paddling a canoe. A man paddling a canoe may seem very symmetrical and very harmonious in relation to the elements. He is, in fact, a servo mechanism. The better adjusted he is to that paddle, the more a servo mechanism he is. That doesn't mean it isn't fun. The danger, however, of becoming a servo mechanism of our own environment by adjustment is headed off by the artist who creates violent new images to dislocate our sensibilities. The job of the artist is dislocation of sensibility to prevent us from becoming adjusted to total environments, and to becoming the servant and robots of those environments. That may sound paradoxical.... The job of the artist is to upset all the senses, and thus to provide new vision and new powers of adjusting to and relating to new situations.[6]

The hearing aid is like McLuhan's canoe. It enables the deaf people who stand ashore at the river of sound to climb in the water and paddle in it; but in doing so, it transforms them from shore people into canoers, just like all the other canoers. If all the shore people become canoers, we'll lose the perspective from the shore. If all the deaf people become hearing, we'll lose the perspective of the deaf. If all the schizophrenic people become "sane," we'll lose that sensibility as well.

Neurological diversity requires us to tolerate, value, respect, and accept all neurological dispositions, even the ones that may seem "abnormal" or "dysfunctional." This tolerance should be expanded into the realm of neurological dispositions towards different forms of media. Perhaps we've reached the age of media sophistication when we could admit that forcing children to master forms of media, such as literacy, when their minds are simply not neurologically disposed towards those forms of media, is actually doing more harm than good? Perhaps a better approach would be to help them learn alternate forms of media that they *are* neurologically predisposed to mastering?

The Vulnerability/Stress Model

There's one model of psychopathology that has the distinct benefit of always being correct. This model assumes that every mental disorder is the result of a combination of both biological factors and environmental factors. Every person has a unique set of biological and genetic traits, which means that some people—based purely on their own genetics—will be more vulnerable or predisposed to mental disorder than others. At the same time, everyone experiences a unique environmental life history, with experiences and situations that are exclusive to them. While one person may experience much trauma and stress, another person may experience very little. Therefore, if you take identical twins with identical genetics, the likelihood that one of them will develop a mental disorder will correlate highly with the likelihood that the other one will develop a mental disorder, especially if they grow up in the same household. However, if you enact the unethical "forbidden experiment" of separating these twins at birth and raising them in completely different environments—one environment being high stress and the other environment being low stress—it's likely that the twin in the high stress environment will develop a mental disorder, while the other twin is likely to be spared that fate.

Some mental disorders, such as PTSD, are very much dependent on the presence of trauma or stress. Nevertheless, if a group of people are exposed to the same level of trauma or stress, there will always be some people who develop symptoms of PTSD, while others will be more resilient and will not develop symptoms. Vulnerability is *always* a factor, even with disorders that are primarily precipitated by stress. Similarly, some mental disorders, such as autism, are very much dependent on genetic factors that determine or influence the neuro-connectivity or neurochemistry of the brain. Nevertheless, the environment in which an autistic child is raised will have a critical influence on the symptoms of autism they will display as they develop, to the point where a child who may have an extreme genetic vulnerability or disposition towards autism may, given the proper environment, grow up to be someone who has relatively few or even no symptoms of classic autism. Such is the adaptive power of plasticity in the brain, and such is the significance of the environment as it interacts with the brain. Stress or lack of stress in the environment is *always* a factor.

The vulnerability/stress model has the benefit of always being correct, with the drawback of being entirely unspecific. The media ecology model I will propose in this book has the benefit of being very specific, as it focuses only on the environment, and only on a specific aspect of the environment—media. The specificity of the model itself dooms it to being incorrect in a lot of insistences. However, if it's right in some ways, it could be extremely valuable as a new metaphor for understanding mental disorder. My model is couched within the vulnerability/stress model, as it needs the support of a broad structure that's always true.

So, if a critical reader points out, "*Hey, how could you argue that autism is caused by media, when researchers much more qualified than you in the scientific study of autism assert that autism has a genetic/neurological basis?*" My reply would be, "*Of course, the vulnerability of genetic/neurological predisposition is an integral factor. However, the* *environment is <u>always</u> a factor, and therefore an environmental model of the cause and course of autism, or of any mental illness, is complementary to a biological model."*

In the end, no single model is an appropriate metaphor for any complicated problem. All psychologists need to adopt an eclectic approach, that borrows from a variety of complementary models. So, my media ecology model is not offered as a replacement to any of the models mentioned above, but as an additional metaphor to complement the existing models.

My basic argument in this preliminary chapter has been that the current state of psychological science diminishes the role of the environment in the etiology of mental disorder, as the medical, mechanical, clinical, and neurochemical models all focus single-mindedly on the role of genetics, neuro-connectivity, and neurochemistry. My argument in the succeeding chapters is that the media that saturates both our environment and our minds has critical effects on both the etiology and the developmental course of many, if not most, mental disorders.

The Media Ecology Model

In a sense, the model that I'm currently proposing is the reverse image of Freud's. The crux of Freud's argument was that we are unconscious of the "dark continent" within ourselves that molds our behavior and shapes our thoughts, and that this unseen force is at the root of all neuroses. My model flips the image. I argue that we are unconscious of the dark continent *outside* of ourselves, the invisible media atmosphere that saturates our environment, that seeps into our minds to mold our behavior and shape our thoughts. As an important distinction, I'm not saying that the content of our media is invisible (other than spoken words, which are literally invisible). I'm saying that the effect of the media themselves are invisible to us. We don't notice the effect of the medium of information, because we're focused on the content of the medium, the information itself. To borrow yet another of McLuhan's metaphors, we can visualize the content/medium duality by analogizing it to the figure/ground duality in a picture. When looking at a picture, we're likely to miss elements of the background, because we're focusing on the figure in the foreground. The ground of our perception fades into invisibility as our attention is drawn to the figure, the focal point of our perception. Similarly, we don't notice the effect of the medium of information, because we're focused on the content of the medium, which is the information itself.

In his infamous adage, "The medium is the message," McLuhan was merely stressing the fact that at a societal level, the effect of the media themselves have a much greater impact on our thoughts and behaviors than the specific content of the media.[7] For instance, as you read these words, you're focusing on the meaning of the words, and how they fit together to compose the argument I'm making. You're *not* focusing on the effect that the medium of literacy has on your thought process, the fact that it demands and creates a thought process that is sequential, linear, logical, abstract, and detached. Though the content of my words might have some effect on the content of your thoughts, it's the *medium* of literacy itself that actually shapes and molds your thought processes, into the sequentially thinking, literate-minded, logical individual that you are. Similarly, Freud's focus on the psychological effects of the unconscious on neurosis was an attempt to shift attention from the conscious figure or *content* of our thoughts, to the unconscious ground of our existence.

My focus in this book is on the psychological effects of media on mental disorder. It's an attempt to shift our attention away from the psychological effects of the *content* of media (e.g., violent videogames or pornographic images), to the much more invasive and overwhelming effects of the *media* themselves (e.g., gaming platform technology or the internet).

The message of this book is the medium...

• Two •

Language, Literacy
and the Leftward Shift

*This very heart of mine will forever remain indefinable to me.
Between the certainty I have of my existence and the content I try to
give to that assurance, the gap will never be filled. Forever I shall be
a stranger to myself.*

—Albert Camus (1955)[1]

Humans, as far as we know, are the only creatures who question the nature of their own existence. *"Man is a problem to himself."* Just to understand the existence of this problem requires an ability to reflect upon oneself objectively, as if "I" and "me" were separate entities, able to examine one another with the distance necessary to analyze and interpret. There seems to exist a *split* in the human psyche, enabling us to look inwardly, and to gaze upon the person within us, who is both our self, and the one observing our self. Certainly, this ability gives us the power to understand our selves and our world in ways that other less reflective animals can never dream of doing.

Nearly every field of study—philosophy, psychology, theology, neurology, medicine, anthropology, sociology, history, etc.—is, to some degree, a branch of the most fundamental endeavor, the endless attempt to understand ourselves. Yet, at the same time, the peculiar ability that engenders self-reflection also enables self-estrangement. The deep-seated duality of our thought processes condemns us to a cerebral hall of mirrors, in which every thought, feeling, urge, and desire is subject to endless reflection and inspection. Ultimately, we reach a point of essential uncertainty as to who we really are. Am I the "real me," or the reflection of "me." Is there even a "me" at all, or only endless reflections? Thus, as Camus said, we become "strangers" to ourselves.

As if to taunt us with our own self-doubt, Nature has provided an answer to the problem of duality in an object that is so demonstrably

37

dualistic that it seems too obvious to be true. The brain, the seat of consciousness and all mental activity, the physical home of the mind, is clearly divided into two halves. The physical duality is apparent even to the naked eye. Could the division of the brain into left and right hemispheres be the actual root of human duality, or is it just a mirage, a cruel practical joke? The answer, it seems, is both. The duality of mind is almost certainly rooted in the duality of the brain, the twin hemispheres that seem to function simultaneously and somewhat independently as parallel processing units. Yet, the more we try to understand how these two brains unite to create one mind—one sense of self—the more complicated and elusive the solution becomes. Like an organic babushka doll of infinite intricacy, the more layers of the brain we reveal, the more puzzles we uncover.

Fortunately, for you and for me, there is a guide to this maze of the mind. Iain McGilchrist, a world-renowned scholar, practitioner, and researcher, published a landmark book in 2009 that may turn out to be the most significant book of the century. *The Master and His Emissary: The Divided Brain and the Making of the Western World*, summarizes the relevant neurological research on hemispheric differences in the brain and their effect on human behavior (a gargantuan task in-and-of-itself). The book goes on to speculate how these neurological differences in perception and cognition have molded the ways that humans have thought about the world and themselves over the past few millennia, and especially over the past few centuries. The gist of McGilchrist's epic tome is that human thought has bit-by-bit become dominated by the brain's left hemisphere, as input from the right hemisphere has become inhibited and largely shut off. The significance of this shift towards left hemispheric cerebral dominance will be addressed in this book in the following ways:

1. How the leftward shift in cerebral dominance could be understood as neurological adaptations to different forms of media.
2. How these neurological adaptations to media in the form of changes in hemispheric dominance are *directly responsible* for the emergence of some mental disorders, such as schizophrenia and autism.
3. How the *environments* that arose to facilitate the use of these media created pressures that are *directly responsible* for the emergence of mental disorders such as dyslexia and the other learning disabilities, as well as ADHD, and some forms of intellectual disability.
4. How the new environmental pressures of our evolving

media environments continue to influence our mind and behavior, especially in relation to the disorders mentioned above, as well as other conditions such as anxiety, depression, and some personality disorders.

Language and Lateralization

If language is the defining feature of the human species, the adaptation that enabled us to think, communicate, and cooperate within a dimension far more sophisticated than any other animal in nature, then the evolution of language in the human brain is key to understanding human nature itself. In his 1991 book, *Origins of the Modern Mind: Three Stages in the Evolution of Culture and Cognition*, neuropsychologist Merlin Donald asserts that the evolution of the human brain must be understood within the context of the evolution of human communication. The first great leap forward in communication came when humans began to use abstract symbols to communicate, rather than simple signs and signals, such as the grunts and growls of apes and monkeys. In a communication system based on simple signs that everyone understands, new ideas cannot be communicated, because every sign that's expressed must be understood by the recipient *before* it's expressed. If I have a sign that means "apple," for instance, I can only share the message "apple" with you if you know the sign for "apple" before I express it to you.

This communication system then, is extremely limited, as it's circumscribed by the finite number of signs that people can share, and isn't open to the expression of new, original expressions. In a communication system based on abstract symbols, however, the thing that is shared by everyone is not the signs themselves, but the shared symbols that are used to *create* signs. In this system, new ideas can be expressed, because new signs can be created and understood, as long as both the sender and the recipient of the message share the same system of abstract sign-creating symbols. As Chomsky and others pointed out, it's the infinite "generativity" of a communication system based on abstract symbols that distinguishes it as a "language," as opposed to a simpler and extremely limited communication system based on signs.[2]

Donald argues that the first true language ancient hominids shared was a "mimetic" language using body movements and vocalizations, but relying primarily on hand signals. The evolution of mimesis as a protolanguage was a natural development that grew out of the increased manual dexterity Paleolithic hominids evolved in order to master tool use and fire-making—manual skills so complex that they could not be re-discovered and re-invented by each individual—skills that had to be passed down or "communicated" from one individual to another.

The modern mimetic languages known as "sign languages," commonly used by the deaf and mute communities, bear witness to how mimesis could be used to communicate quite proficiently. Indeed, the innate ability for people to learn and use sign language as a substitution for oral language could very well be a neurological artifact of the mimetic stage of language evolution. Furthermore, the fact that our visual information processing rate for images and visual symbols greatly exceeds our auditory processing rate for speech, "suggests that our information-processing capacity evolved before a modern vocal-tract morphology."[3] That is, humans evolved the capacity to express and comprehend visual symbols *before* they evolved the capacity to use auditory symbols such as spoken words.

This leads us to wonder if the Paleolithic cave paintings dating back to as much as 64,000 years BCE, were made by archaic preverbal humans whose primary means of communication were mimetic hand signals and gestures, punctuated by the typical grunts and growls of our primate ancestors. More significantly (for my theory), the evolution of the mimetic medium in the Paleolithic era explains why language function was originally lateralized in the left hemisphere of the brain.

Each hand is controlled by a different hemisphere of the brain in a contralateral fashion, so that the right hand is controlled by the left hemisphere, and vice versa. The lateralization of hand control in the opposing hemispheres is an extremely important adaptation, as it enables each of our hands to function independently of the other, thereby exponentially increasing our ability to perform sophisticated manual tasks. Imagine playing the piano, for instance, if your left hand was unable to function independently of the right. It would be impossible. However, while independent hand function is crucial, it's also adaptive for people to have a "dominant" hand, a *master* hand, rather than two hands that always function completely independently of each other.

The dominant hand, the right hand in the vast majority of people, serves to focus one's manual attention very specifically on a task, when such focus is necessary. In a high-focus-required task, the master hand takes over, and the subdominant hand recedes to play a subservient role to the master. Imagine trying to make a fire or stone tool by striking two flint stones against each other. If each hand was striking its stone independently onto the other, the effect would be unfocussed and un-precise. It's far more efficient to subdue one hand's motion (the left hand, for most of us), and to use this subdominant hand to merely hold one stone still; while the other hand, the right or "master" hand, makes precision strikes onto the stone to effect the precise sparks or chips you need to create your fire or hand-axe. This need for focus and dominance explains why right hand dominance was originally lateralized in the left hemisphere, and why this leftward lateralization has continued since the Paleolithic Age, following the ever-increasing species-wide demand for focused attention.

As McGilchrist explains comprehensively in his book, the left hemisphere specializes in taking a focused approach to stimuli, while the right hemisphere specializes in a more holistic, "gestalt" or "big picture" approach. Working together, the left and right hemispheres complement each other perfectly, not just for manual dexterity, but for language, and also for our entire approach to engaging with our environment. Bradshaw and Nettleton (1981) argued that the "left hand delineates the *frame* into which the right hand inserts the *contents*, a concept with overtones of a right-hemisphere global-holistic and a left-hemisphere serial-analytic dichotomy."[4]

Donald's theory provides a parsimonious explanation for how human language developed gradually during the Paleolithic. Most importantly, it explains how language evolved from preexisting skills, rather than suddenly emerging from primitive primate vocalizations. It's hard to imagine oral language—a medium so sophisticated and complex—popping up suddenly and de novo in history, the firstborn child of the primitive grunts and growls of our primate relatives.

Though counter-intuitive at first, upon reflection, Donald's argument that oral language actually evolved from mimetic communication makes more sense than the hypothesis that oral language evolved from grunts and growls. Donald's theory also explains why language was initially lateralized in the left hemisphere, as it evolved out of the mimetic language that was lateralized in the left, due to the right hand dominance of most humans. It also explains why language is not completely relegated to only the left hemisphere, but is processed with input from the right hemisphere, though with the left hemisphere retaining clear dominance.

Manual dexterity is aided by handedness, the dominance of one hand, but it's still important for both hands to work together, with both mutual independence and mutual cooperation. So too, language is aided by the single-minded focused approach of the left hemisphere, as the primary function of language is the ability to express our ideas very specifically, with pinpoint focus on the exact words that express the precise meaning we need to convey. At the same time, language also needs to be open to metaphor, to portray big pictures in broad brushstrokes, to express poetic fancies that by their very nature need to be deliberately vague and undefined. In short, language needs to be a whole-brain process, but in order to function effectively, it needs to be dominated—lateralized—by a strict master, which for most of us is the left hemisphere.

Another reason why language must be lateralized in one hemisphere has to do with "callosal transmission," the transmission of neural messages across the hemispheres via the corpus callosum—the thick band of neuronal fibers that connects the two hemispheres of the brain; most high order interhemispheric communication in the brain is carried out though this neural highway. There's a very brief time delay of 25 milliseconds involved in callosal transmission. That may not seem like a lot of time, but when we're dealing with language, 25 ms to transmit a word would seem way too long. The verbal thought function in the brain translates complex thoughts into sophisticated combinations of abstract symbolic sounds known as words, in a process that seems so instantaneous that the very fabric of thought seems to be language itself—though we know that words are merely the symbols or representations of thought.

Therefore, 25 ms is an unacceptable delay, which means that in order for verbal thought to function automatically and instantaneously, it must be lateralized completely within one hemisphere.[5] At the same time, we know that language and thought are whole brain processes, and we also know that language is comprehended and produced in both hemispheres. So, how is it possible that language must be lateralized in a single hemisphere in order for it to work—but at the same time—language is and must be processed in both hemispheres? The answer, incredibly, is that both hemispheres have their own language function, and that they both produce their own versions of verbal thought. That is, each hemisphere is independently conscious, and each hemisphere has its own stream of verbal conscious thought. The remarkable truth is, behind the illusion of unity, there is a duality of independent, fully conscious hemispheres.

"*Homo duplex, homo duplex!*"[6] Each one of us is two!

Research done on "split-brain" patients (epileptics whose corpus callosa were surgically severed), revealed that both hemispheres seem to experience consciousness in their own ways, independently of each other. Dr. Roger Sperry, who received the Nobel Prize for his pioneering research on split-brain patients, noted that each hemisphere is "a conscious system in its own right, perceiving, thinking, remembering, reasoning, willing, and emoting, all at a characteristically human level ... both the left and the right hemisphere may be conscious simultaneously in different, even in mutually conflicting, mental experiences that run along in parallel."[7]

So, if the brain creates two streams of consciousness, why are we aware of only one? The answer is inhibition. The left hemisphere of the brain, the dominant hemisphere during the waking state, is usually inhibiting a great deal of the thought process of the subdominant hemisphere, the right hemisphere, from entering the dominant stream of verbal consciousness, which is situated in the left hemisphere. McGilchrist cites a plethora of research revealing that many of the connections in the corpus callosum, possibly a *majority* of the connections, serve an *inhibitory* purpose.[8] This inhibition is absolutely necessary in order to maintain a sense of mental unity. Our sanity depends on there being only one voice of consciousness within the mind, not two.

Oral Language and Linearity

Returning to Donald's model, the evolution of language beyond mimesis proceeds in a parsimonious manner. One can imagine being a proverbial "caveman" in the Paleolithic, trying to teach a friend how to make a fire, when your language is based on hand signs. It would be impossible to simultaneously demonstrate the method of fire-making, while also explaining the technique, because you'd have to put down the flints in order to talk with your hands. (I'm reminded of the old joke: "How do you get an Italian to shut up.... Put him in handcuffs." Seriously, though, we all talk with our hands—it's our evolutionary heritage.)

In the Paleolithic world, to facilitate communication while simultaneously demonstrating a manual task, one would naturally fall back on an earlier, more primitive medium, vocalization. Thus, vocalization would be supplementary to mimetic language, but over the course of much time—quite probably the entire course of the Middle Paleolithic (300,000 to 45,000 years ago)—the vocalizations, and the physical and neural abilities to vocalize, would gradually increase in sophistication, until the point when they could actually supplant the mimetic signs themselves, leaving the hands free to work. Thus, we have the very first "hands-free" communication system! When ancient humans shifted from mimetic language to oral language during the Middle Paleolithic, the structures in the dominant hemisphere that facilitated mimesis were functionally duplicated within areas in the dominant hemisphere that evolved specifically for oral language—Broca's area and Wernicke's area.[9]

This evolutionary neurological adaptation, which took hundreds of thousands of years to achieve, formalized the lateralization of language in the dominant hemisphere, which is the left hemisphere in 96 percent of right-handers, and in 75 percent of left-handers. Since right-handers comprise 89 percent of the population, that means that about 95 percent of the human race have brains that are lateralized for language dominance in the left hemisphere.[10] As we'll see, the consequences of language lateralization for the capacities of thought and speech and nearly every other aspect of cognition are so far reaching and extensive, that they merit the aphoristic pronouncement of renowned geneticist and biologist, Theodosius Dobzhansky: "Except in the light of lateralization, nothing in human psychology and psychiatry makes any sense."[11]

The transformative effect that language has on thought is in its sequential linear form. Donald refers to pre-linguistic thought as "episodic." Without concrete symbols to categorize thought, animals—including preconscious and unconscious humans—simply live from moment to moment, from episode to episode. That doesn't mean that the pre-linguistic mind is a blank. It just means that the thoughts in the mind are proceeding in a formless or directionless manner, because there's no symbolic structure to categorize thoughts, and therefore no system with which to process thoughts in a way that would be sequential or linear. Rather than experiencing thought as a continuous line of words spoken to and heard by oneself, thought would be a continuing sequence of visual episodes, like a dream or a never-ending movie. A quotation from Aeschylus, in *Prometheus Bound*, recalls the state of humanity before the gods blessed them with language:

> *Senseless as beasts I gave men sense, possessed them of Mind...*
> *In the beginning, seeing they saw amiss, and hearing heard not,*
> *   but, like phantoms huddled.*
> *In dreams, the perplexed story of their days; Confounded.*[12]

Episodic thought proceeds via association—one thought is linked to another by some sort of remembered connection, analogy, or similarity that associates one thought with the other—and then a third association is conjured, and a fourth, and so on. The order of thought is not relevant, because the associative links are relatively random. One thought does not logically or systematically follow from, lead to, or build upon the previous or next thought. Dreams provide an excellent example of this daisy chain of associative thought. While dreaming, experience follows thought in a rather haphazard way, with one thing happening after another in a stream of associations that just keeps on going. While dreaming, it all seems to make sense, because at any given moment, it's clear that the present thought has come to us through an association with the previous thought, and that the succeeding thought is clearly linked with the present thought. But when we awake and try to make sense of the dream, it seems impossible, because there's no logic in the dream, no coordinating or sequential line of thought in which one thing logically follows from another. The dream is just a collection of non sequiturs—loosely connected associations—that have no definitive form or meaning.

Dreams, for most of us, are expressions of right hemispheric processing.[13] When we awake, we abruptly shift back to left hemispheric processing, which is dominated by a language that is sequential, linear, and "log-ical" ("log" from the Greek root, *logos*, "word"). Words cannot adequately define, understand or interpret the primarily visual and illogically associated episodes of a dream, so our grasp of the dream just fades away, which is why we forget the majority of the content of our dreams so soon after waking. Other examples of nonlinear thought can be heard in the adorable but nonsensical ramblings of very little children, the psychedelic "far-out" descriptions of LSD trips reported by hallucinatory drug users, and the tangential, disorganized, derailed, loose associations of schizophrenics, often referred to as "word salad."[14]

When humans took their first great cognitive leap from episodic thought to mimetic language, their thought process became sequential and linear, because a complex message is only comprehensible—for both the sender and the recipient—if each part of the message follows a deliberate sequence, in which one part logically follows the previous part and then logically leads to the next part in a linear fashion. A clear message must be a straight line of thought, leading directly towards a specific meaning or point. The next great cognitive leap, from mimetic to oral language, creates an even more linear structure to language and thought. As the "father of 20th century linguistics," Ferdinand de Saussure, explains: "...a primary characteristic of the spoken sequence is its linearity.... In itself it is merely a line, a continuous ribbon of sound."[15]

This "continuous ribbon of sound" describes not only speech, but the stream of consciousness that evolved from internalized speech. It's difficult to imagine the stream of consciousness as a "continuous ribbon" of imagined mimetic hand signals. The transformation of language into phonetic oral language increases its ability to flow endlessly, which in turn necessitates a more linear structure, so that the "ribbon" of verbal thought doesn't twirl, spiral, and collapse upon itself into illogical nonsense; but rather proceeds linearly, logically, and sequentially, one thought building upon another and another and another, a straight, sequential, continuous *line* of thought.

Literacy and Linearity

Returning once more to Donald's model, we reach the last stage of his theory, in which oral language is supplemented by a "theoretic" medium of communication. Ancient humans in the Middle Paleolithic were learning to speak as their primary mode of communication, though probably at a glacial pace. Their hands, however, molded by millions of years of evolution to be deft and nimble at toolmaking and fire-making, and already specialized for mimetic communication, were to "grasp" at language once again. Oral language, while an excellent form of communication in the present here and now, is not a good medium for information storage, because heard words must be stored in the brain as memory. Repetition of information within one's head via verbal thought is the only way a person limited to oral language can engrain verbal information into their memory banks. That method of memorization was both inefficient and insufficient for the amount of information humans needed to master their environments and to succeed in their ever-increasingly sophisticated societies. Therefore, according to Donald, the hands of the Middle Paleolithic "cavemen" got busy creating "external memory systems."[16]

The primary benefit of an "external memory system" is that it doesn't rely on human memory. Ancient cave paintings dating back from at least 28,000 to as much as 64,000 years ago are evidence of the first human uses of external memory. The paintings seem to be records of hunts and also, possibly, spiritual/fertility rituals. The fact that we can see these paintings so many millennia later is testimony to the other great benefit of an external memory system—its independence from time. Unlike spoken words, the paintings are not confined to the here and now. The ancient cave painters could return to their work and recall the past events recorded in them, giving them a tangible sense of personal and cultural history. The images, when focused upon, become engrained in memory in ways more lucid and concrete than oral words can be remembered.

So, as oral language proceeded to develop, ancient humans also proceeded to use their hands to record memories in cave paintings and with other "visuographic inventions," such as engravings on stones, clay, and bones, as well as ritualistic piercings and body paintings (tattoos), most of which are lost to time.[17] The evolution of external memory systems begins with the early pictorial representations of the Middle and Upper Paleolithic, which evolved into the more specific pictographs of the Mesolithic, which further evolved into the ideograms, hieroglyphs, and cuneiform number systems of the Neolithic, and then at long last, into the phonetic alphabet.

The invention of the alphabet was a true revolution in communication, probably the most important media revolution in history. The alphabet merged the oral medium of language with the visuographic medium of images by breaking down the sounds of words into phonemes (letters representing specific sounds), and then combining the letters to create visual words (writing), that could later be deciphered as oral language by others (reading). Please note that Chinese pictographs and other writing systems that use ideograms or symbols to represent whole words rather than specific sounds, are not considered alphabets, because an alphabet, by definition, is a string of letters, with each letter referring only to a sound, and not an entire word or idea. The effect phonetic-alphabet-based literacy would have on the mind of the Western world is profound.

When we learn to read, we read aloud, translating the images of the letters into the sounds of words. In transfiguring the auditory process of language into a visual process, we're "literally" rewiring the function of language in the brain. In infants and small children, who are preliterate, language is processed primarily in the right hemisphere.[18] Reading and writing, however, are processed primarily in the left hemisphere.[19] Each aspect of literacy represents another leftward shift of language functioning in the brain. When we teach small children to read and write, we take an experience that is spoken and heard, and turn it into an experience that is drawn and seen. The linearity of language, implicit in the spoken word, becomes explicit in the written word, as the child "literally" sees and draws *lines* of letters, that spell out words in *lines* of sentences. This mechanical, linear, assembly-line consumption and production of words in a sequential and logical pattern is very much the specialty of the left hemisphere. The spontaneity and instinctiveness of oral language is lost when it's transfigured into literacy, as the written medium is inherently concrete, regimented, and fixed.

Grammar, the rules that fix a specific order or "syntax" within language, is implicitly understood in oral language, even by very young children; hence Chomsky's observation of an apparent "universal grammar" in humans, that's genetically inherited and "hardwired" in the brain.[20] Grammar, in the written word, is anything but implicit. The rules of grammar in writing are countless, extremely explicit, and nearly impossible to master for children (and most adults). Grammatical writing, in this sense, is the epitome of left hemispheric functioning, as it requires extensive focusing on details, the application of logical rules, and the meticulous separation and rearrangement of the elements of language into individual mechanical parts. Writing refashions a task that is, in the oral medium, natural, instinctive, and spontaneous, into a task that is reflective, deliberate, purposeful, logical, and sequential. To quote McLuhan, *"Nobody ever made a grammatical error in a nonliterate society."*[21]

The cerebral dominance of the left hemisphere in the use of language is the critical point that I've been leading up to. Language is inextricably tied in with verbal thought, which in turn is inextricably tied in with consciousness. In the transitions drawn out by Donald, we can discern a pattern in which language becomes increasingly more specific, increasingly more linear, and increasingly more sequential. In terms of language processing in the brain, each of these steps requires a further lateralization of language towards the hemisphere that specializes in focused, linear, and sequential tasks, making the left hemisphere more dominant at each step. When we made that first initial leap from "episodic" experience to mimetic communication, an associative thought process that was entirely nonsequential and nonlinear needed to adapt to a medium of communication that was necessarily sequential (one sign at a time).

The physical medium of mimesis—hand gestures—is also related to leftward lateralization, as the dominant right hand is contralaterally controlled by the left hemisphere. Upon proceeding from mimetic to oral communication, language becomes more sequential and linear still, as words replace signs in a more fluid and streamlined flow of ideas, Saussure's "continuous ribbon of sound." In the next great leap from oral language to literacy, words in the visual format become concretized as physical visual objects on the page. In this format, words must be explicitly grammatical, requiring a much more reflective and deliberate processing of language, in order for the output to conform to preset standards and rules of syntax, rules based on the logic, sequence, and linearity of word and sentence structure. The leftward lateralization of language happened linearly and sequentially over the course of evolution, and it proceeds likewise through history and through the ensuing media of the modern world: print, electronic, and digital media.

Cognitive Distance

The frontal lobes of the brain are referred to as the "neocortex," indicating that the majority of the frontal lobes represent recent evolutionary additions to the anatomy of the brain. The frontal lobes process higher order "executive functions" such as language and verbal thought. In considering the evolution of the brain, we must avoid teleological thinking, the idea that the brain has some sort of plan or end goal that it's working towards. Instead, we must remember that the brain is always adapting to its current environmental pressures. In terms of evolutionary direction and momentum, the brain is always being pushed ahead by present pressures, never pulled forward by future goals. So, in hindsight, we must observe the pressures imposed upon the brain over time, in order to discern how and why certain parts and certain connective configurations of the brain evolved.

One well-documented observation is that the brain has evolved certain significant asymmetries between the hemispheres, and that functional and anatomical studies of these asymmetries lead to the conclusion that they developed in order to accommodate the ever-increasing neurological need for language processing capacity, especially since language is involved in both communication and in private thought.[22] McGilchrist has argued that these hemispheric asymmetries are further proof that our brains have become more lateralized in their respective functions—each hemisphere has become more mutually independent of the other—because if the brain as a whole increased in capacity as a function of increased whole-brain processing, then we would have seen symmetrical increases in brain size, rather than asymmetrical increases.

Simply put, asymmetries in the hemispheres of the brain are recent evolutionary adaptations that serve to further lateralize language and verbal thought in the left hemisphere.[23] Furthermore, the asymmetries increase the left hemisphere's ability to function autonomously, by inhibiting the right hemisphere's input. In doing so, the left hemisphere, which deals more with the cogitating of abstract symbols and the close analysis of specific details, is able to distance itself from the right hemisphere, which experiences the world more holistically and intuitively.

One of the related functions of the frontal lobes is to inhibit immediate instinctive reactions to our environment, in order to allow us to think before we react, a distinctly human trait that certainly gives us a major adaptive advantage. The inhibitory function of the frontal lobes, to quote McGilchrist, "allows for a distance in time and space in order to cogitate upon a considered action." It gives us that distinctly human trait of suspended judgment. But where does this "necessary distance" come from? We cannot assume that the brain teleologically foresaw the tremendous advantage of suspending judgment, which arises from cognitively distancing oneself from a situation in order to abstractly consider our best reactions. Rather, we must assume that some earlier ability created this sense of "distance," as an accommodation to an existing environmental pressure.

Once "distantiation" as a trait proved itself adaptive, the brain would continue to expand the sense of cognitive distance between individual and environments, strengthening the trait and extending the distance, as long as it was evolutionarily advantageous to do so. One may even expect that at some point, the progressive genetic adaptation for distantiation would go "a bridge too far," leading to a pathological level of distantiation, and a genetic disposition that creates too much cognitive distance between the individual and their environment, making them act and feel disconnected from others, alien to Nature and to their surroundings, and estranged even from their own sense of identity and being.

Cognitive distance begins with language. A nonlinguistic animal, such as a dog, engages directly with its environment. Without cognitive symbols with which to represent objects in its environment—such as a bone—or subjects in its environment—such as a cat—the dog can have no "ideas" about bones and cats, only memories of experiences ("episodes"), of once having a bone and once chasing a cat. Like Aeschylus, we can imagine the mindset of the dog and the cat as a dreamlike experience, or perhaps like a movie, in which episodic memories are triggered and recalled via association with whatever happens to be going on. The animal has no "conscious" control of the episodes they're remembering or imagining, because they're not "conscious" of their own thought processes in the way that we are. Their ability to be aware of their own awareness, to think about their thoughts and manipulate them purposefully, is circumscribed by their inability to think abstractly because of the lack of abstract symbols in their thought process. When the dog interacts with a cat, it has no idea about the cat to cogitate upon—no cognitive distance from the cat—it merely responds intuitively and instinctively towards the cat, with no forethought for what it should do, and no afterthought about what it should have done.

When we add language to the mix, we mentally represent the cat with an abstract symbol such as the word "cat," and now there is cognitive distance, because long after the cat runs away, we can abstractly recall the symbol of the cat, and therefore the idea of the cat, and we can cogitate upon the idea of what the cat *could* do, and what we *could* do in response to the hypothetical cat's hypothetical action. The abstract symbol of the word is a cognitive tool with which we can grasp our mercurial thoughts very firmly, allowing us to adroitly manipulate them into an infinite variety of hypothetical cognitive models.

Hand tools such as a hammer and a pair of tongs enhanced our ability to grasp and shape metal objects so greatly that they actually created new forms of labor, such as metal forging, which in turn created entire new ages of human experience, the Copper Age, the Bronze Age, the Iron Age, and so on. Similarly, the cognitive tool of verbal language enhanced our ability to grasp and shape thought so greatly that it created entire new dimensions of thinking, including objective thought, and conscious awareness of our own thought process. When the abstract symbology of verbal language is internalized as verbal thought, the "voice of consciousness" is born. *It is the voice of consciousness that creates and fills in the distance between our experience of the world and our participation in it.* The substance of that distance filler is forethought and afterthought. But how is language actually internalized as verbal thought, and what do we mean by "thought," anyway?

A thought is a hazy thing. What exactly is a thought, other than the circular definition of thought as the product of thinking? Thoughts as discrete objects don't exist in the brain. I believe that the closest thing we may have to "pure thought" are the sounds and visions that stream through our awareness in dreams. Those "thoughts" have no discrete beginning and no discrete end. They refer to many things in general but to nothing in particular. They have almost no relation to the specific thoughts we may have while awake, specific thoughts about our tax bill or about our checking account balance or about what to make for dinner. Thought, in its pure unrepresented state, is a process in-and-of-itself, not the product of a process. In fact, in order to have a discrete and specific thought about any one thing, we must be able to label and categorize that thought with a specific symbol.

In the case of verbal thought, words are those symbols that we use to objectify thought. So we can say with some certainty that once oral language is "hardwired" into the brain, we have the necessary groundwork for internalized verbal thought. But the process doesn't end there. In fact, it just begins there. Oral language alone doesn't necessarily confer cognitive distance. Very small children, for instance, are extremely verbal, yet they lack the cognitive distance to think before they act or react. Not only are their frontal lobes not fully developed, their capacity for objective thought is not yet fully developed either.

It is, in fact, *literacy* that truly drives forward the *objectification* of thought. When learning to read, the child transfigures the sight of words on a page into the sounds of words in his mind. The words on the page are objective, physical, tangible, visible objects. At first, the child reads aloud, transforming the visible sights into audible sounds. But soon, the child stops reading aloud, he or she even stops moving their lips, as the objects of thought on the page stream seamlessly into symbolic objects of thought in their mind. The objectification of thought, and the internalization of verbal thought, are not necessarily created by literacy, but the processes are without doubt propelled and accelerated by literacy.

In reading—and even more so in *writing*—we are forcing our minds to be more "conscious" of its own use of language, and in response, our minds become more "conscious" of their own verbal thoughts. Our thinking becomes "self-conscious," and oftentimes, "hyperconscious" of its own thought process. Literacy drives linguistic thought forward, but inwardly. In a 1997 neurological study entitled "What the reader's eye tells the mind's ear: Silent reading activates inner speech," Abramson and Goldinger found that "inner speech" in reading is "heard" in the mind in the same way that overt speech is heard.[24] The practice of reading silently and hearing the sound of our own voice saying the words in our head, serves to amplify the volume of the internal voice of consciousness.

Once objectified into their linear, sequential and logical forms, words in the written format become inherently more logical and more objective, and since these very same words are imbibed by literate minds, becoming the very fabric of conscious thought, it stands to reason that the literate mind itself will invariably become more distanced, more objective and more logical. In reading, words as objects are internalized as thoughts; and then in writing, thoughts are objectified as exteriorized words. "It is certain," wrote Edgar Allan Poe, "that the mere act of inditing tends in a great degree to the logicalization of thought."[25]

Another mental trait garnered from literacy is *abstraction*, thinking of something hypothetically, outside of its context, in order to analyze it narrowly, objectively, and with a focused perspective one can only gain by distancing oneself from the context of the matter. John Locke famously stated—*"Beasts abstract not!"*—to which Bishop Berkley agreed, but with the reminder to Locke that many "*men abstract not*" as well. Both points are true. *My* point is that abstraction is a specialization of the left hemisphere, a necessary affiliate of the abilities to objectify and distantiate, and similarly a byproduct of literacy. All other media prior to the phonetic alphabet retain meaning in their symbolic forms.

Pictorial representations, hieroglyphs and ideograms use images that look similar to or analogous to the things they represent. Mimetic signs mimic the things they represent visuo-spatially; while oral words, though abstract, still each represent a specific thing, so each word in-and-of-itself has a meaning that is related directly to something. Furthermore, oral words often have an onomatopoeic origin—they sound like the things they refer to, like "cuckoo" or "drip." To the contrary, the symbols in the phonetic alphabet—the letters—have no actual meaning, other than representing specific sounds, which in-and-of-themselves are meaningless until arranged and composed into words. To quote McLuhan again, "...our alphabet ... dissociates or abstracts, not only sight and sound, but separates all meaning from the sound of the letters, save so far as the meaningless letters relate to the meaningless sound.... By the meaningless sign linked to the meaningless sound, we have built the shape and meaning of Western man."[26]

It's quite telling that while little children love to sing and to learn songs, the first song we actually require them to sing and to learn, the first song they're forced to repeat aloud until set to memory, is the "Alphabet Song," which has no meaning, just a list of meaningless sounds linked to a set of meaningless signs. The overall significance of this process of abstraction is that a mind trained to learn and to think by means of literacy, is a mind that will by force of habit abstract information and experience from their context, in order to enable the extremely efficient mode of thinking known as "hypothetical-deductive reasoning," which Jean Piaget designated as the hallmark of "formal operational thought," the highest level of cognitive development in his model, and a stage reached only by individuals who master literacy. As UNESCO's Report on Literacy stated, "...the illiterate man's thought ... remains concrete. He thinks in images and not in concepts. His thought is, in fact, a series of images, juxtaposed or in sequence, and hence it rarely proceeds by induction or deduction."[27] As the process of reading and writing are processes of abstraction, it follows that the literate mind proceeds in thought by abstraction, as literacy is an extension of thought.

Yet another way that literacy creates a sense of mental distance is by its transcendence of time and space. Oral language is always in the present. Excepting the use of modern electronic equipment, the things you or I say exist fleetingly in the moment that we say them, in the place that we say them, and then they're "gone with the wind." Oral words exist only in the present time and in the present space. Not so with the written word. Once a word is visualized and objectified onto a page, the written word can exist indefinitely, to travel anywhere and anyplace, to be read by anyone at any time. The de-contextualization of language from the present afforded by literacy is profoundly abstract, and has a profound effect on the mind. The verbal thought of consciousness that is derived from literacy will likewise be de-contextualized from time and space. The narrative voice of consciousness, the ongoing internal story we tell ourselves about ourselves, is also remarkably independent of time and space. The inner voice can travel backwards in reverie and forwards in fantasy at will. It can leap continents, travel to outer space, or even to imaginary lands only conceivable to ourselves... "My mind to me a kingdom is; such present joys therein I find; / As far exceeds all earthly bliss, which God and Nature hath assigned."[28]

Though we can conceive of this total freedom of mind as liberating, it can also be inhibiting, for despite our capacity for whimsical flights of fancy, in the end, we're still physically in the context of this world at this time. The "kingdom of mind" that we so often retreat to has ramparts and motes that distance us from others beyond the kingdom walls. "The more literate people become, the more they tend to become detached from the world in which they live," wrote Marshall McLuhan.[29] At the end of this process of distantiation, abstraction, de-contextualization and objectification, we observe the effect on the thinker himself. The objective thinker, in self-reflection, becomes an object to himself. The distanced thinker who creates "necessary distance"[30] between himself and his world, and between himself and others, in order to be objective and thoughtful in his words and deeds, becomes distant from himself. "That literate man," according to McLuhan, "when we meet him in the Greek world, is a split man, a schizophrenic, as all literate men have been since the invention of the phonetic alphabet."[31]

Print

Gutenberg's invention was nearly as important to literacy as the invention of the phonetic alphabet. Before the printing press, all books were handwritten manuscripts. Books were exceedingly rare, as were people who had access to them and were able to read them. The printing press changed the economics of literacy, making it possible, cheap and efficient to mass produce books. Demand grew in proportion to supply. With cheap and accessible books and pamphlets on hand, more people educated their children to read, creating more demand for the supply of new books. *While the phonetic alphabet gave rise to literacy, typographical print gave rise to literature.*

Print was the first mass medium. Just as the automobile and the subsequent invention of the assembly line by Ford created a supply of automobiles that in turn gave rise to nations of drivers, the alphabet and the printing press created a supply of literature that gave rise to a culture of readers. So, while the neurological consequences of literacy affected many individuals in the early days of alphabetic literacy, beginning about 3,500 years ago in the Near East, the number of literate people actually living in these ancient societies was a tiny fraction of 1 percent of the population. Indeed, there weren't even any real books, as we know them, until the Romans.[32] Only after the printing press did we see the beginning of *mass literacy* and the inception of *mass education* to create and increase mass literacy. Therefore, any discussion about "modern society" and the environmental pressures that exist in modern society must acknowledge the foundational influence of print, the technology that gave rise to the modern world.

In his book *The Gutenberg Galaxy* (1962), McLuhan made the point that in order for reading to truly engrain the process of internalized verbal thought in the brain, the speed of reading would have to approximate the speed of oral language.[33] When we think in words, we don't do it slowly, one word at a time, like a small child first learning to read. We think quickly in words, in great lightning-fast streams of words, as quick if not quicker than the words that pour out of our mouths when we speak, the "continuous ribbon of sound." However, prior to print, in the ancient and medieval worlds, all reading was done aloud.[34] Manuscripts were thick scrolls typically made of parchment. They were unwieldy, nonportable, difficult to handle, and often brittle and fragile.

The script was written with ink and quill, so the pages and writing were oftentimes faded with age, and the ink was often blotched, blotted, or smudged. Scribes all wrote in their own peculiar styles, using idiosyncratic scripts, and their own personal spellings, grammars, and lexicons. Early scribes did not use vowels or punctuation and often didn't place spaces between words, making the content extremely difficult to read, unless the reader was entirely familiar with the text before reading it. The standardization of spelling, grammar, and lexicon came well after the print revolution, as a means of furthering the standardization of the written word, to make reading quicker and easier. Since manuscripts were hard to read, even for scribes, the script readers read slowly and aloud, like a small child learning to read.

Furthermore, most scripts were holy scrolls, and most readers and scribes were clergymen. The process of "reading" these holy scrolls was not at all similar to the secular and casual process of a modern reader reading a modern book. Each word in the holy scrolls was a sacrament. The sages, priests, rabbis, imams and monks were taught to recite each holy word aloud, in a slow and reverent chanting melody, in order to induce a prayer-like state of spiritual meditation. *Lectio*, "reading," was a "spiritual exercise," as nearly all reading was *lectio divina*, reading the holy scriptures.[35] The purpose of the "reading carrels" in medieval libraries was not to insulate the reader from outside noises, but to *isolate* the reader from other readers, as all of the readers were reading, indeed *singing*, aloud.[36]

Print changed everything. Printed books on paper presented a uniform typography, set in perfectly straight lines in precise order, in spelling, grammar and vocabulary that were increasingly standardized, all packaged neatly in a portable product that was easy to carry and exponentially easier to read than the manuscripts that preceded them. While

Gutenberg's first product was his famous bible, his invention was soon employed to print secular literature, a product that quickly led to the democratization and secularization of reading. So, while literacy was necessary for the internalization of verbal thought, it was print, with its "mass production of exactly uniform and repeatable type,"[37] that accelerated the speed of reading to the point where it reached the same velocity as speech. The increased speed of reading and the spread of reading to the masses made reading aloud too slow for practicality, and too loud for classrooms and libraries now filled with readers. Silent reading to oneself became the expected and the required norm. With the silencing of the outer voice came the amplification of the inner voice. The inner voice we hear when reading silently is the same voice we hear when thinking. Reading *print*, therefore, is not necessarily the mother of conscious thought, but the godmother that gives conscious thought its volume and its range.

The amplification and engraining of the inner voice of consciousness, and the "democratization of literacy"[38] via the advents of mass literacy and mass education, both furthered the process of leftward language lateralization in the brain. By the 19th century, the Western world is quickly becoming a world populated by literate individuals, each with a private "kingdom of mind" of their own conscious making, and each with an analytical mind able to think objectively and dispassionately, able to distance itself from others and from the world and even from itself. The narrow lines of sequential text in the books that literate individuals read sculpted minds that mirrored the medium. The literate mind, like the books being read, focused narrowly on sequential lines of thought. To quote William Blake, "*We become what we behold.*" Furthermore, we behold what we've become, creating a new world in our own image. Behold the post-industrial world begotten by the mass product of the first assembly line industry and the first mass medium— the world empowered by easily accessible, easily transferable, easily understood, easily expressed, and easily shared information. It's a world of lines. Lines of railroads and highways going across. Lines of skyscrapers and telecom towers going up. Telephone lines and power lines crisscrossing the air, lines of airplanes crisscrossing the sky, lines of electrons shooting down from satellites in space, transmitting lines of information through our screens and into our brains...

Electronic Media and Digital Media

"Electronic media" is a blanket term applied to all media that use electricity. Thus, the media themselves are extremely varied, with extremely varied effects. The first truly electronic medium was the 19th century telegraph, which was, in essence, an extension of literacy, as the messages sent and the messages received were both written words. Hence, the effect on the literate mind was not in-and-of-itself transformative, but the direct effect of the telegraph line as a driving force in the modernization and linearization of the industrial world was profound.

The minute that information could travel vast distances at the speed of light was the minute that the individual person became connected via information to everyone else in the world. In the pre-telegraphic past, it was none of my concern if forest fires raged in California, or if typhoons blew in Southeast Asia, or even if senators and presidents stole and lied in Washington. It was none of my concern because I had no way of knowing about it in the present moment. I was blissfully ignorant and therefore unconcerned and unconnected with the rest of the world. McLuhan relates a statement recorded in the minutes of a meeting held by President George Washington, in which the president remarked that they hadn't heard from Mr. Pinckney, their ambassador to England, in over a year; "Someone should write him a letter."[39]

In a world in which information is slowly dispersed, expectations for information are much more laid back. Patience, in the old world, was a true virtue. But in the telegraphic world, when all news of everyone from around the world becomes instantly accessible, the problems of the world are laid at my feet, and this becomes my concern, and my burden. Furthermore, the access to instant information creates an expectation for instant information. The telegraph created a world in which information travelled at the speed of light, which quickly turned into a world where people expected information at the speed of light, a world of people who are frustrated when they cannot get their information at the speed of light. The electronic medium did not change the substance of thought, but it accelerated the *velocity* of thought, resulting in a modern world of instant everything. And thus the "Age of Anxiety" was borne not of the printing press but of the telegraph.[40]

The electronic age is a world marked by, driven by, and suffering from a pathological level of impatience. As the march of newer and more sophisticated electronic media developed—radio, film, television, etc.—the anxiety that arose from a world of instant infinite information grew. Instantaneity of information breeds impatience, both with others and with oneself. When one gets information instantly, one begins to expect information instantly, even information about the future. Anxiety, as an emotional response to the unknown future, is experienced as a state of dread. Dread that doesn't arise from *knowledge* of an awful future event, but from the *lack* of knowledge.

I have anxiety over a lecture I'm delivering tomorrow, for instance. My anxiety stems from a sense of dread that the lecture *may* go dreadfully wrong. The anxiety is not about my knowledge about whether or not the lecture will go wrong, it's about my *lack* of knowledge, my complete uncertainty. If I knew for certain that the lecture would go wrong, I'd simply decide not to do it, or barring that, resolve myself to my fate. In either case, my anxiety would be allayed. But since I *don't* know what will happen tomorrow, my expectations are left precariously dangling in mid-air, my fears are left hanging, leaving me in a state of dread about a potential fall, rather than an actual fall. The actual feeling of anxiety or dread is a feeling of *impatience.* I desperately need to know what will happen, but the information is not coming to me in the manner that I've become accustomed to, which, in a post-telegraphic world, is instantaneously. Therefore, my impatience just grows and festers.

My brain (more specifically, the left hemisphere), perseverates hyperconsciously on what it doesn't know, trying desperately to deduce via detailed abstract analysis of hypothetical futures what it can never truly know ... because the future is inherently unknowable. And so we see that the modern world—a world in which nearly a third of all people suffer from severe anxiety at one point in their lives[41]—is a world where media consumption and production has shifted the dominance of the mind's focus, once again, towards the left hemisphere of the brain.

Electronic media are varied in form, and have various effects, some of which are converse to the leftward hemispheric shift I've been explaining. For instance, while the telegraph could be seen as an extension of literacy, the succeeding technology, the telephone, reversed the communication medium from a literary form into an oral form. When the telephone was invented, people began to speak to each other via long distances, rather than sending long written letters or brief telegraphic messages to each other. In other words, the effects of electronic media are complicated and multidirectional, and influence hemispheric lateralization in both directions.

Digital media is a form of electronic media, but it's also extremely varied in its form and its effects. Like the telegraph, digital media increases the velocity of information, but it also increases the volume or density of information being sent, the total amount of information in a message. The telegraph, for instance, was an excellent way of transmitting "headlines" across vast distances, but it was not expedient for sending entire news stories. With digital media, however, we can send and receive an entire newspaper full of stories with much greater ease than it once took to telegraph one word. Furthermore, the volume of digital media allows it to subsume virtually all other forms of media: television, film, radio, telephone, photography, telegraphy, print, oral communication, mimetic communication, etc.

In short, the effects of electronic and digital media on the mind and behavior are so complex and multidirectional that they cannot be summarized here. The further effects of both electronic and digital media on a variety of psychopathological conditions, and their relation to the leftward shift of cerebral dominance, are covered in depth in subsequent chapters.

A final note on the topic: social media (e.g., Facebook, Twitter, Instagram, etc.), rather than being extensions of a particular thought within a specific medium—such as literacy or language—are extensions of our entire selves. A Facebook page, for many people, expresses almost everything about their identity: their appearance over time, their family, their friends, their educations, occupations, and personal background, their political opinions, their religious beliefs, their favorite movies and music, their likes and dislikes, everything... Therefore, in a way that is infinitely more powerful than a spoken or written message, a social media app extends our individual identities outward into the ether as visual objects representing ourselves. For the vast majority of people we may deal with via social media, (our thousands of Facebook "friends,") the only interactions we'll have with each other is via these "objects" of "virtual identity."

Many people take their virtual objects of identity extremely seriously, as if they were not just extensions of their selves, but their *actual* selves. Disagreements, insults, nasty comments, negative ratings, "dislikes," and "unfriends," are taken very personally, just as much as if their actual selves were disparaged, and even more so, because the virtual disparagement is enacted in a worldwide public forum for the whole world to see, and recorded digitally so that it exists forever. Thus, digital media in general and social media in particular further the leftward shift process by pressuring us to objectify ourselves through media, fostering a sense of distance from our personal identities, as we increasingly perceive ourselves as virtual representations of our own identities.

The modern media environment creates an extremely objectified, depersonalized, and dissociated sense of self, a world in which our own identities and the identities of others are deconstructed by the left hemispheric mind into cybernetic digital bytes, and then reconstructed by the same hemisphere as objective virtual representations of ourselves. The digital media we consume also consumes us. Recalling William Blake, "We become what we behold." If what we behold all day, every day, are screens projecting images reflecting ourselves, then we become both the source and product of those screened images. And if those screens are wired to digital machines that think objectively, abstractly, sequentially, and linearly, then, as McGilchrist said, "We are busy imitating machines."[42]

The Forest of Mirrors

To summarize the evolution of the leftward shift so far: the initial shift began in the Lower Paleolithic, when manual manipulation of tools and fire-making necessitated the neurological lateralization of handedness in order to establish a dominant hand (typically the right hand). The leftward shift proceeded as mimetic communication duplicated functions already being used for tool use, and already situated in the left hemisphere, into functions used for language. As mimetic communication evolved into oral language, the shift towards the left continued, with the left hemisphere further specializing in abstract symbols and linear thought, which are the defining features of oral language. The advent of language also initiated the function of internal verbal thought, which would also be lateralized in the left hemisphere, with necessary right hemispheric input being controlled and inhibited, so as to retain a sense of cognitive unity—a singular voice of consciousness. As literacy evolved, the leftward shift picked up steam, as the requirements of literacy included an even more detailed and linear mode of thinking, depending even more on abstract symbols, and focusing more and more singularly on symbolic representations of the world, as opposed to actual experiences of the world.

Print technology pushed the leftward shift even further, via the deliberate training of silent reading in child populations, a process that invokes the inner voice of verbal thought. Print technology also heralded revolutionary changes in the environment of the Western world. The Renaissance, the Enlightenment, and the Industrial Revolution are all attributable to the advents of mass education, mass literacy, and the ability for new information to be speedily distributed across populations, which are all directly attributable to the advent of print technology. In the modern world, electronic and digital media accelerate the velocity and density of communication, creating a media environment marked by information overload, media saturation, and a culture of instantaneity, that interact with the "left hemispheric mindset" to create pathological levels of impatience, hyperconsciousness, perseveration, and anxiety.

The left hemisphere's analytical, sequential, and linear focus on specific details creates a mindset that is prone to conceptual myopia.

The brain is dependent on the right hemisphere for context, for seeing and experiencing the world as a whole, for seeing people as whole beings rather than as collections of personal details, for seeing the forest composed of trees. The left hemisphere has been specialized by evolution to process abstract symbolic representations. Without proper input from the right, the left cannot see the world, it can see only what it *re-presents to itself* as the world. Without the right, the left cannot see the forest for the trees. It is, indeed, like Narcissus, forever gazing at a reflection that it does not recognize as himself. Able to see only reflections, and incapable of seeing the forest beyond the reflecting trees, the modern mind is increasingly finding itself lost in a forest of mirrors.

Cerebral Dominance and the Sickle Cell

The left-hemisphere shift model presumes that environmental pressures stemming from the media that we use to express and process language and verbal thought, evoke adaptations at the genetic and "epigenetic" levels. That is, over thousands of years, our genes have adapted to the media environments we live in by predisposing our brains towards cerebral dominance for language and verbal thought, towards one hemisphere or the other. Furthermore, as each of us develops in our own individual media environments our brains—which are extremely "plastic" or adaptable to their environments—adjust themselves epigenetically by modifying the expression of the genes responsible for cerebral hemispheric dominance. In this sense, epigenetic changes are tantamount to real-time evolutionary adaptation, as the "switching on or off" of the expression of existing genes allows for adaptation in each individual, through the course of his individual development.

Thus, how we think and use media at the neuronal level, is an expression of both our genetic inheritance (which predetermines our neurological dispositions), and our individual epigenetic adaptations to the particular media environments that we grow up in. So, hypothetically, if identical twins (who share 100 percent of the same genes), are separated at birth and raised in different media environments, it's likely that the way they process language and verbal thought will be very similar, due to their shared genetic inheritance; but it's also likely that there will be significant differences in the way they process language and verbal thought, as each of their brains would make different epigenetic modifications to the expression of the genes that control language and verbal thought processes, in response to the different media environments in which they were raised.

Before proceeding further in describing a model in which genetic and epigenetic variations in hemispheric dominance cause various mental disorders, it's necessary to discuss briefly how a variety of seemingly disparate disorders—schizophrenia, autism, dyslexia, ADHD, anxiety, depression, etc.—could arise from different variations in the expression of the same genes. Specifically, a number of genetic studies have inculpated the deletion of the 22q11.2 gene on the 22nd chromosome, as a common association linked to a variety of psychiatric disorders, including autism and schizophrenia.[43] To facilitate this discussion of genetic "pleiotropy"—the influence of one gene on multiple phenotypic traits—I'll make an analogy with the gene for the sickle cell.

Over the course of evolution, primarily in Africa and Asia, an adaptation to the deadliest disease in the history of the world—malaria—arose in the form of a mutated hemoglobin cell in red blood cells, which has a "sickle" shape. Genes for the sickle cell perpetuated in the population for millions of years because carriers of this trait are resistant to malaria. However, the trait also causes sickle cell diseases such as sickle cell anemia, which is often fatal. The evolution of the sickle cell is probably the best-known example of an evolutionary trade-off, in which a gene that confers both advantages and disadvantages perpetuates, because on average, the evolutionary advantage is greater than the disadvantage.

People carry two genes for hemoglobin. A heterogeneous sickle cell carrier is someone who has one normal hemoglobin gene and one sickle cell gene. This person is resistant to malaria. A noncarrier, someone who has two normal hemoglobin genes, is not resistant to malaria. Someone who has two sickle cell genes is resistant to malaria, but will also have a sickle cell disease, which is even deadlier than malaria. So, in a simple example, if two heterogeneous carriers of the sickle cell gene have a child, they will each pass down one of their genes for hemoglobin to their offspring. That child, via the calculation of Mendelian inheritance, will have a 50 percent chance of being homogeneous for the hemoglobin gene (having either two normal or two sickle genes). He or she will also have a 50 percent change of being heterogeneous for the hemoglobin gene (having one of each).

Being homogeneous is unlucky, because that means the child will either have two normal genes, making them vulnerable to malaria, or the child will have two sickle cell genes, resulting in sickle cell disease. Being heterogeneous, however, is very lucky, because that child will have no sickle cell disease, and will also be resistant to malaria. The evolutionary trade-off perpetuates the inheritance of a deadly gene, because, when evenly distributed across a population, it conveys a distinct adaptive advantage to 50 percent of the population (heterogeneous carriers), no advantage to 25 percent of the population (homogeneous noncarriers), and a very harsh disadvantage to the remaining 25 percent of the population (homogeneous carriers of the sickle cell gene). This scenario is also a good example of the principle of "hybrid vigor," the fact that genetic heterogeneity (aka "diversity"), is oftentimes extremely evolutionarily adaptive.

Applying this analogy to the hypothesized gene for cerebral dominance, we must first acknowledge that having two independently functioning cerebral hemispheres is adaptive. This principle is very well established. Secondly, we must also acknowledge that cerebral dominance for language in one of the hemispheres is also adaptive for many reasons, including the need to preserve a unity of consciousness. This principle is not necessarily established, but it's not too hard to accept prima facie, for the sake of argument. Thirdly, we must acknowledge that genetic traits when observed in the population are generally expressed along a continuum or spectrum of variation, and that this diversity is generally adaptive for the species as a whole over vast stretches of time, though specific variations may be quite maladaptive for specific individuals. This is a basic principle of evolution, of which the sickle cell gene is a lucid example.

So, in the analogy, the gene for cerebral dominance, like the gene for the sickle cell, perpetuates in the population, because it bestows great advantages to the vast majority, even though it may convey serious disadvantages to a minority of the population. Furthermore, just as the sickle cell gene is expressed in an array of genetic variations—heterogeneous carrier, homogeneous carrier, noncarrier—the cerebral dominance gene would also be expressed in an array of variations, due either to the heterogeneity or homogeneity of the genes involved, or to other epigenetic factors.

As in the expressions of the sickle cell trait, it's likely that the most adaptive expression of cerebral dominance would be a heterogeneous as opposed to a homogeneous expression. That means that, *in general*, mild or moderate hemispheric dominance in either hemisphere is more adaptive than severe or profound hemispheric dominance in either hemisphere, as the mild and moderate patterns maximize flexibility and adaptability in thought and behavior. And finally, just as the variations expressed by the sickle cell gene result in an array of conditions—malaria resistance, malaria nonresistance, sickle cell diseases—the variations expressed by the hemispheric dominance gene would also result in an array of conditions.

The Hemispheric Dominance Model of Mental Disorder

The theory proposed in this book suggests three categories of variation of hemispheric dominance, based on three possible forms of dominance (left hemispheric, right hemispheric, and neither, i.e., "nondominance"). Each category is broken up into four different levels of degree of dominance, modeled after the four levels of severity that the DSM applies to the variations of intellectual disability (mild, moderate, severe, and profound). The resulting 12 hemispheric types are there:

1. Mild left hemispheric dominance
2. Moderate left hemispheric dominance
3. Severe left hemispheric dominance
4. Profound left hemispheric dominance
5. Mild right hemispheric dominance
6. Moderate right hemispheric dominance
7. Severe right hemispheric dominance
8. Profound right hemispheric dominance
9. Mild hemispheric nondominance
10. Moderate hemispheric nondominance
11. Severe cerebral nondominance
12. Profound cerebral nondominance

Our media environments, over the course of evolution, have exerted pressures that created a dominant left hemisphere for language and verbal thought in the brains of most people. Verbal thought, the voice of consciousness, is an adaptive benefit, because it allows us to distance ourselves from our environment, in order to think objectively and logically about our problems, and to respond to the challenges of our environment with forethought, rather than instinct. The downside to this mode of thought is that we as a species tend to get cognitively stuck in the mode of forethought, always thinking about the future rather than the present, always calculating what could happen in the future, leaving us in a state of constant and pervasive dread of the future, a state of anxiety.

The condition of most modern people, I suggest, would be a state of mild left hemispheric dominance, making us, as a species, prone to anxiety. This theory coalesces with what we currently know about anxiety disorders, which is that they are "the most common mental disorders in the United States," and that nearly a third of all people "develop one of the disorders at some point in their lives."[44] Furthermore, many more than the diagnosed third of all people suffer in silence, self-medicating their anxiety with alcohol, marijuana, comfort foods, pills, or binging on various forms of media as a way of tuning out the anxiety ridden thoughts in their heads. Moderate left hemispheric dominance would therefore relate to a higher, more pervasive, and chronic state of anxiety. The topic of anxiety, as well as its ugly stepsister, depression, is covered in depth in Chapter Five.

Severe and profound left hemispheric dominance would represent the logical endpoint of the leftward shift process, a state in which the left hemisphere is pathologically dominant, resulting in excessive inhibition of right hemispheric input into the thought process. The symptoms related to left hemispheric over-dominance would include over-focusing on details to the exclusion of the big picture, a preference for repetitive tasks that can be analyzed and mastered to the exclusion of new stimuli, an inclination towards interacting with the parts of things rather than dealing with whole beings—such as people—who are unpredictable and can't be broken down into component parts, and as a consequence of these predilections, a tendency towards severe shyness and aloofness, in which the individual is overly content to be alone. In short, severe and profound left hemispheric dominance would be related to the autism spectrum. This topic will be covered in depth in the next chapter.

Moving to the other side of the brain, mild right hemispheric dominance is less common than left hemispheric dominance, and would be associated with thought patterns and language use that diverge from the norm. Eccentricity as a character trait may be related to mild right hemispheric dominance. In his book, *Eccentrics: A Study of Sanity and Strangeness* (1995), David Weeks' description of the "Eccentric Personality" coalesces perfectly with the right hemispheric approach to stimuli in the environment. While eccentricity (as a function of mild right hemispheric dominance), is positively correlated with high functioning and positive psychosocial adjustment; moderate right hemispheric dominance, on the other hand, may relate to depression.

The topic of depression is also covered in depth in Chapter Five, but the main argument revolves around research that suggests that the right hemisphere has a more realistic as opposed to optimistic perception of reality, ostensibly because the right hemisphere tunes into the world as it appears, as opposed to the left hemisphere, which tunes into the world as it is represented by abstract thought. Furthermore, the right hemisphere is known to be more involved in sad emotions and reactions. It tends to dwell on negative memories from the past (as opposed to the left hemispheric focus on the future). Negative past-oriented thoughts are suppressed by the future-oriented consciousness of the left hemisphere, relegating them to the more "unconscious" thought process of the right hemisphere.[45] This means that people whose minds are significantly more right hemispheric dominant are also more likely to be prone to depression.

The left hemisphere has been the dominant hemisphere for communication for millions of years. Our ability to understand and express extremely detailed and complicated messages with an extremely high degree of clarity arises from the left hemisphere's spectacular ability to deconstruct and analyze abstract symbols, to focus on details, and to express sophisticated ideas by stringing together a massive amount of information in sequential and logical lines of thought. Severe right hemispheric dominance, therefore, would inhibit someone's ability to think, speak, and understand language in the analytic, detailed, deeply-focused, linear, sequential, and logical ways necessary for the mind to master literacy and literacy-based tasks. In short, severe right hemispheric dominance would relate to learning disabilities such as dyslexia, as well as attention deficit disorders and mild intellectual disability. Profound right hemispheric dominance would relate to more severe deficits in language and thought, in which the individual has difficulties understanding and expressing oral language, and verbal thought is impaired, indicated by more severe disorders, such as language disorder and intellectual disability. These topics are covered in depth in Chapter Six.

The final category of hemispheric dominance is a state of "nondominance," in which neither hemisphere has clear dominance of the functions of language and verbal thought. As mentioned before, if both hemispheres simultaneously process language and verbal thought, it is absolutely crucial that verbal thought is experienced or "heard" in only one dominant hemisphere, as the existence of two simultaneous streams of consciousness would shatter the sense of cognitive unity that we all must maintain for our own sanity. Nevertheless, since hemispheric dominance for language and verbal thought is determined by genes that are expressed in a spectrum of variation, some people, by fluke of nature, will fall right in the middle of the spectrum, having brains that are predisposed towards hemispheric nondominance.

The lucky ones will experience mild hemispheric nondominance, which would result in patterns of language and thought that are more open to making loose associations and unconventional connections between seemingly unconnected areas, as input from both hemispheres would be relatively uninhibited. This type of "out-of-the-box" thinking could be advantageous, as it inspires creativity and ingenuity, and would be similar to or even the same phenomenon as mild right hemispheric dominance.

As we approach moderate hemispheric nondominance, however, the unwanted and uncontrolled spillover between the dual streams of consciousness will result in the symptoms of psychosis experienced by people on the schizophrenia spectrum, such as auditory oral hallucinations (hearing voices), delusions, and disordered thought. Severe and profound hemispheric nondominance would result in full-blown psychosis, the agonies of the tormented schizophrenic, whose mind is split in two. This is the topic of the fourth chapter.

The topic of the next chapter is autism. I am by no means the first person to suggest that the etiology of autism lies in the hyper-dominance of left hemispheric function, resulting in the over-inhibition of right hemispheric function. McGilchrist stated as much in his book, published in 2009:

> Then there is autism, a condition which has hugely increased in prevalence during the last fifty years ... marked by clinical features strongly suggestive of right-hemisphere hypofunction, and the resulting picture is one of left-hemisphere dominance. There is in autism an inability to tell what another is thinking (lack of "theory of mind"); a lack of social intelligence—difficulty in judging nonverbal features of communication, such as tone, humour, irony; an inability to detect deceit, and difficulty understanding implicit meaning; a lack of empathy; a lack of imagination; an attraction to the mechanical; a tendency to treat people and body parts as inanimate objects; an alienation from the self (autistic children often fail to develop the first-person perspective and speak of themselves as "he" or "she"); an inability to engage in eye contact or mutually directed gaze; and an obsession with detail. All these features will be recognizable as signs of left hemisphere predominance.[46]

If the current chapter is read as a narrative—the story of how cerebral dominance in the human brain has been shifting leftwards over the past 50 millennia or so—then the end of the story is a brain that is so imbalanced in terms of cerebral dominance that it's dysfunctional. In this sense, the logical endpoint of the leftward shift is autism.

• THREE •

Autism and
the Inhibited Mind

It is possible that evolution might actually promote the disconnection of certain brain functions from others. For instance, along certain paths of cerebral evolution, perhaps in emerging branches of the human species, there may be an increasing disconnection of cognitive from emotional processes. This may be the path of autism in its various forms....

—Jaak Panksepp (1998)[1]

It was once presumed that the brain was composed of various modules, each one specializing in specific neurocognitive functions, such as language, memory, learning, etc. We now know that the brain is much more "plastic" than once conceived, and that the brain as a whole can mold or adapt itself to many different functions, depending on the individual's experience and environment. Nevertheless, there are some areas that do seem specialized for specific functions, such as Broca's and Wernicke's areas in the left hemisphere, which are specialized for language and speech. Furthermore, if we step back and consider the brain as a whole, we see that the two hemispheres of the brain work in tandem, each with its own specialty in terms of perceiving and interacting with the world.

In a very general sense, it's fair to say that the left hemisphere specializes in understanding the world by focusing on details, taking a deconstructive, analytical approach. The right hemisphere, on the other hand, specializes in understanding the world by seeing the big picture, perceiving entireties or whole entities in a broad "gestalt" approach. I will momentarily sacrifice absolute accuracy for conceptual clarity, in saying that the left hemisphere specializes in specialization itself, fragmenting the world into detailed bits, while the right hemisphere's function is to integrate these detailed bits into entireties, so we can appreciate the whole.

Imagine a child working on a connect-the-dot coloring book figure. The process of perceiving each individual dot and methodically connecting each dot to the one specific correct dot in the sequence of dots could be perceived as a left hemispheric task. However, at the same time, the child is aware of the whole picture that is being drawn—the right hemisphere's contribution to the undertaking. Both hemispheres need to be working in tandem in order for the process to work. The focus on details—the individual dots and how each one connects with the other—is absolutely necessary, and is, in fact, the primary work being done. However, an awareness of the whole picture is integral and absolutely necessary.

When focusing only on the dots, the child is apt to lose sight of the big picture, as the process of focusing in and of itself produces a sort of tunnel vision of perception, in which the individual dots become extremely clear, but the overall pattern, the big picture, is lost. The child must occasionally step back and orient himself to the overall pattern in order to remind himself of what he's doing in the first place—the grand purpose of the overall task—which is to make a picture, not just to connect specific dots to each other. Whereas the left hemisphere does the lion's share of the work, without the persistent contribution of the right hemisphere, which constantly reminds us of the big picture and of the grand purpose of connecting all the dots, the entire enterprise would lack meaning and cohesiveness.

Indeed, if a child could not perceive the pattern of a whole picture within the jumble of scattered dots, she would not venture to start connecting the dots in the first place. In conceiving the internal image of a big picture, the right hemisphere provides the impetus to start connecting dots, the guiding vision to continue connecting dots, and the denouement of achieving a sense of meaningful wholeness—the big picture—out of what was once a seemingly random assortment of unconnected dots. Thus, the integrative function of the right hemisphere and the fragmenting function of the left hemisphere are both absolutely necessary, so much so that each function would be *dysfunctional* without the other.

When working in tandem, the twin hemispheres complement each other perfectly, allowing us to investigate matters deeply by focusing on isolated details, while still maintaining an appreciation for the matter as a whole thing. When the hemispheres are not working in tandem, the experience of the world becomes unbalanced, and in some cases, unhinged. When the left hemisphere is damaged or over-inhibited, we can still appreciate the entireties of phenomena, but with a deficit of detailed understanding of what we perceive, an inability to dig into the phenomena and analyze them critically by observing in isolation their constituent parts. When the right hemisphere is damaged or over-inhibited, we lose the ability to appreciate the wholeness of things, perceiving the details but not the big picture. We lose sight of the forest for the trees.

Thus far, I've contended that the human brain, as a necessary adaptation to the environmental challenges of language, literacy, and an increasingly intellectual and technological world, has been gradually shifting the neural balance of power towards the left hemisphere. The "Left Shift Hypothesis" explains the "dominance" of the left hemisphere as an accommodation to a changing media environment. Whereas humans once controlled our environments through the physical mastery of the land via farming and gathering, and the physical mastery of animals via hunting and domestication, we now control our environments through the intellectual mastery of technology and information. The leftward shift in cerebral dominance is both the cause and effect of our increasingly technophilic and information-based existence. The process continues and will continue to continue, because it's a positive feedback loop. A brain that is adapted to a world in which success depends primarily on the ability to focus on details, to deconstruct and analyze data, will further its cause by becoming even more detail-oriented, even more analytical. In doing so, the individual contributes to the ongoing creation of a world of detailed information, making it that much more detailed, and that much less cohesive. As a species, we are busy building and connecting more and more and more dots, even as our sight of the big picture becomes increasingly lost amid the massive jumble of infinite dots. We're losing sight of the big picture for the dots. Losing sight of the forest for the trees.

If the broad function of the brain is to adapt itself to the demands of our environment, then we can discern a clear pattern of adaptation over the past 50,000 years. First, the means of communication between humans switched from a full-body means of communication reliant on mimetic physical movements, expressive gestures, and vocalizations, to linguistic speech, which is a much more specialized and fragmented means of communication, dependent completely on the use of words, which are abstract symbols associated with specific things. Language is the first fragmenter of thought, dividing whole ideas into individual words that, like the dots in a connect-the-dot picture, must be strung together in the correct sequence in order to create meaning. The cognitive tool of language empowered humans to analyze their environments critically, in order to develop new methods and tools for mastering their environments. The brain of each new generation of humans was then obliged to adapt itself to the use of these new methods and tools, making itself more and more specialized for specific tasks.

The work of the farmer, for instance, is more specialized than the work of his evolutionary predecessor, the hunter-gatherer, because of the number of tools required to do the job, and the number of details required in order to do it properly. The work of the blacksmith, in turn, is more specialized than the work of the farmer. The work of the electrical engineer is more specialized than the work of the blacksmith, and the process of increased specialization continues and increases as each generation creates more methods and tools that are necessarily more specialized and detailed than their predecessors. This positive feedback loop, in which each new generation begets a newer environment of even more specialized tools and work, is the invisible force that pushes cerebral dominance further and further towards the left.

But at what point does the leftward shift fall in upon itself, collapsing of its own weight? At what point does the page of ever-increasing dots cease to be the ground for a meaningful pattern or big picture, becoming a jumble of dots so complex and so unintegrated that there is no discernible pattern at all, just an infinite chaotic mishmash of unrelated dots? I would say that this critical endpoint of leftward cerebral dominance arises when the brain of the species as a whole becomes so fragmented from adaptation for specialization, that the people possessing this brain are no longer able to perceive whole patterns. Such a person, whose brain is so specialized for detailed focusing that they cannot discern the big picture, has become so adapted to specialization that they've become *maladapted* to that which is unspecialized: the world as a whole, experience as a whole, and other people, who are un-relatable unless intuitively conceived as whole beings.

The brain of such a person has become so detail-oriented that it cannot see the whole pattern embedded within the jumble of dots, and so it becomes disinterested in the task itself, as the endeavor of connecting endless random dots is pointless if one cannot intuit the underlying big picture hidden within them. With the integrative function of the right hemisphere overly inhibited by a hyper-dominant left hemisphere, the individual becomes unintegrated from anything that must be experienced as a whole, which includes the experience of other people, and the experience of life itself. While life can certainly be lived as an experience of one detailed phenomenon after another, the essence of life—the *meaning* of life—can only be discerned and appreciated as a whole experience, in which each detail merely serves the larger purpose of creating the illusion of a cohesive whole.

At the far end of the spectrum, at the point where the leftward shift falls in upon itself and the adaptive process of specialization becomes maladaptive, we find a person who is *dis*-integrated. A person who cannot relate to others, because they cannot perceive the wholeness of other persons, but rather sees them as a collection of details, a page of unconnected dots. This dis-integrated mind, this mind that sees dots but not pictures, this mind that is adept at specialization but inept at integration, this mind has detached itself so far from the integrating function of the mind that it has become functionally *fragmented*. This mind, imprisoned in a perceptual labyrinth of unintegrated fragments, a network of parts without a whole, is, in a word, "autistic."

Autism as the Endpoint of the Leftward Shift

In 1912, the Swiss psychiatrist, Eugen Bleuler, struck at the very heart of the issue when he coined the term "autism." Derived from the Greek root "autos" for self (as in *auto*-matic), "autism" refers to a personal system that functions within itself without need for or reference to input from outside sources. In light of the current model being revealed, the term is exceptionally apt, as it could refer to the left hemisphere's over-reliance on itself, to the over-exclusion of input from the right hemisphere. If autism, as I and others suggest, is related to a mind that is so left hemispheric dominant that right hemispheric input is overly inhibited to the point of pathology, then the autistic mind would represent the endpoint of a leftward shift in hemispheric dominance that probably began over a million years ago. The renowned neuroscientist, Jaak Panksepp, suggested how such an evolutionary shit in cerebral lateralization could occur:

> The level of integration between brain areas may be changing as a function of cerebral evolution. One reasonable way for cortico-cognitive evolution to proceed is via the *active inhibition* of more instinctual subcortical impulses. It is possible that evolution might actually promote the disconnection of certain brain functions from others. For instance, along certain paths of cerebral evolution, perhaps in emerging branches of the human species, there may be an increasing disconnection of cognitive from emotional processes. This may be the path of autism in its various forms.[2]

Why would an entire species evolve towards "an increasing disconnection of cognitive from emotional processes," that is, a diminishing connection between thought and feeling? Well, one could say that the story of human neuro-evolution over the past few hundred thousand years has been the story of a beast whose behaviors were ruled by his own instincts and feelings. This beast developed the ability to create and manipulate tools, which in turn led to the development of cognitive tools such as language, which eventually created the ability for the beast to listen to and direct his own thoughts. Once the beast became self-aware of his own thoughts, he found that he was no longer an unknowing beast, controlled by instinct and emotion, but a self-aware and reflective person—*Homo sapiens sapiens.* Now, instead of responding to environmental challenges with instinctual reflexes or emotional reactions, humans could think about their possible actions *before* acting.

The Promethean gift of language, when used privately, became the reasoning consciousness of private thought. To further exploit the gift of private thought and consciousness, the brain would need to inhibit and subdue the "more instinctual subcortical impulses"—instinct, intuition, and emotion—in order to allow for a detached and impassive reasoning style that would be cool and calculating rather than heated and impulsive. The increasing inhibition of the more intuitive and emotional hemisphere by the now dominant left hemisphere is an ongoing evolutionary process, engendered by the continuing shift of cerebral dominance from right to left.

The initial shift began in the Lower Paleolithic, when manual manipulation of tools and fire-making necessitated the neurological lateralization of handedness in order to establish a dominant hand (typically the right). The leftward shift proceeded as mimetic communication duplicated functions already being used for tool use (and already situated in the left hemisphere), into functions eventually to be used for language (Broca's and Wernicke's areas in the left hemisphere of the brain). As mimetic communication evolved into oral language, the shift towards the left continued, with the left hemisphere further specializing in abstract symbols and linear thought, which are the defining features of oral language.

The advent of language also initiated the function of internal verbal thought, which would also be lateralized in the left hemisphere, with necessary right hemispheric input being controlled and inhibited, so as to retain a sense of cognitive unity, the singular voice of consciousness. As literacy evolved, the leftward shift picked up steam, as the requirements of literacy included an even more detailed and linear mode of thinking, depending even more on abstract symbols, and focusing more and more singularly on symbolic representations of the world, as opposed to actual experiences of the world. "Literate man undergoes much separation of his imaginative, emotional, and sense life," Marshall McLuhan wrote in 1964. "If Western literate man undergoes much dissociation of inner sensibility from his use of the alphabet, he also wins his personal freedom to dissociate himself from clan and family."[3]

Print technology pushed the leftward shift even further, by amplifying the effect of verbal thought as the singular voice of consciousness, via the deliberate training of silent reading in child populations, a process that invokes the inner voice of verbal thought. Print technology also heralded revolutionary changes in the environment of the Western world: the Renaissance, the Enlightenment, and the Industrial Revolution are all attributable to the advent of mass education, mass literacy, and the ability for new information to be speedily distributed across populations.

The modern world of human thought is an environment molded from the literate mindset. In order to adapt to the intellectual challenges of this literate world, a world that requires humans to think in a highly logical and sequential pattern of thought, the human brain on a species level has become more literate. One of the consequences of this adaptation, as we shall see, is the far side of the spectrum, in which neurological modifications that make the species as a whole more adaptive to its media environment, when expressed in the extreme, unfortunately result in pathological modes of engagement that constitute the principal symptoms of autism.

The Displacement Effect

In his book *The Symbolic Species* (1997), neuroscientist and evolutionary anthropologist Terence Deacon argues that the "reorganization of the brain for language brought with it many indirect consequences including ... a susceptibility to such mental disorders as schizophrenia and autism."[4] The process behind this reorganization—and the process behind its "indirect consequences"—is a combination of lateralization and displacement. As mentioned previously, as language and verbal thought gradually became more and more important, the brain evolved to accommodate the increases in these forms of cognition by devoting more and more neural space and connectivity to linguistic thought. Since, for most of us, linguistic thought is dominated by the left hemisphere, this lateralization of hemispheric dominance moved in a leftward direction. However, just as water in a bathtub will be displaced by an addition of a body into the tub, neural connectivity and neural activity in the brain will be displaced by the addition of a new mode of cognition (such as language). Deacon explains how the displacement effect works at the level of the individual neuron:

> I call this evolutionary mechanism *displacement*. In general terms, relative increases in certain neuronal populations will tend to translate into the more

effective recruitment of afferent and efferent connections in the competition for axons and synapses. So, a genetic variation that increases or decreases the relative sizes of competing source populations of growing axons will tend to displace or divert connections from the smaller to favor persistence of the larger.[5]

In other words, nothing can change in one part of the brain that won't directly or indirectly cause changes in other parts of the brain, because the brain is completely interconnected and organic—a living and changing organism—constantly adapting itself in real time to its environment. When the brain accommodates a particular mode of cognition by increasing neuro-connectivity in one region, the brain is obliged to displace or reduce neuro-connectivity in other regions to a proportional degree. Hence, increased abilities in one cognitive domain are likely to correspond to decreased (or "displaced") abilities in another domain. The displacement effect doesn't necessarily decrease neuro-connectivity in neighboring regions of the brain, and it doesn't necessarily affect other regions at random. The brain's bi-hemispheric form and function enable dual-processing of many cognitive tasks (especially language), so when displacement occurs, it's likely to affect the complementary region of the brain within the *opposing hemisphere.* In the case of language and verbal thought, increased neuro-connectivity in the linguistic regions of the left hemisphere may happen at the cost of decreased neuro-connectivity in the linguistic regions of the right hemisphere.

The displacement effect doesn't just happen once and then it's over. Displacement, like evolution and development, is a constantly ongoing process. So, the larger and denser a region becomes, the more likely it will continue to grow, as Deacon explains:

> The relative enlargement of one structure with respect to another may give the larger some sort of competitive advantage in the battle for influence over target synaptic activity. In other words, if one brain structure is relatively enlarged compared to another, this should translate into both displacement of connections during development and displacement of computational influence in adulthood with respect to other competing inputs from other brain structure. More inputs equals more votes influencing the computational outcome. Parcellation is a zero-sum game. When one structure becomes partially enlarged, another is reduced.[6]

To put it simply, a neural region is like the monstrosity in the movie *The Blob* (1958). The bigger the blob gets, the more powerful it becomes, enabling it to absorb even more and more stuff around it, which makes it bigger, which it makes it even more powerful, which makes it even bigger, and so on. It's a positive feedback loop. As long as the increase in neuro-connectivity within a particular region is reinforced by an environmental demand for the cognitive ability engendered by the brain region, the neuro-connectivity will continue to increase. To accommodate those increases, neuro-connectivity in opposing regions will continue to be displaced. In terms of language function, the more we use language, the more our brain wires itself for language, at the cost of other cognitive functions. The more environmental demands placed on language—such as the rigorous demands for increasingly sophisticated speech, comprehension, reading, and writing placed on young people in school—the more the brain will accommodate this increased demand by increasing density in certain linguistic regions, at the cost of displacing neuro-connective density in other regions. The loop continues to swirl.

We must always remember that the process explained above does not happen in a vacuum. The brain makes adaptations and accommodations to its environment; while the environment changes in response to the new cognitive abilities displayed by its inhabitant; which in turn evoke even more neural adaptations and accommodations. It's like playing a videogame that has "dynamic game difficulty balancing," in which the game itself is constantly gauging the gamer's ability, and automatically increasing the difficulty as the player improves. Because the game is automatically increasing the level of challenge, the gamer is constantly improving his skills, which in turn causes the game to further increase the challenge, which in turn causes the gamer to improve, and so on. The integrated system of gamer and game creates a circuit or positive feedback loop, in which the game is constantly accommodating itself to the gamer's skill level by becoming more difficult, and the gamer is constantly adapting himself to the game by becoming more skillful.

Another example of how brain/environment adaptations can create a positive feedback loop, and one that's more relevant to the topic, is the well-known "Flynn effect" on IQ scores. IQ tests must have standardized scoring in order for the results to be meaningful at a population level, therefore the test themselves must be calibrated in terms of difficulty so that the average score of the population is always 100. Intelligence researcher James Flynn pointed out that for most of the 20th century, IQ tests had to be recalibrated every so often, because the average scores tended to rise a few points each year. (In America, the average rise was about three points per decade.)

There are many possible reasons for the Flynn effect. One primary reason, and the one I will focus on for this example, is the increasing levels of education and literacy in most developed and developing societies that took place in the 20th century. Since IQ scores generally test for scholastic aptitude and basic literacy skills, a population of people who are increasingly better educated, with children who start schooling earlier and earlier in childhood, and who are exposed to literature and literacy earlier and to larger degrees, it makes sense why average IQ scores tended to drift upward.

To put the pieces of this example together, let's consider the academic and cultural demands for increased education and literacy as a constant evolutionary pressure towards increased linguistic reasoning. Let's then consider the neurological adaptations in the brain for linguistic reasoning as neural accommodations for this evolutionary pressure. By the time these neural accommodations are spread evenly across the population, the initial environmental pressure for a standard level of linguistic reasoning has increased, prompting the brain to accommodate even more neural processing space for linguistic reasoning.

Let's say that Jack is an average five-year-old boy taking the IQ test in 1950. Since he is "average," he will score a 100 on the test. Now, let's say we clone Jack so that his genetic identical twin is born in 1955 and takes the IQ test in 1960. Given the exact same genetic makeup, Jack II is just as average as Jack I; however, because he grew up in the 1950s instead of the 1940s, he was likely to be exposed to more literature and to more literate people than Jack I, and he was also more likely to start school earlier than Jack I. Therefore, when given the exact same IQ test that Jack was given in 1950, Jack II, in accordance with the Flynn effect, will score 103, rather than 100. If we repeat the process and clone a third Jack, when Jack III takes the same exact IQ test in 1970, he will score 106.

The Flynn effect on increasing IQ scores demonstrates how environmental pressures for a certain mode of cognition can evoke neural adaptations in the brain, and how these neural adaptations can spread across a population, causing an ongoing *increase* in the same environmental pressures, which in turn evoke even more neural adaptations, and so on. In the 20th century, the environment and the brain, working in tandem, created a positive feedback loop, pushing our brains and our media environments further and further in the direction of perpetually increasing linguistic sophistication.

Lateralization, in Deacon's view, is a "zero-sum" game, because any increase in connectivity in one region of the brain will inevitably come at the cost of a proportional decrease in connectivity in an opposing part of the brain. Since every brain region is in some way associated with a neurological function, we can say that every functional increase will also beget a functional decrease, and vice versa. These functional trade-offs are apparent, even in the case of neurological damage or disorder: "When a structure is damaged, not only is there a loss of function, but there is also inevitably a gain of function—though not an improvement—in the form of "released" behaviors, which appear to be disinhibited by the removal of competing influence."[7] Deacon argues that the cognitive strengths displayed by autistic people and—most saliently—by autistic savants, are the results of these "functional trade-offs" that occur in the brain.

Autism: Epidemic or Epiphenomenon?

Prior to 1966, autism was considered an extremely rare disorder, in large part because it was so obscure that most people—including pediatricians and child psychiatrists—had never heard of it. Between 1966 and 1991, the diagnostic rate of autism in the general population was 4.4 per 10,000, making it a "rare" disorder. Then, in the following decade (1992–2001), the rate tripled to 12.7 per 10,000, raising the alarm. Autism was now considered a new "epidemic," as the epidemiology of the debilitating developmental disorder continued to skyrocket. A decade later, in 2012, the diagnostic rate had tripled again, to 1 per 88. By 2014, just two years later, the rates had risen once again to 1 per 68. By 2018, the rates had risen to 1 per 60, and at the time this sentence was written (April 2020), the CDC's official diagnostic rate was 1 per 54.[8] The rates keep rising, with no end in sight. Clearly, we are living in the middle of an autism epidemic ... or are we?

Epidemiologists know for certain that the drastic rise in diagnoses over the past six decades is primarily due to increased awareness of the disorder among parents, teachers, pediatricians, psychologists, and psychiatrists. If people don't know about a disorder, it will not be detected, diagnosed, and reported. That's not to say that prior to 1966, children with severe autism passed for normal with nobody blinking an eye at their pathology. These children were diagnosed with other disorders, such as mental retardation (now referred to as intellectual disability), and childhood schizophrenia (now a defunct disorder, partially replaced by a disorder called "childhood onset schizophrenia"). It's also quite certain that most children with relatively mild autism, prior to the 1990s, were not diagnosed with anything at all. Since their autistic symptoms were mild and their intelligence relatively unimpaired, they were just considered eccentric or odd, but not disordered or pathological.

What happened, beginning in the 1980s, was a broadening of the way psychological disorders were perceived, resulting in a steep increase in the diagnosis of all psychological disorders, especially in children. Autism was and still is at the vanguard of this broad approach to diagnosis, so that a hypothetical child with the same level of autistic symptoms in 1990 would receive a diagnosis of autism, while the same exact child with the same exact symptoms back in 1960 would not be considered disordered at all, and would therefore receive no diagnosis.

The broadening trend in psychiatric diagnosis that's been going on since the 1960s is too big an issue to cover here. Suffice it to say that the "pathologization of normalcy"—the narrowing of the lines that demarcate "normal" from "abnormal"—and the resulting diagnosis of nearly all variation of human behavior as some sort of psychopathology, has caused a dramatic increase in the diagnosis of nearly all types of psychological disorder, with autism standing out as the most potent example.

Furthermore, the diagnostic criteria for autism have broadened immensely. Whereas in order to get a diagnosis of autism in the 1960s, a child had to be completely mute and totally unreceptive to social engagement, in the 1980s, children began getting diagnosed with autism even if they were highly verbal, and even if they engaged socially with others. In 2013, the DSM-V replaced the old diagnosis of autism with the new diagnosis of "autism spectrum disorder." In perceiving the disorder as a spectrum, we now allow for a diagnosis of ASD, even if the symptoms are relatively mild.

The "spectrum" model of diagnosis is the broadest conceivable model of mental disorder that still assumes a qualitative difference between normal and abnormal behavior. So, one could argue that the autism "epidemic" is just an artifact of increased awareness of the disorder, better detection and interpretation of the symptoms, and much broader diagnostic criteria. By this reasoning, once awareness, detection, and diagnostic criteria for autism stabilize, we should expect the diagnostic rates themselves to stabilize and plateau.

Unfortunately, seven years after the application of the broad spectrum model of autism, diagnostic rates continue to rise, even though everyone at this point in the 21st century is extremely aware of autism and on the lookout for it. Many researchers argue that the continuing epidemic-level rise of diagnostic rates cannot be fully accounted for statistically by increased awareness, detection, and broader diagnostic criteria alone. Many suspect the influence of an environmental factor. Clearly, I am one of those suspicious researchers. My argument in this chapter is that the media environment of the modern world places an environmental pressure on the brain towards left hemispheric dominance, and that autism represents the endpoint of this "leftward shift," which has been going on for millennia; but has certainly increased over the past few centuries, and especially over the past few decades, due primarily to the relatively new societal demands for increasingly analytical and literate modes of thought.

In short, the argument I am laying out is that autism is not so much an epidemic as it is an *epiphenomenon*—a canary in a coalmine—indicating that the evolutionary trend towards increasingly analytical and detail-focused mental engagement that's been influencing our entire species for the past 50,000 years has an endpoint, and that endpoint is autism. An epiphenomenon is a secondary phenomenon that exists as a result of a primary phenomenon, even if the primary phenomenon is obscured. Oftentimes, we're aware of an epiphenomenon because it's more salient, leading us to acknowledge the existence of the epiphenomenon and dwell upon it, while the primary phenomenon that actually causes the condition remains silently unrevealed.

A simple example of an epiphenomenon is seen in the way that we used to think of asthma. In the "old days," asthma was considered a form of neurosis or anxiety disorder, with the characteristic symptom of wheezing as an externalized physical expression of feeling psychologically stifled within, which is why (we believed) asthmatic symptoms generally emerged under stressful conditions. Now we know that asthma is actually caused by chronic inflammation of the bronchial tubes in the lungs, i.e., the "primary phenomenon." The fact that asthmatic symptoms only become apparent in times of stress (when we start breathing faster), is a secondary phenomenon—an "epiphenomenon"—which is not directly related to the actual cause of the disorder. For many years, asthma was considered a "nervous disorder" and treated as such because the epiphenomenon of stress-induced symptoms was so salient, and the primary phenomenon of chronically inflamed bronchial tubes was invisible to the naked eye.

Similarly, my argument is that autism is an epiphenomenon of the leftward shift in cerebral dominance that's been going on for millennia. The leftward shift itself is just an invisible idea, and the genetic/neurological processes behind it are largely invisible, existing only in the microscopic neuro-connections hidden deep within the recesses of the brain. These neuro-connections are hidden because they function by cross-hemispheric inhibition—the left hemisphere's inhibition of input from the right hemisphere. So it's not that the left hemisphere is more connected and active while the right hemisphere is less connected and less active, they both will appear the same. The issue is that the left hemisphere is often actively inhibiting the right hemisphere's input, making the hemispheric differences in functioning appear less salient from the perspective of a researcher gauging hemispheric neural connectivity and activity.

Autism, however, is quite salient. We all see it, we all know about it, and we all know someone who has it, or someone who is related to someone who has it. The salient epiphenomenon of autism has grasped our attention and we're more than curious to know the cause. The salience of autism as an "epidemic" that's critically afflicting millions of children (and adults) may be blinding us to a deeper truth, which is that the brain of the human race has been becoming more and more left-hemispheric dominant since the Paleolithic Age. The human brain and the human race has been in the process of becoming more and more "autistic" since archaic times, and the process has been speeding up over the past few centuries, and especially over the past few decades. Autism stands out as the epiphenomenon of a much larger and much more universal evolutionary trend. It's the canary in a coalmine, because just as the suffering of the canary provides coalminers with proof of the existence of deadly invisible fumes in the mine, the suffering of the children provides us all with salient proof of the existence of invisible pressures within our environment and within our brains, that are affecting us all.

Genetic Causation of Autism

The leftward shift in cerebral dominance is pushed forward from generation to generation by both increasing environmental pressures and genetic inheritance. Significant genetic causation of autism is well established. Neuro-genetic researchers now refer to the "broader autistic phenotype (BAP)" when discussing autism, referring to the well-known finding that autism runs in families, and that it's quite common for relatives of autistics to display "autism-related" personality traits such as obsessive interests or asocial behavior.[9] All the way back in 1943, Leo Kanner (the psychiatrist known for "discovering" autism in America), observed that "For the most part, the parents, grandparents, and collaterals are persons strongly preoccupied with abstractions of a scientific, literary, or artistic nature, and limited in genuine interest in people."[10]

Relatives of autistic people are much more likely to be on the spectrum as compared to nonrelatives in the general population, with the concordance rate between identical twins at 60 percent.[11] Furthermore, recent studies have shown that the specific genes associated with autism have been in the gene pool for millions of years. In a 2014 article in Nature Genetics entitled "Most genetic risk for autism resides with common variation," Gaugler et al. used cutting edge methods in genetic research to show that the genetic clusters that indicate statistical risk for autism are not "rooted in rare de novo mutations," but rather stem from "common variations" in "very old genes that are shared widely in the general population." This suggests that autism "is not a product of modern civilization" but "is a strange gift from our deep past, passed down through millions of years of evolution."[12] Autism, as a neurocognitive trait, appears to be a very old and deep-seated aspect of humanity.

Marian Annett, a renowned neurologist, espouses a "right shift theory," which suggests that there are specific genes that determine cerebral hemispheric lateralization. Because her theory is based on studies of handedness, a "right shift" refers to a lateralizing shift of dominance towards the right hand, indicating a shift in cerebral dominance towards the left hemisphere (making it somewhat confusing for our purposes, as Annett's "right shift" in handedness corresponds with my "left shift" in cerebral hemispheric dominance). Annett's "RS+" gene would foster left hemispheric lateralization, and the "RS+" would foster right hemispheric lateralization.

Annett believed that there may be a mutant variation of gene expression that would be "agnosic for left versus right," that is, a gene expression that does not distinguish between input from the left hemisphere and the right. This mutant gene expression would only be problematic when it affects both hemispheres. In her model, a genetic expression in which there was an agnosic gene affecting both hemispheres—a double dose of the agnosic gene—could result in a near total inhibition of one hemisphere of the brain, typically the "sub-dominant" right hemisphere. According to the gene risk calculations in her model, "the frequencies suggested that a double dose of the agnosic gene would occur in about 4 in 10,000 cases, about the rate estimated for strictly defined autism."[13]

Though our understanding of the genetic underpinnings of autism is still rudimentary, in terms of how genetics fit into the current theory, it's clear that autism has a very strong genetic link, that the genes in question are not new mutations or variations but extremely old and widely distributed in humans, and there's tantalizing evidence that the specific genes in play may be related to the process of hemispheric lateralization.

Intellectualism and Autism

In 1943, Leo Kanner, then a psychiatrist at Johns Hopkins University Hospital, published a paper entitled "Autistic Disturbances of Affective Contact." He borrowed the term "autistic" from Bleuler, who coined the term to describe the inward, asocial, detached affective styles of many of his schizophrenic patients. Kanner coined the term "infantile autism" to describe similar symptoms in his child patients. Meanwhile, in Europe at around the same time, the Austrian pediatrician Hans Asperger coined the term "autistic psychopathy" to define the symptoms of some of his child patients. Ironically, Kanner and Asperger—two clinicians who lived on different sides of the world and who never met each other or read each other's work—simultaneously discovered a new developmental psychopathology, and they both used the same term, "autism," to refer to it.

However, if autism is expressed along a spectrum of symptomatic behavior, then Kanner and Asperger were focusing on opposite sides of the spectrum. Kanner's patients were extremely asocial, almost completely uncommunicative, and entirely obsessed with repetitious and restricted behaviors and interests. These children with "Kanner's syndrome" (the condition now referred to as "classic autism") were extremely dysfunctional, and lived a solitary life inside their own minds, immersed in their private fantasy worlds, islands unto themselves. Kanner described the children he observed as having an "*inability to relate themselves* in the ordinary way to people and situations" and they displayed "an *extreme autistic aloneness* that, whenever possible, disregards, ignores, shuts out anything that comes to the child from the outside."[14]

Asperger's patients, on the other hand, were bright, loquacious, and often gifted with excellent memories and intellectual skills. He referred to them as his "little professors," because they would talk on-and-on about their specific hobbies and interests, lecturing like academics, without seeming to care or even realize that their listeners were bored or uninterested in hearing an hour long lecture from a nine-year-old about the reproductive strategies of honeybees. So, while children with "Kanner's Syndrome" represented the very low functioning end of the autism spectrum, the children with what was eventually to be called "Asperger's Syndrome" represented the very high end of the same spectrum. The traits that they shared in common were their tendency towards aloofness (being overly content to be alone), and their obsessions with repetitive and restrictive interests.

While Kanner's patients spoke very little if at all, Asperger's patients had no overt language deficits, but the content of their speech was non-pragmatic. They had one-sided monologues rather than real social conversations, and their manner of speech was often stilted or odd in terms of their volume, tone, lack of emotional affect or gestures, etc. (Asperger's Syndrome no longer exists as a disorder in the current edition of the DSM, having been subsumed by the broad spectrum of autism. Someone with what used to be called Asperger's would now simply be called "on the spectrum," but very high functioning).

One specific observation made by both Kanner and Asperger was that their child patients tended to be quite intelligent, even if their intelligence was overshadowed by their dysfunctionalities, and that their parents tended to be highly educated and very intellectual as well. The latter observation—intellectual parents—made by both Kanner and Asperger, as well as many other clinicians to follow them, later became controversial. Kanner spoke of the parents of his autistic patients as cold perfectionists who were too interested in their intellectual pursuits to really care about their children, whom they "kept neatly in a refrigerator that didn't defrost."[15]

In 1967, Bruno Bettelheim, a child psychologist, published a book called *The Empty Fortress: Infantile Autism and the Birth of the Self*, in which he made similar observations regarding the highly intellectual parents of autistic children. Rather than just noting the correlation, Bettelheim drew a faulty line of causation, arguing that the intellectual parents actually caused their children to be autistic, by withholding love and affection and by being so cold and distant that their children could not form an attachment with their mothers, resulting in their emotional retreat inward, into their "empty fortress" of autistic isolation. Bettelheim referred to these cold and intellectual mothers as "refrigerator mothers," and an entire generation of parents of autistic children—especially mothers—were put to blame for their children's condition.

In some cases, autistic children were taken away from their parents and placed in hospitals and group homes, safely sequestered from the icy frost of their refrigerator parents. The painful legacy of Bettelheim's blunder was so vast and long-lasting that it became taboo to mention parental involvement in any way in relation to autism. Thus, the many observations that drew correlations between intellectualism in parents and autism in their children were seen as either biased, incorrect, or coincidental. Thankfully, enough time has passed since the dark days of Bruno Bettelheim and "refrigerator mothers" for us to take another look at this correlation.

As mentioned above, many clinicians have noted that their autistic patients tended to have intellectual parents. Kanner (1943) noted in particular that his autistic patients tended to come from families with high levels of education as well as income, and he noted the same tendency in his other patients within the same practice. Even Bernard Rimland—a harsh and vociferous critic of the ill-conceived "refrigerator mother" theory—who championed the theory in the 1960s that the causes of autism were primarily genetic and neurological, noted that both autistic people and their relatives tended to be highly intelligent.

Clinical observations, however, are not necessarily empirically valid, because the observations are made without control groups to balance for observational bias. Maybe the observations regarding intellectual parents resulted from the fact that in the early days of autism research, the clinicians all worked in university hospital settings, and therefore their patients tended to come from areas neighboring universities where intellectuals were more likely to live. Also, since autism was virtually unknown prior to the 1960s, parents seeking assessment from specialists in the rare condition known as autism, must have been relatively well-read and educated in order to even know that such a thing as "autism" existed.

Since then, however, much empirical research has been done in the field of autism, and a lot has been learned about the parents and relatives of autistic people. For one thing, we now know that autistic traits seem to run in families, and that autism itself has a strong genetic component, as revealed by twin studies and hereditability studies. Empirical studies have also revealed that there is a strong positive association between autism and higher maternal education. In the largest study up to that date on socioeconomic factors in autism, Croen et al. (2002) surveyed millions of families and "observed a fourfold higher rate of autism in children whose mothers had had postgraduate education, compared with those who had not completed high school. Adjusted for race, birth place, maternal age, birth order, and other factors, the excess of autism in highly educated families was twofold." Similarly, a 2003 Viennese study found that the fathers of autistic people were significantly more likely than control group fathers to be employed in technical professions, especially electrical engineering.[16]

While we may cautiously surmise that education, intellectualism, and technological proficiency are positively associated with autistic people and their relatives, correlation does not imply causation. Nevertheless, if the hypothesized "leftward shift" is driven by neurological adaptations made primarily to accommodate the cognitive challenges of language, literacy, logical-mathematical thinking, and the other intellectual requisites of our increasingly cerebral and technological media environments, then the strong associations between these variables would support the leftward shift hypothesis in regards to the rising prevalence of autism. Simply put, for the past few millennia, and especially for the past few centuries, our world and its inhabitants have become ever-increasingly more literate, more educated, and more intellectual, in order to adapt to our increasingly intellectual media environments.

At the same time, for at least the past half-century, we've seen an alarming increase in the prevalence of a disorder that is marked by intellectual obsessions, extremely focused and analytic cognitive styles, and a tendency towards highly literal and literate approaches to mental tasks. Furthermore, the same people afflicted by this disorder tend to come from families of people who are highly educated, extremely literate, and very intellectual. And finally, the disorder falls out along a spectrum in which the upper end of functionality is inhabited by people who are extremely intelligent, hyper-analytical, and prone to intellectual obsessions. So, although there's no "smoking gun" pointing to a causational link between intellectualism and autism, the associations mentioned above clearly point to a common denominator between these two cognitive-behavioral traits.

What Kanner and Bettelheim and their cohort noted in their patients' parents were *not* the causes of autism but were hints of an underlying socio-genetic variable associated with the autistic neurological disposition—intellectualism—which is a product of both a genetically determined predisposition towards literacy and an analytical mindset, as well as environmental pressures within modern society towards ever-increasing analytical and intellectual cognitive abilities. Rimland hypothesized that autism was primarily transmitted via genetic inheritance, which explains the shared cognitive similarities in families with autistic people. He also made the bold conjecture that autism represented something of a detour on the genetic "road to high intelligence," which "lies along a knife-edged path," so that "the higher the potential intelligence, the steeper and more precarious the slope." More simply put, autism represents a situation in which genetic causation for intellectualism can result in cognitive pathology in some individuals, a case of "brightness gone awry."[17] Rimland's conjecture is supported by recent (2016) findings by Scottish researchers that "genes associated with autism are also associated with higher levels of cognitive ability."[18]

Weak Central Coherence

As autism increases in prevalence, various movements in favor of a stance of neurological diversity towards all people—even those diagnosed with mental disorders—have criticized the use of terms such as "weak central coherence" in describing autistic symptoms. The idea is that our use of terms indicating deficits overshadows our entire concept of people, so that all we see are deficits rather than differences, symptoms rather than diversity, and weaknesses rather than potential strengths. In other words, "weak central coherence"—an inability to see the central core or "big picture" in a situation due to a sustained deep focus on the details—could just as easily be referred to as "detail oriented" or "close focused."

I agree wholeheartedly with this approach, as the underlying premise of my leftward shift hypothesis is that nearly all mental "disorders" could be perceived as being different strands along the vast and broad spectrum of neurological diversity. Nevertheless, because the current literature on autism is comprised primarily of the research and reports of clinicians who deal with deficits for a living, and because these research articles and reports rely on the currently used terms of deficiency, I feel it necessary to use the same terms, in order to avoid confusion.

Uta Frith, a renowned expert and researcher in the field of autism, is known for championing the theory that "weak central coherence" is the core symptom of autism, the root from which all other symptoms stem. Her theory is supported by empirical evidence that points to the tendency of autistic people to overly focus on details, and to rely too heavily on analytical approaches to information processing, as opposed to holistic or gestalt approaches. Specifically, autistic people reliably score better than "neurotypicals" in controlled embedded figure task experiments, in which the subject must find hidden shapes within drawings. In order to find the hidden shape within the drawing, one must suppress the tendency to see the big picture, and actually ignore the picture itself, in order to focus narrowly on unrelated shapes embedded within the drawing.

Similar tendencies have been found in autistics when performing conflicting letter tasks, in which the subject is shown an image of a large letter, that's actually composed of a lot of very small letters. The subjects are then asked to state the name of the small letters that comprise the image of the large letter. Since the big letter is the overall pattern, that choice represents a gestalt perspective; and since the small letters are the "details," they represent the nongestalt perspective. In the task, when the small letters and the big letter they compose are consistent, neurotypicals and autistics score the same; but when the letters are inconsistent, neurotypicals are more likely to mistakenly name the large letter, while autistics are more likely to correctly name the small letters that combine to make the big letter.[19] These results are interpreted as a "local bias" in autistics (seeing the trees), and a "global bias" in neurotypicals (seeing the forest).[20]

Frith believes that while neurotypicals tend to intuitively search for "meaning" in things, autistics don't, or at least are not as motivated by an intuitive drive for meaning or "central coherence." Hence, an autistic child working on a jigsaw puzzle will attend to the shapes of the pieces as opposed to the overall picture that the pieces are supposed to create. Similarly, while neurotypicals are better at remembering lists of words that have related meanings as opposed to lists of unrelated words, autistics tend to perform at the same level, regardless of whether the words on the lists are related.[21]

Significantly, for the leftward shift hypothesis, weak central coherence is associated with the tendency to process information sequentially rather than simultaneously, a cognitive strategy that facilitates analytical and logical thinking, and which is detail-focused. In order to perceive a whole, or a gestalt, one must process multiple salient factors simultaneously, such as in the recognition of a face or a picture. Processing information sequentially—one detail at a time—hinders one's ability to intuitively and instantly perceive a whole thing, whether it's a picture or a place or a person. The significance here is that language in general, and literacy in particular, as well as any task that relies on logical or linear reasoning, all depend on sequential processing—processing one word, or one number, or one symbol at a time.

The increased ability of our species as a whole to think logically and intellectually may, at the far end of the spectrum, result in brains that are cognitively stuck in the sequential processing mode, resulting in deficits whenever gestalt processing is required. For autistics, this would mean a preference towards repeating specific serial or sequential tasks over and over again ad infinitum, matched with difficulties in dealing with big pictures or whole beings, which require simultaneous processing of multiple factors. These preferences and deficits correspond with the hallmark symptoms of autism: "restrictive and repetitive behaviors and interests" and "deficits in social interaction."[22]

Similarly, weak central coherence would support a preference for activities and stimuli that are well-known and predictable, as opposed to new activities and stimuli, which would be more difficult to process sequentially, as our initial understanding of any new stimulus depends on an initial gestalt process, our mind's way of figuring out what in general something is, before trying to break the thing down into detailed bits and pieces. The social deficits of autism, which Kanner saw as the core symptoms of the disorder, could be the byproduct of a brain stuck in the sequential processing mode, because people are not collections of details, but whole beings who must be experienced holistically. People, in fact, would represent the polar opposite of the kind of stimuli preferred by a mind stuck in the sequential processing mode, because people are whole beings rather than collections of parts. Also, people—unlike objects—are prone to emotional and illogical behaviors, making them unpredictable. Is it possible that autistic isolation, Bettelheim's "empty fortress," is merely a pattern of preference towards stimuli that, unlike people, can be understood as repetitive and predictable patterns of sequential details?

Let's imagine an autistic child with weak central coherence. The child enjoys predictable stimuli, such as spinning disks and computer games. Now imagine this child encountering an unknown person. The process of trying to comprehend who and what this person is would be compromised by the autistic child's sequential processing style. The person, if not perceived as a whole being, must then be perceived as a collection of infinite details that all have to be sequentially analyzed and put together. That's too much information for anyone to process within the time restraints of a real-time social interaction. Like a computer overloaded with too much data to process, the autistic child's mind would become overloaded with too much information, leading to intense anxiety. In response to this state of information overload and the anxiety it creates, the autistic child is likely to either shut themself off from the new stimulus, in order to defend their senses; or else they will breakdown, that is, have an emotional meltdown. Either of these typically autistic ways of dealing with the stress of a social encounter with a new person could be explained using Frith's model of weak central coherence.

Marshall McLuhan observed of the modern individual in the world of electronic information: "When faced with information overload, we have no alternative but pattern-recognition."[23] That is, when the left hemisphere's sequential processing style is compromised by too much information, the brain will switch perspectives by seeking overall patterns of data to get a sense of the big picture, which is the right hemisphere's processing style. Some theorists have postulated that autistics are better than neurotypicals at seeing sequences of information, but are worse at perceiving "social patterns."[24] Boucher quoted "John," one of her autistic patients, a "high functioning" autistic adult, as an example of how autistics seem to process stimuli sequentially, attending to details, as opposed to holistically, attending to the central core or overall meaning of the stimulus:

> My way of perceiving things differs from that of other people. For instance, when I am confronted with a hammer, I am initially not confronted with a hammer at all but solely with a number of unrelated parts: I observe a cubical piece of iron near to a coincidental bar-like piece of wood. After that, I am struck by the coincidental nature of the orin and the wooden thing resulting in the unifying perception of a hammerlike configuration. The name "hammer" is not immediately within reach but appears when the configuration has been sufficiently stabilized over time. Finally, the use of a tool becomes clear when I realize that this perceptual configuration known as a "hammer" can be used to do carpenter's work.[25]

One could imagine the difficulty an autistic person would have if they perceived people in the same way they perceive things, by attending to details as opposed to the whole. There's a substantial amount of evidence—both empirical and anecdotal—that this is exactly what's going on with autistic socialization. Many studies confirm that autistics do poorly as compared to neurotypicals on facial recognition tasks. Again, if you attend to details rather than a whole, a face is just a collection of details ... a nose in the middle, a pair of eyes above it, etc. Recognizing a face for neurotypicals isn't a process of putting facial pieces together, it's an intuitive act of recognition of the whole face, which we either immediately recognize, or we don't. When looking at a face, there's an intuitive "aha!" moment when we recognize it, usually within the first second of exposure. After that first moment, if there's no recognition, you can stare at the face for hours, studying each facial part in detail, but no matter how long you study the parts of the face sequentially, you won't recognize it, because that's not how we process whole stimuli, like faces, which can't be broken down into detailed parts.

Facial recognition deficit (aka "prosopagnosia,") is common among autistics. Temple Grandin deals with her prosopagnosia by falling back on her cognitive strength of attending to visual detail. When addressing several people at a meeting, she makes mental notes, such as "Sam is the one in the red jacket," or "Sue is the one with the blue scarf," to help her remember who is who.[26]

We could imagine the state of an autistic child meeting another person that they don't know. While a neurotypical would get an intuitive feel for the person as a whole, the general sense of who and what this person is; the autistic child, whose sense for gestalt impressions is inhibited, will be overloaded with sensory information about this person, but unable to organize it into one cohesive unit, a whole person. Faced with information overload of the social variety, the autistic must fall back on his cognitive strength, the sequential processing of sensory details, in the hope of recognizing some sequence that will help put all the pieces together. If this is truly what's going on, then "weak central coherence" as a result of right-hemispheric over-inhibition would explain both the social deficits apparent in autism, as well as their preference for nonsocial, restrictive, and repetitive stimuli. Limiting or avoiding social interaction could be seen as a defense mechanism among autistics, because social experiences—especially with new people—result in information overload, and people, unlike objects, are hard to reduce into sequential patterns of recognizable details.

According to McGilchrist, the right hemisphere attends to living beings, picking up on and expressing empathic and emotional cues, and processing social relations. Inhibiting the right hemisphere would impair the ability to relate to others. "The right hemisphere has by far the preponderance of emotional understanding. It is the mediator of social behavior. In the absence of the right hemisphere, the left hemisphere is unconcerned about others and their feelings."[27]

Intense World Syndrome

Another symptom of autism, listed in the DSM-V under the category of "restrictive, repetitive behaviors, interests, or activities," is extreme hypersensitivity to certain sensory phenomena. Boucher argues that the hypersensitivity experienced by autistics may be a symptom of the autistic mind's tendency towards hyper-focusing on details (in this case, sensory details), combined with the similar autistic tendency to perseverate on stimuli, to remain focused or cognitively "stuck" on certain stimuli that most other people will begin to ignore or not even notice after a little while. Thus, two cognitive strengths of autism—heightened attention to detail and sustained attention—become psychosocial deficits—hypersensitivity and perseveration—when the autistic is confronted with the kind of sensory stimuli that can't be processed by hyper-focusing on details.

Boucher suggests that autistic people's "over-focused" attention causes them to narrow their field of attention to just one stimulus at a time. When confronted with too much sensory information, or when forced into a situation of multiple sensory inputs (such as being forcibly hugged and kissed by an over-affectionate aunt), the autistic will display the "defense reaction of shutdown," retreating physically and mentally into themselves, into their safe but isolated "empty fortress."

Related to the symptom of hypersensitivity to certain sensory stimuli is the autistic symptom of self-stimulatory sensory behavior, commonly referred to as "stimming." Autistic children often engage in hand-flapping, rocking, spinning, and other behaviors that seem to perform the function of stimulating their nervous systems in a self-soothing way. Oftentimes, stimming behaviors are the most noticeable and the most dysfunctional symptoms of the disorder. Temple Grandin relates her own experiences with hypersensitivity and stimming as follows:

> This ties in with earlier studies concerning the inability of autistics to handle simultaneous stimuli and being able to attend to only one aspect of a compound visual or auditory stimulus. Today, even as an adult while waiting in a busy airport, I find I can block out all the outside stimuli and read, but I still find it nearly impossible to screen out the airport background noise and converse on the

phone. So it is with autistic children. They have to make a choice of either self-stimulating like spinning, mutilating themselves, or escape into their inner world to screen out outside stimuli. Otherwise, they become overwhelmed with many simultaneous stimuli and react with temper tantrums, screaming, or other unacceptable behavior. Self-stimulating behaviors help calm an over aroused central nervous system.... The autistic child self-stimulates to calm himself....[28]

There's always been a shroud of mystery surrounding autism, in part because the people with the most severe form of the disorder are usually completely silent, so they can't tell us what they're thinking and feeling. Another mystery is the existence of apparently contradictory sets of symptoms. Autism is a neurocognitive disorder, yet many autistics are extraordinarily bright. Autism is related to severe language deficits, yet many autistics are extremely verbal and literate, and oftentimes are excellent lecturers and writers. And also, autism is indicated by the symptom of hypersensitivity to certain sensory stimuli, yet it's also indicated by *undersensitivity* to certain sensory stimuli.

In a 2007 *Frontiers in Neuroscience* article entitled, "The Intense World Syndrome—an alternative hypothesis for autism," Markram, Rinaldi, and Markram suggest that autistics suffer from "excessive neuronal processing" that "may render the world painfully intense." "Intense world syndrome," is the result of a cognitive trend to focus on stimuli so deeply and so intently and so fixatedly that the stimuli themselves becoming overwhelming. Imagine, for instance, trying to fall asleep, but there's an amorous cat out in the yard meowing longingly for a mate. You shut the window, you bury your head in the pillows, you pull the blankets over your head, but no matter how hard you try, you can't "unhear" the annoying cat. If only you had "earlids" to shut![29] Though the meowing itself isn't particularly loud, the stimulus has somehow engaged your attention in such a way that you can't ignore it. In fact, the harder you try to ignore it, the more your brain seems to perseverate on the annoying sound, quite against your own conscious will.

This rather banal experience may be similar to what autistic hypersensitivity to certain sensory stimuli is like. Other noises—the wind and rain on a stormy night, the drone of traffic in the distance, the mechanical grind of a running air conditioner—are easily ignored, but this one specific noise, for some reason, cannot. Markram et al. believe that the autistic brain experiences this kind of hypersensitivity all the time, and that their conditioned response might be "to rapidly lock down" their sensory world "into a small repertoire of secure behavioral routines that are obsessively repeated," providing a safe sanctuary from invasive sensory stimuli that they may be hypersensitive to. In other words, they retreat inwards, into Bettelheim's "empty fortress."

Thus, to the naked eye of the observer, autistics often seem "under-sensitive" to certain sensory stimuli, but this is an illusion. What's actually going on, according to proponents of "intense world syndrome," is that autistics have developed conditioned responses to the stimuli they're hypersensitive to, allowing them to completely tune out—not just to tune out the specific stimuli they're hypersensitive to, but to tune out *everything* (except for the specific self-stimulating stimuli that they've learned to perseverate on in order to drown out the unwanted stimuli). Thus, the "fortress" remains "empty," because for the autistic mind, there could be no stimulus more stressful than that of an unwelcome person trying to invade his sensory space, because people—inscrutable, unpredictable, irreducible people—are surely the most intrusive and annoying stimuli in the world.

Theory of Mind

Simon Baron-Cohen and his colleagues have put forth what is possibly the most famous model of autistic cognition, commonly referred to as "theory of mind," which is the implicit understanding that other people are conscious beings, just like ourselves, and therefore have their own private worlds of thoughts and feelings. Baron-Cohen argues that autistics lack a proper theory of mind for others, making it difficult or even impossible to truly empathize with other people, because they cannot project their own sense of consciousness into the mind of someone else.[30] In order to test if a child has a fully developed theory of mind, a simple hypothetical scenario is depicted. The child is shown two dolls, Sally and Ann. While Ann is watching, Sally places a piece of candy under a pillow and then leaves the room. While Sally is away, Ann takes the candy and hides it in her pocket. Sally re-enters the room. The experimenter then asks the child observing the scene: "Where does Sally think the candy is?" A child without theory of mind (such as a pre-school aged child), would say that Sally thinks the candy is in Ann's pocket, because he cannot comprehend that Sally has a different point of view than his own. A child with theory of mind (a school-aged child), will correctly say that Sally thinks the candy is under the pillow, even though he knows that it's actually in Ann's pocket—demonstrating that he can adopt Sally's perspective. Autistic school-aged children, however, usually say that Sally thinks the candy is in Ann's pocket. The implication is that autistics don't develop a theory of mind like nonautistic children, because they don't intuitively adopt Sally's point of view. Baron-Cohen calls this condition of autistics "mind-blindness," because they are blind to the minds of other people.[31]

Mind-blindness in autistics would cause them to perceive other people as beings without "minds," like androids or living robots, which will naturally foster social deficits such as social withdrawal, because what would be the point in creating a personal connection with a machine? According to the theory of mind model, compensatory preferences for solitary activities would arise, including a preference for repetitive activities that require detailed focus and memorization, to the exclusion of activities that require social interaction and novel experiences. While theory of mind, and the lack thereof, goes a long way to explain autistic deficits in social behavior, it doesn't explain its own existence—why the deficit in attributing consciousness to others exists in the first place. The model drawn out in this chapter, based on the leftward shift hypothesis, explains the existence of theory of mind deficits in autistics as a symptom of a much deeper and wide-ranging issue, an issue related to two completely divergent ways of attending to the world—the divergent ways of the twin hemispheres.

The left hemisphere evolved specializations for the mastery of tool use and for the processing of abstract linguistic symbols as linear sequences of objective thought. A mind in which the left hemisphere is overly dominant will show a clear preference for physical objects over human beings, an interest in parts of things rather than whole systems, and a preference to repeat already mastered skills and memorized facts ad infinitum over discovering new skills or fresh knowledge. As McGilchrist noted, "the *self-referring* nature of the world of the left hemisphere ... deals with what it already knows, the world it has made for itself."[32] Similarly, with its hyper-focused attention to details, "the left hemisphere has difficulty disengaging."[33]

Thus we see in a mind with an overly dominant left hemisphere, the basis of the narcissistic nature of autism, not in terms of self-grandiosity, but in terms of "self-referentiality," the single-minded focus on what one already knows, the perseveration of thought on a single well-tread track, seen in the "restrictive and repetitive behaviors and interests" that are one of the hallmarks of autism. The other hallmark of autism, lack of social interest, arises from the inhibition of right hemispheric engagement, a natural corollary to the left hemisphere's cerebral dominance over the stream of consciousness. Like Pete Townshend's autistic icon "Tommy," whose interests are restricted to the repetitive single-player game of pinball, and who gazes only into the mirror and sees only himself, the autistic mind reflects a perspective situated from within a hall of mirrors, a perspective that's incapable of looking outwards.

"Theory of Mind" is a metaphor for the self-awareness of one's wholeness of being, the entirety of conscious experience, as it exists in ourselves, and in others. The mind (unlike the brain), cannot be dissected and deconstructed into bits and pieces, to be analyzed and understood in terms of its detailed structure. The mind, like the soul, comprises the essence of a person. The experience of mind in this way, and the knowledge of this experience in oneself and in others, is an elemental experience. It can only be conceived of as a gestalt—a whole phenomenon—and any attempt to break down the experience into bits and pieces of detailed data is not only pointless, but impossible.

The term "theory of mind" is somewhat misnamed, I believe, because the word "theory" evokes associations with abstract scientific exposition—a complicated detailed explanation of a complex phenomenon—such as the chapter you're reading right now. In this sense, one might presume that theory of mind is a left-hemispheric function, when, in fact, it's exactly the opposite! The experience of the phenomenon is really quite basic, elemental, and entirely intuitive. It is the opposite of theoretical! The experience is that of intuitively feeling that someone else is a sentient being just like you, and that you can relate with that other person, who thinks and feels just like you. Newborn babies do this within weeks after birth when they gaze into our eyes and offer us the "social smile." Dogs do this when they cuddle and play with us, or when they beg for attention. Small children push this entirely intuitive and not-at-all theoretical "theory" to the limit when they project minds and souls into their teddy bears and dolls.

Theory of mind gives us a sense of other beings as whole entities with whom we can engage and relate. In this, it is the epitome of right hemispheric functioning. If theory of mind was truly a "theory"—a process of deliberate abstract deduction—then it would almost invariably emerge from the left hemisphere, yet brain imaging studies have located the seat of theory of mind processing in the temporo-parietal junction of the right hemisphere.[34]

If theory of mind were truly a "theory," then it would be a truly "autistic" way of conceptualizing others. If, from the hyper-focused, detail-fixated perspective of an over-dominant left hemisphere, another person is perceived as a puzzle, a collection of details that need to be deconstructed and then reconstructed in order to be understood, then communication and interaction would invariably breakdown at the onset, as it does in classic autism. For a person is not a collection of puzzle pieces to be put together, nor is she a collection of details that need to be collated and explicated. If one sees someone else as a puzzle, then there will always be missing pieces, and the puzzle will never be solved, because a person is more than the sum of her parts. The essence of a person—her body, mind, heart, and soul—must be appreciated and experienced as a gestalt—a whole being. This happens intuitively, pre-cognitively. Indeed, the entire notion of trying to cognitively construct the mental concept of another person's mind by applying some abstract "theory" is, in itself, an extremely disjointed and "autistic" way of con-ceptualizing interpersonal relation.

Imagine a toddler asking you, "What's a frog?" Would you take the child to a lab and there, for the child's edification, dissect a frog, so they could see the thing in all its detail, and thus construct an accurate and detailed "theory of frog?" I wouldn't. I would take the child to a pond, where there is a living frog, and there revel in its prodigious leap and stentorian croak. To the child, the essence of the frog is not to be found in its liver or gallbladder, the essence can only be found in the whole living being, and the experience of the frog is not achieved through theorizing, but through interaction. The frog is only meaningful on a personal level, as is every other being. If, due to a neurological disposi-tion, one is compelled to conceptualize another as a collection of details that need to be put together, then one faces the ungainly task of trying to put together a puzzle without the guidance of a picture on the box top of the whole image being represented, and without the crucial corner and side pieces that ground the whole image into one. Autism, indeed, is a confounding puzzle, both to us who try to understand it, as well as to those who experience it firsthand.

Language Deficits

Language deficits in autistics invariably involve the semantics and pragmatics of speech. Even when the autistic individual is linguis-tically fluent, as in Asperger's Syndrome (aka very high functioning autism), there will still be deficits in understanding the meaning of phrases, especially when nuanced interpretations of nonverbal ges-tures and illocutionary intent are required, and there will still be defi-cits in mastering the social aspects of language, such as how to engage in "small talk," or how to know when you're boring your listener, or how to politely change the subject when the person speaking to you is being boring.

There's an irony apparent in the left shift hypothesis, in that lan-guage—the primary driving force behind the shift—is deficient in autis-tic people, the same people who theoretically represent the "endpoint" of the shift. The irony is resolved when we remember that language is primarily a *social* behavior, and is only privatized as silent thought *after* it's been thoroughly acquired developmentally and neurologically. If the core deficit of autism is a failure to desire or create meaningful social interactions and relationships, then a person suffering from "classic autism" would show "little or no interest in interacting with others at any level or by any means, including language."[35] Whetherby and Prutting (1984) found that even when autistics are verbal, their language differs from those of "neurotypicals," in that it tends to be bereft of social content. As compared to "language-matched normally developing children," verbal autistic children are

> ... unimpaired in their use of language for requests for objects or actions, protests, and self-regulation.... Yet certain speech acts were completely absent. These included comments, showing off, acknowledging the listener, and requesting information. These findings are consistent with several other studies (e.g., Loveland et al., 1988). The speech acts missing from the conversations of children with autism all have in common an emphasis on *social* rather than environmental uses of language.[36]

Hans Asperger, reflecting on his work with his "little professors," who were quite verbal, despite being autistic, noted that while the technical aspects of their language were perfect, the children lacked "pragmatic" or social etiquette in their speech. They spoke in monologues rather than dialogues, delivering lectures on the topics they were obsessed with, regardless of whether or not their listeners were interested in the subjects. They interrupted often, abruptly changed conversation topics, broke off conversations abruptly, avoided eye contact, and generally lacked the social graces of interactional language. The ability of people with Asperger's Syndrome to master the phonological, morphological, and syntactic aspects of language, demonstrates that the neurological condition of autism in-and-of-itself does not entail deficits in the "hardware" of language. Many high functioning people on the spectrum, in fact, excel in lecturing and writing, especially on scientific and intellectual topics. The deficits apparent in highly verbal autistics appear solely in the social use of language. It's therefore presumed that language deficits in autistic children arise from an innate lack of interest in social interaction, which would necessarily exhibit itself in a lack of interest in engaging in our primary form of social interaction ... conversation.[37]

Language processing development is lateralized in the right hemisphere in the early years of life, and proceeds leftwards with age and education. This makes sense, as language is at its genesis a means of social engagement, which is a right hemispheric specialty. The severe language delays that are common among autistic children, and which—in "classic autism"—was a requirement for diagnosis, fit in well with the leftward shift hypothesis. If the right hemisphere's language function is inhibited in the autistic brain, then early language development would be inhibited as well, even though eventually, in due time, language processing will be strongly lateralized in the left.

The irony here is that the adaptations in the brain that in most people create a more robust and dominant linguistic intelligence, have the opposite effect in autism, because the over-inhibition of the right hemisphere in early development results in language deficits so profound, that the left hemisphere doesn't have the opportunity to pick up where the right hemisphere leaves off, because language processing is stunted right from its origin. This phenomenon also explains why autistic children who do somehow overcome their early language delays oftentimes become excellent writers, especially in technical subjects, while they still lack much of the "pragmatic" skills involved in oral language (such as polite conversation). For these people, left hemispheric language, which is technically proficient, is dominant; while right hemispheric language, which is inherently social, is lacking. Temple Grandin, the most famous autistic person in the world, who writes copiously about her autism, is a prime example. While her language skills are perfectly adapted for the detail-oriented, logical, and sequential style of thinking necessary for writing in the sciences, her pragmatic conversational skills are still profoundly deficient.

Language development follows an ontogenetic path from right hemispheric to left hemispheric processing, beginning with the gestalt of language—the general idea that speaking is about relating to others on a personal level. Perceiving the gestalt of a situation, understanding another person as a whole and sentient being just like oneself, and having the impulse to relate to that other person, to communicate, are all right hemispheric specialties. These are the basics of pragmatic language. Further elaboration from those basics, things that fall under the umbrella of social etiquette and polite conversational skills, are merely window dressing on the basic premise that language is our primary means of social engagement. In this light, it makes perfect sense why someone with an inhibited right hemisphere will show deficiencies in language pragmatics at both the most basic level, and the most sophisticated.

The leftward shift is engendered by the increasing need to focus on linguistic details as we grow older. First, we must learn how to put words together and understand their proper uses (morphology), as well as their correct pronunciations (phonology). Details. Then we must learn the different meanings of thousands of words (semantics), and the implicit rules for how they fit together grammatically in sentences (syntax). Even more details. Though all of these components of language are grounded in the terra firma of "whole language" (language as a social phenomenon), there's a point where language can be cut off from its pragmatic grounding and propelled into the realm of pure abstraction, in which language is used technically and proficiently, but not socially (as in the way I'm using language right now, to write about an extremely detailed and technical subject). Literacy provides this cut off point, as the written word fosters private verbal thought, and both reading and writing are activities best done alone, or at least in silence, without direct social interaction. Thus, for people like Temple Grandin, literacy becomes their primary mode of linguistic expression. The problem is, how to get a nonverbal autistic child to engage in oral language, because literacy stands on the shoulders of oral language—the former cannot exist without the latter.

Delays in language acquisition and language deficiencies would arise in autistics not because of neurological impairment in Broca's or Wernicke's areas in the brain, but because language is a whole brain function. Though most of the physical processing of language is performed in the left hemisphere, there still needs to be a recipient for language outside of the self in order for language to even get started, whereas the autistic individual is indisposed towards relating with others. First we learn to speak to others, then we learn to speak to ourselves, then we silence that private conversation and it becomes subjective verbal thought, the voice of consciousness. If there is a serious delay at that very first step of language development—learning to speak to others—every other step in that sequence will also be delayed, possibly to the point of never developing at all. In "classic" or severe autism, this is exactly what happens. The mind turns in upon itself so entirely that it completes a defensive ring, walling off the outside world of others and pulling up the drawbridge of social language into a private castle of inward fantasy and outward silence. The outwardly focusing "social brain" is thus trumped by the inwardly focusing autistic consciousness. The "kingdom of mind" in autism becomes a cold and empty "fortress of solitude."

"Autistic Intelligence"

Hans Asperger was relatively unknown during his lifetime, but in retrospect he's now regarded as a clinician, theorist, and researcher who was at least a half-century ahead of his time. Not only did he recognize and identify autism as a disorder that is different, discrete, and independent of other known childhood disorders, he also perceived autism as more of a personality style or cognitive trait, and like all other styles or traits, autism presents itself along a "range" or spectrum, on which any behavioral symptom can be expressed within a broad scale ranging from extremely severe to practically nonexistent. Since autism, in Asperger's perspective, is an innate cognitive/personality feature (a "natural entity"), it cannot be regarded as merely a developmental disorder, because it's not limited to childhood. Asperger considered autism to be a distinct condition that is "unmistakable and constant throughout the while lifespan." And finally, unlike his contemporary across the pond, Leo Kanner, Asperger did not perceive autism as a condition that purveys only deficits, but as a variety of human experience that is as rich and diverse as any other human experience, purveying both deficits and advantages, depending on the individual and his environment.[38]

While Kanner—focusing on deficits, as per his wont—regarded deficient social behavior as the core feature of autism, Asperger focused on the potentially positive aspect of "autistic intelligence" as the condition's core feature, the tendency for his "little professors" to focus single-mindedly on their chosen pursuits: "In everything these children follow their own impulses and interests ... regardless of the outside world."[39] In describing his construct of "autistic intelligence," Asperger noted the broad spectrum that is now—75 years later—acknowledged by the majority of the field: "The range encompasses all levels of ability from the highly original genius, through the weird eccentric who lives in a world of his own and achieves very little, down to the most severe, contact-disturbed, automaton-like mentally retarded individual."[40] Asperger also noted the specific strengths of "autistic intelligence" that are expressed in "clusters of enhanced ability in music, memory, art, mathematics, science, and technology,"[41] and how they are beneficial not only for individuals, but for society as well:

> Abstraction ability, for instance, is a prerequisite for scientific endeavor. Indeed, we find numerous autistic individuals among distinguished scientists.... It seems that for success in science and art, a dash of autism is essential. For success, the necessary ingredient may be an ability to turn away from the everyday world, from the simply practical, an ability to rethink a subject with originality so as to create in new untrodden ways.[42]

In the 1960s, Rimland suggested that eccentric geniuses such as Einstein and Newton represented autistic intelligence in its most productive formation...

It may not be too far amiss to suggest that some autistic individuals are incipient geniuses whose eccentricities are so severe and incapacitating that all but minimal participation in the "normal" world is precluded.[43]

Deducing that autism was at some level a genetically determined neurological predisposition, Rimland proposed that autistic people inherited "a double dose of the extreme ability to concentrate—to narrow their attention to a very fine point, like a searchlight, to illuminate with great intensity a very small matter."[44]

Following Asperger's and Rimland's viewpoints, Boucher noted that "spared cognitive abilities" (cognitive strengths in autistics), including "rote memory, fitting and assembly tasks, and mechanical reading," are all directly related to their highly selective and focused attention to detail.[45] Autistic savants tend to excel at tasks involving the exact reproduction from memory of complicated patterns. J. Langdon Down, the 19th century British doctor known for first describing both Down syndrome and Savant syndrome, wrote of a patient who could recite verbatim the entirety of Edward Gibbon's weighty tome *The Decline and Fall of the Roman Empire*, by heart.

In a 2011 article in *Nature* entitled "The power of autism," Laurent Mottron argued that "autism can also be an advantage," especially in the field of "scientific research."[46] Though "autistic brains operate differently," he stressed, "this redistribution of brain function may nonetheless be associated with superior performance ... a growing body of research is showing that autistics outperform neurologically typical children and adults in a wide range of perception tasks, such as spotting a pattern in a distracting environment."[47] In his clinical studies, Mottron found that autistics do better in "Raven's Matrices, a classic intelligence test in which subjects use analytical skills to complete an ongoing visual pattern ... autistics completed this test an average of 40% faster than did nonautistics."[48]

Even more recent studies have shown that "polygenic risk" for autism is "positively correlated with general cognitive ability."[49] Oliver Sacks, quoting and paraphrasing his colleague, Uta Frith, found in Sherlock Holmes the perfect example of autistic intelligence:

... Sherlock Holmes with his oddness, his peculiar fixations—his "little monograph on the ashes of 140 different varieties of pipe, cigar and cigarette tobacco," his "clear powers of observation and deduction, unclouded by the everyday emotions of ordinary people," and the extreme unconventionality that often allows him to solve a case that the police, with their more conventional minds, are unable to solve. Asperger himself wrote of "autistic intelligence" and saw it as a sort of intelligence scarcely touched by tradition and culture—unconventional, unorthodox, strangely "pure" and original, akin to the intelligence of true creativity.[50]

"Homo Aspergerus" and "Geek Chic"

In his book *Neurotribes* (2015), Silberman noted that Asperger was "prescient in insisting that the traits of autism are 'not at all rare.'" According to Silberman's calculations, given the current [2015] estimates of prevalence, "autistic people constitute one of the largest minorities in the world. There are roughly as many people on the spectrum in America as there are Jews."[51] Silberman's demographic comparison was, perhaps, carefully chosen, because just as Jews have been discriminated against because of their cultural differences, autistics have been discriminated against because of their cognitive differences. Also, just as the Jewish faith is associated with the genocide in Europe during World War II, there's a rising movement of "anti-cure" activists in the autism community who believe that an actual "cure" for autism, if implemented broadly, would be tantamount to neurological genocide ... the destruction of an entire category of people because of their variation from the cognitive norm.

While the term "Asperger's Syndrome" is no longer in the DSM, it's still widely used, oftentimes with pride, as it represents the highest functioning group of people on the spectrum. And while the term didn't enter the popular vernacular in America until the 1990s, it was discussed in other terms well beforehand. In 1984, Jean Hollands, a psychotherapist, published a book entitled *The Silicon Syndrome*, as a guide for the wives and girlfriends of "sci-tech" men who work in Silicon Valley. "Sci-tech" men were emotionally distant, somewhat asocial, intellectually gifted, obsessed with their jobs, and were exceedingly logical and literal in their approach to everything. Hollands' description of the "Silicon syndrome" was practically a verbatim description of Asperger's syndrome.[52]

In a 2006 article in *Locus Online* entitled *"Homo Aspergerus:* Evolution Stumbles Forward," science fiction author/scholar and self-diagnosed autistic, Gary Westfahl, suggested that Asperger's Syndrome represented the vanguard of a new and improved model of the human race:

> ... Asperger's Syndrome should not be regarded as a handicap or as a debilitating condition; rather, it is a tremendous asset, a set of beneficial traits that may someday be recognized as the characteristics of a new, and superior, form of humanity.... We are moving toward a world ... where Asperger's Syndrome will no longer be a liability, and instead will become only an asset.... Perhaps, as advanced forms of artificial intelligence become significant participants in the human community, people who long for human contact will be disadvantaged while people with Asperger's Syndrome—who traditionally preferred the company of machines to the company of people anyway—will get along just fine.

Perhaps, instead of science fiction's *Homo superior*, the dominant new form of humanity in the future will be the unanticipated *Homo aspergerus*. Perhaps, then, we will someday live in the world of E.M. Forster's "The Machine Stops" (1909), where people live out their entire lives in enclosed individual chambers while they virtually interact with other people and machines when and to the extent that they choose....[53]

Westfahl's argument, while tongue-in-cheek, represents a new cultural movement among people on the spectrum (whether officially diagnosed or not), to be proud of their autistic intelligence, and to consider it as an advantage rather than as a disorder. The "autistic pride" movement is directly related to a parallel cultural movement, oftentimes referred to as "geek chic."

The term "anorexic chic" has been used for decades to refer to a manner of advertising that glorifies and glamorizes the "super-thin" look among models and actresses. In order to emulate the super-thin look, teenage girls starve themselves, becoming anorexic as a self-destructive fashion choice. "Anorexic chic" therefore refers to both the glamorization of the super-thin look that inspires anorexia as well as the actual practice of anorexia in order to match one's body to the look. The irony is that a term created to describe a psychopathology has somehow been co-opted by a subgroup of society, and used to glorify and glamorize the same condition, making the deadliest psychiatric disorder[54] seem fashionable, cool, and "chic."

Though anorexia and autism are completely dissimilar conditions, the same ironic scenario is playing out in popular culture. The kids who used to get picked in on school for being "nerds" or "dorks" or "geeks," have taken ownership of those terms (sort of like the way many people in the African American community have taken ownership of the "n-word"), and now they use the same terms proudly in reference to themselves. To be sure, it's not chic to be severely autistic, but in some circles (especially in Silicon Valley), it's chic to have all of the symptoms of Asperger's syndrome.

The technophilic digital age has created a new sort of hero, a champion of coding and engineering. The path to great success which was once paved with outgoing personality features such as extroversion, popularity, and athleticism, has changed course. To be a great success in the digital age, one must be technologically oriented, a master of binary code, and analytically minded. The heroes of the Millennial generation are the Mark Zuckerbergs, the Bill Gates, the Steve Jobs—all "geeks"— and all unusually successful. "Asperger's chic" refers to the fact that people at the very high end of functionality on the autism spectrum seem to have the inside track on the road to success in the digital arena. What was once a stigmatic disorder has now become a status symbol. Now that the nerds have had their revenge, they've begun to self-proclaim their own preeminence by taking ownership of the "Asperger's" label and its recent cachet, and wearing it as a badge of honor.

In a 2011 article in *Nature* entitled "Scientists and autism: When geeks meet," Lizzie Buchen noted that the tech industry in Silicon Valley seems to be dominated by people (mostly men), who have all the symptoms of Asperger's. Others have made the same observation. Silberman quoted a supervisor from Microsoft who told him: "All of my top debuggers have Asperger syndrome."[55] Asperger's has often been referred to as the "engineers' disorder" and the "geek syndrome," and it seems to be grossly overrepresented in tech industries. Temple Grandin, in reference to "autistic spectrum disorder," wrote: "At one end of the spectrum, you might find the severely disabled. At the other end, you might encounter an Einstein or Steve Jobs."[56] In reference to Asperger's, Grandin wrote:

> Half the employees at Silicon Valley tech companies would be diagnosed with Asperger's if they allowed themselves to be diagnosed.... I've been to their offices; I've seen their work force up close. Many of the hits on my home page come from Silicon Valley and other areas with a high concentration of tech industries. A generation ago, a lot of these people would have been seen simply labelled as gifted....[57]

The density of people in Silicon Valley who apparently have Asperger's-like personalities and thinking styles has become a matter of great concern. If Asperger's truly represents the upper end of functionality on the autism spectrum, then the valley of tech kings is over-populated with the "broader autistic phenotype," which means that couples who share the same phenotype are at much greater risk of having children who are on the spectrum. In a study of autism epidemiology done in Eindhoven, a technology hub in the Netherlands, Simon Baron-Cohen concluded that "children living in the town were 2 to 4 times more likely to be diagnosed with autism than were children living in two other Dutch towns of similar size."[58] In an interview with Buchen, Baron-Cohen remarked: "I do think that when these geeks marry each other, that's bad news for the offspring."

Asperger's chic is not just a Silicon Valley phenomenon. Pop culture figures once regarded as alien have become figures of identification for legions of fans, especially in the sci-fi genre, which has always been associated with the "geek" subculture. (Silberman argues in *Neurotribes* that the entire genre of science fiction, and the geek sub-culture that has grown around it, has always been populated predominantly by people on the spectrum). In an interview with Oliver Sacks, Temple Grandin admitted: "I can really relate to Data," referring to the android character on *Star Trek*. Sacks noted that "A surprising number of people with autism identify with Data, or with his predecessor, the ultra-logical Vulcan, Mr. Spock."[59] People on the spectrum, according to Sacks, identify with these alien/android characters because they feel alienated themselves. In a world where happiness is related to being outgoing and overtly social and emotional, autistics at any point in the spectrum seem like misfits, "freaks and geeks" who will forever be on the outside looking in.

Like Data and Mr. Spock, who are fascinated with human emotionality and sentimentality and desperately want to feel the way that humans feel, autistics are aware of their differences, but cannot change their own personalities and cognitive traits in order to fit the mold. The tide is turning, however. Remembering her school days, Grandin recalled: "And then there are the geeky, nerdy kids I call Steve Jobs Juniors. I think back on kids I went to school with who were just like these kids but who didn't get a label. Now they would."[60] The "label" of Asperger's or, in the current nomenclature, the high-functioning end of the autism spectrum ("HFA"), used to carry a stigma that was incontrovertibly negative. Now, in the era of "geek chic," the label has positive connotations as well.

Some tech companies actively and overtly recruit people on the spectrum. Grandin visited these companies:

> Aspiritech, in the Chicago suburb of Highland Park, and Specialsterne in Copenhagen, both employ primarily high functioning autistics and individuals with Asperger's to test software. Their brains—wired to endure repetition, to focus closely, to remember details—are just what the job requires. The son of Aspiritech's founder was diagnosed with Asperger's at the age of fourteen, and as an adult he was fired from his job as a grocery bagger. But when it comes to testing software, he's the go-to guy.[61]

The recruitment of people on the spectrum by tech companies, however, carries with it a potential risk, as Grandin noted in an interview with Silberman:

> Grandin also noticed how many parents at autism conferences were gifted in technical professions. "Early on I met a family with two severely nonverbal kids. Dad was a computer programmer and Mom was a chemist. Both super-smart.... I saw lots and lots of cases like this. I started to think of autistic traits as being on a continuum. The more traits you had on both sides, the more you concentrated the genetics. Having a little bit of the traits gave you an advantage, but if you had too much, you ended with very severe autism." She warned that efforts to eradicate autism from the gene pool could put humankind's future at risk by purging the same qualities that had advanced culture, science, and technological innovation for millennia. The maker of the first stone spear, she observed, was likely

a lone autistic at the back of the cave, perseverating over the subtle differences between various types of rocks—not one of the "yakkity yaks" chatting away in the firelight.[62]

In a 1998 *Atlantic* article entitled "Neurodiversity: On the neurological underpinnings of geekdom," Harvey Blume argued that "NT [neurotypical] is only one kind of brain wiring, and, when it comes to working in hi-tech, quite possibly an inferior one." Is it possible that the tables are turning—pushed by the demands of our technophilic media environment—to the point where being "neurotypical" could be construed as a handicap, and autism as an advantage? Blume quotes a self-diagnosed high-functioning autistic (HFA) who, with tongue squarely in cheek, argued that "Neurotypical syndrome is a neurobiological disorder characterized by preoccupation with social concerns, delusions of superiority, and obsession with conformity." While the sarcasm is amusing, it does point to a true feeling of disenfranchisement that people on the spectrum feel, and a rising movement to stop perceiving autism as a purely deficient mode of thinking and feeling, and to focus on the potential advantages of autistic intelligence. In his article, Blume concludes: "Neurodiversity may be every bit as crucial for the human race as biodiversity is for life in general. Who can say what form of wiring will prove best at any given moment?"[63]

Digital Reflections of the Autistic Self

"In the Information Age," Blume asserts in his article, "geekdom is ascendant, and the Internet the medium and the meeting place of choice."[64] Silberman argues in *Neurotribes* that digital media was in large part created by the somewhat autistic brains of Silicon Valley for communicating with other autistic brains. In her own book, *The Autistic Brain* (2013), Grandin wrote that the "similarity between my brain and a search engine, though, shouldn't come as too much of a surprise. Who do you think designed the original search engines? Very likely it was people whose brains work like mine."[65]

The spread of digitality across the world creates an increasingly hospitable media environment for autistic brains, which may in turn evoke even more epigenetic expressions of autistic traits in the general population. If the brain and its environment can create a positive feedback loop in which autistic intelligence creates a more autistic world, which in turn creates more autistic intelligence, then we can see digital media playing a crucial role in the ongoing process of leftward hemispheric lateralization. On the topic of the internet, Silberman quotes

Carolyn Baird, an autistic mother of four and an advocate for autistic children, who said: "For many of us, this medium has given us the opportunity to be accepted for the first time in our lives as being just like everyone else, and gives us our first hint at what it feels like to be accepted on the quality of our thoughts rather than the quality of our speech."[66]

The internet mitigates autistic people's socialization issues, but it also exacerbates them. Modern e-communication is, in its own way, quite autistic. This should come as no surprise, if we follow Grandin's suggestion that the internet was created by autistic people, and if we accept Silberman's argument, that the internet was created by autistic people as a means of fostering communication with other autistic people. In addition to the basic fact that e-communication enables isolation by allowing people to function without real in-person social interaction, e-communication, like texting, is lacking in the "pragmatic" or social dimension of communication.

Texts and emails are detached from the social context of speech, just like autistic speech. They are devoid of eye contact, facial gestures, vocal intonations—anything that is personal or emotional. E-messages are abstract, distant, disconnected, and depersonalized. People naturally try to compensate for the emotional barrenness of e-communication by making up and using acronyms that impart emotional superlatives, such as "lol" or "omg," but the banality of the acronyms themselves seems to only add to the problem. The lack of real-time interaction diminishes the reciprocity of communication, making it feel like one-way messages being sent and received, as opposed to the natural flow of a real two-way conversation in real time. Metalinguistic nuances such as sarcasm, irony, metaphor, and humor are difficult if not impossible to impart via text messages, without being misconstrued. The language we now use for the bulk of our correspondence, once filtered through digital media, is clearly autistic. If the modern brain has been molded over many millennia by our species' mastery of language, how will the brain change in response to our changing use of language? Will the adoption of an autistic medium of communication influence our brains to become even more autistic than they already are?

William Blake's aphorism "We become what we behold" is certainly truer now than when he wrote it, back in 1804. If what we behold all day, everyday, are computers displaying digital information, then we are rapidly becoming a species of beings that are interconnected so completely with our computers that we've begun to think and even feel like them. As McGilchrist warned, "We are busy imitating machines."[67] A brain that perceives the world as becoming more and more of a virtual reality inhabited by computer generated icons and dissociated robotic figures, will adapt to this new world by becoming more computer-like and robot-like itself. It will inhibit emotional processes by disconnecting them from cognitive processes. Could the product of this hyper-adaptive neuro-evolution be a brain that is ultimately incapable of conventionally human socio-emotional responses? Is the evolution of media technology leading the human race to the inevitable end point of "Homo Aspergerus"?

Four

Schizophrenia, Dual Consciousness and the Split Mind

Schizophrenia may be a necessary consequence of literacy.
—Marshall McLuhan (1962)

In discussing the duality of mind in a 1917 essay, Freud famously remarked, "The ego is not master in its own house."[1] Less than a century later, the title of Iain McGilchrist's 2009 book *The Master and His Emissary* alludes to another type of master. The title of McGilchrist's book on the cerebral hemispheres refers to an allegory found in Nietzsche involving a "wise spiritual master," who ruled a land that flourished and spread so greatly that the master himself could no longer oversee all of its villages, so he relied on trusted emissaries to rule in his stead, while he provided insights and judgments from afar. One particular emissary became hungry for power and used his position to increase his influence above all others. He cultivated the illusion among the people that he was not an emissary, but the master, until he reached the point where he and he alone ruled the land, while the judgments of the true master went unheeded and ignored. The emissary became the master, but lacking the wisdom and spirit of the true master, he misguided the people, and the kingdom fell to ruins.[2]

For Freud, the master represented the unconscious urges and drives that propel and steer our behaviors, regardless and heedless of the conscious ego's thoughts and preoccupations. For McGilchrist, the superseded master represents the right hemisphere of the brain, the perspective-taking ground of our perceived reality. The usurping emissary represents the left hemisphere, the primary seat of language and the dominant voice of consciousness. The masters in these two metaphors point to the same underlying truth. Intuitively, we must believe that there is an internal state of unity in our minds, a stable singular identity that maintains peace and harmony between the two sides of our selves. We must believe that "I" am one. In actuality, this sense of unity is a carefully crafted chimera, as Carl Jung argued: "The so-called unity of consciousness is an illusion ... we like to think that we are one, but we are not."[3]

The master—if there is one—is merely the aspect of our mind that cultivates the *illusion* of a master ... the illusion of unity. The clearest evidence of this illusion of unity can be seen in the very many examples of people living among us whose inner masters have been dethroned— people with schizophrenia, and also people whose cerebral hemispheres have been surgically disconnected, so-called "split brain patients." The evidence of dual consciousness can be seen in their experiences, thoughts, and behaviors, which reveal the true state of disunity within, the dualistic, conflicted, split mind.

In the interest of proceeding with my own model about media and mental illness, I must forgo a full discussion of dual consciousness, beyond noting how and when the phenomenon ties in with my own theories. I encourage the curious reader, if he or she hasn't already done so, to read the books of Oliver Sacks and V.S. Ramachandran, for excellent examples and discussions on the topic from neurological perspectives, as well as the journal articles of the scientists who performed split-brain patient research, such as Roger Sperry, David Hubel, Torsten Wiesel, Michael Gazzaniga, Joseph DeLoux, and Joseph Bogen.

A.L. Wigan wrote a very speculative but extremely interesting and prescient book on the subject way back in 1844, entitled *The Duality of the Mind*, which was republished in 1985, on the heels of the popular interest in dual consciousness raised by the Nobel Prize–winning research in split-brain patients. In his book, Wigan asserted that each hemisphere is a fully functioning brain, that each hemisphere produces its own stream of consciousness, and since each hemisphere can have "opposing volitions," one hemisphere must be dominant over the other, in order to maintain a sense of unity in both mind and action. These notions (bolstered by modern research findings and newer theories), will compose some of the core hypotheses in this chapter.

A very popular and influential book—though quite speculative and controversial—was published by Julian Jaynes in 1976, entitled *The Origin of Consciousness in the Breakdown of the Bicameral Mind*. In the book, Jaynes suggested that consciousness in ancient humans was split between the two hemispheres, with one hemisphere acting as the commander and the other as the listener. The listening hemisphere experienced the verbal commands from the opposite hemisphere as the "voices of the gods." Jaynes suggested that schizophrenia was a "vestige of the bicameral mind."[4] The argument developed in this chapter is essentially the opposite, that schizophrenia results from a pathological melding—not separation—of the dual processing of verbal thought in the two hemispheres of the brain. Iain McGilchrist's aforementioned book is also filled with interesting ideas about the duality of mind. And finally, my previous book, *The Digital God* (2015), discusses the topic at length.

Schizophrenia as an Aspect of Human Nature

Just as he did with the term "autism," Eugen Bleuler struck at the very heart of the issue when he coined the term "schizophrenia" in 1908. The term is derived from the Greek roots: "schizein," split—and "phren," mind. Bleuler based his original term on extremely incisive observations of his psychotic patients' core state of mind. Their minds, it appeared to him, were "split" in two. The mind of the psychotic did not recognize its own thoughts, which appeared strange and alien to itself. The schizophrenic's internal duality is laid bare for himself to see, but not understand. The schizophrenic is a *stranger* to himself.

In his seminal 1997 article—"Is Schizophrenia the price that *Homo sapiens* pays for language?"—renowned neurologist and psychiatrist Timothy Crow summarizes the research and principles underlying his revolutionary genetic theory of the etiology of schizophrenia. The main points of Crow's theory will form the basis of the media model of schizophrenia that I draw out in this chapter. One point that Crow makes is that "there are no categories of psychosis, but only continua of variation."[5] As per the most recent revision of the DSM in 2013, published 16 years after Crow's article, schizophrenia and other psychotic disorders—schizoaffective and schizophreniform disorders, schizotypal personality disorder, and delusional disorder—as well as other conditions that overlap with schizophrenia—paranoid and schizoid personality disorders—are now generally regarded as disorders that fall within a spectrum of conditions indicated by schizophrenic symptoms. In light of Crow's genetic model, the schizophrenia spectrum can be seen as a product of the spectrum representing the variations of the expression of the gene responsible for language lateralization in the brain.

Schizophrenia is known to affect about 1 percent of the population of the world, and is seen cross-culturally and across all demographics.

Studies showing high concordance rates within families and among twins, indicate a strong genetic component at play. Specifically, identical twins (who share 100 percent of the same genes), have a 48 percent concordance rate for schizophrenia, while fraternal twins (who only share 25 percent of the same genes), have a 17 percent concordance rate, demonstrating that the incidence of schizophrenia is tied directly to genetic inheritance, possibly by as much as 90 percent, though other environmental and epigenetic factors are also at play.[6]

The general prevalence of the disorder across the world suggests that the gene or genes at work in schizophrenia were present in archaic hominids *before* Homo sapiens as a species disseminated around the world. Therefore, according to Crow, the gene in question is likely to be related to a "speciation event"—a genetic change that "defined the species." Furthermore, Crow argues that since schizophrenia is a debilitating disorder that often hampers successful reproduction in its victims, there must be a balancing adaptive advantage to the species involved with the gene, in order for the gene to perpetuate in the gene pool, despite the "fecundity disadvantage."[7]

A gene related to the evolution of language emerges as the most likely suspect, as language is a universal trait found in all humans. It's considered a species-defining genetic adaptation that arose before the worldwide dissemination of *Homo sapiens*, and it bestows a considerable evolutionary advantage to the species. According to Crow, the "anatomical connexions" that separated ancient hominids from the apes "are associated with the speciation characteristic of language." Specifically, the interhemispheric neural connections that remain "plastic" during development through childhood and adolescence are the ones most likely to be shaped epigenetically by environmental pressures for language acquisition and use.[8]

Schizophrenia, simply put, can be understood as a disorder of *language*.[9]

Many of the principal characteristics that define schizophrenia and distinguish it from other disorders (such as Kurt Schneider's "first rank" or "nuclear symptoms" of schizophrenia) are directly related to language function. These symptoms include oral auditory hallucinations, derailment and loose associations in speech and verbal thought, and paranoia and delusions related to the content of thought.[10] These nuclear symptoms, in Crow's theory, "reflect a breakdown of bi-hemispheric coordination of language." That is, symptoms such as the hearing of voices that are not recognized as one's own voice of consciousness, the perpetual derailment of one's train of verbal thought in favor of loosely associated tangents, the intrusion of verbal thoughts into consciousness that one does not recognize as one's own thoughts, the sense that one's thoughts are being "withdrawn" from one's mind by an external source, and the distinct feeling that one's thoughts are being "broadcast" and monitored by an external listener, all can be traced back to a malfunction of the processing of verbal thought.

According to Crow, the nuclear symptoms "constitute a pathology of the relationship between thought and language."[11] So, if schizophrenia is inextricably linked with language at the genetic level, and if language is considered to be *the* defining human trait, then the schizophrenia spectrum is understood to be just another expression of genetic variation in the human species. The key distinction is that the duality of the brain is veiled in nonschizophrenic minds by an illusion of mental unity, an illusion that is unveiled in schizophrenia, resulting in a mental state of disunity, a split mind.

Schizophrenia as a Byproduct of Language

The nuclear symptoms of schizophrenia indicate a breakdown in one's sense of mental unity. Crow's theory explains how this breakdown in unity—this *split* in the mind—is caused by a loss of cerebral dominance for the function of language: "...the findings from anatomical ... and functional studies ... are consistent with the hypothesis that schizophrenia is not a disorder of one or the other hemisphere, but one of the interaction between them, and specifically that there is a failure to establish unequivocal dominance."[12]

Without "unequivocal dominance" of one hemisphere over the other, there is a failure of inhibition of the subdominant hemisphere, resulting in "hemispheric indecision" in thought, speech, and behavior.[13] That is, there is no clear unity of mind and identity, as the product of both left hemispheric and right hemispheric streams of consciousness flow into each other—causing the disorganized thinking, hallucinations, and delusions that are symptomatic of schizophrenia—as well as the loose associations sometimes referred to as the "pathological freedom" of schizophrenic thought.[14] If language as verbal thought is being processed simultaneously in both hemispheres, but only one stream of consciousness is normally recognized, while the other stream is inhibited or "drowned out," then the "nuclear symptoms" of psychosis could be compared to the discordant audio feedback that occurs when the background noise from amplified sound is accidentally re-amplified. A well-tuned PA system cancels out the background noise, so that the audience is not even aware of its existence, while an imperfectly tuned PA system not only fails to cancel out the background noise, it re-amplifies it. The unwanted feedback noise is jarring, it plays over discordantly with the desired sound, and it causes auditory distress and confusion.

Researchers studying hemispheric indecision related to both handedness and language skills, found that "individuals at risk of psychosis" were "pre-disposed to problems in inter-hemispheric integration," and displayed a higher amount of "hemispheric indecision."[15] That is, psychosis seems to be associated with the lack of a dominant hemisphere for thought. A surprising result from anatomical autopsy studies of the brains of chronic schizophrenics discovered that the corpus callosa in schizophrenic brains were, on average, 1 millimeter thicker than the corpus callosa in nonschizophrenic brains, a finding that was both statistically and neurologically significant.[16] Thicker corpus callosa would imply an increased amount of interhemispheric neuronal connectivity, fostering an excess of interhemispheric communication, a condition which would be expected if schizophrenics did not have just one dominant hemisphere for verbal thought, but instead experienced a melding of both hemispheres.

The corpus callosum seems to perform conflicting tasks. On the one hand, it's clearly a bridge of neurons that connects the hemispheres. However, to say that the sole function of the corpus callosum is to transmit communication between the hemispheres is wrong, because much of the time, the corpus callosum is serving to *inhibit* communication between the hemispheres. That is, some of the neural connections transmit signals that activate neural firing, others transmit signals that cause inhibition, and yet others cause disinhibition. Therefore, it would be more correct to say that the corpus callosum *controls* or *manages* interhemispheric communication, but even that statement lacks complete accuracy, because the neuronal signals themselves—whether stimulatory, inhibitory, or disinhibitory—originate from the respective hemispheres. The corpus callosum is merely the medium of the "messages" traveling between the hemispheres. Some of these messages say "Go" (stimulatory), others say "Stop" (inhibitory), others say "Don't stop" (disinhibitory), and others say "Stop not stopping" (dis-disinhibitory), with levels of binary commands going on and on in complexity. The point is, the inhibitory messages transmitted via the corpus callosum are just as important as, and in some cases *more important* than, the stimulatory messages. There is probably no better example of this than the case of verbal thought, which is processed in both hemispheres at the same time (dual consciousness), but which must be inhibited to a large degree, lest more than one voice of consciousness emerge into awareness, as McGilchrist suggests:

If the main effect of an intact corpus callosum is inhibitory, its being compromised will have unpredictable results: either it will prove creatively fruitful, or it will simply be disruptive, by causing premature collapse into unity of elements or processes whose mutual independence needed to be maintained. Research in schizophrenia, using neuropsychological testing, as well as EEG and other measures, demonstrates precisely *a failure of interhemispheric inhibition.* In schizotypy, too, there is known to be intrusion of left-hemispheric modes into right-hemisphere functioning. Many of the phenomena of schizophrenia and schizotypy ... could be explained by such intrusions, including intrusions of right-hemisphere modes into left-hemisphere functioning....[17]

McGilchrist cites a plethora of clinical evidence to support the assertion that as the corpus callosum develops, its function becomes more inhibitory. An "ontogeny recapitulates phylogeny" model could be applied here, if we assume that the corpus callosum evolved in nature initially as a means of interhemispheric communication; but that only relatively late in its evolution did its function evolve to become more inhibitory than stimulatory. If so, then we see a parallel pattern in individual human development, as the cerebral hemispheres of babies and young children are unlike their adult counterparts, because they do not function with nearly as much mutual independence. As children grow, their corpus callosa develop in connectivity, but with a paradoxical effect. "Interhemispheric connectivity grows during childhood and adolescence, with the result that the hemispheres become more independent," McGilchrist writes.[18]

As we mature, our brains, ironically, becomes *less* integrated, rather than more integrated—thought we must admit that the system of independently functioning hemispheres, when it's working properly, results in a well-integrated dual-processing system that's capable of more complex tasks than a single-processing system. Problems arise, however, when the equilibrium of integration and independence, which is balanced via the corpus callosum, errs in either direction: too much integration of both hemispheres (resulting in schizophrenia), or too much independence of either hemisphere (resulting in other disorders, such as autism). McGilchrist quotes *The Upanishads* in order to express the essential and paradoxical function of the corpus callosum: "In the space within the heart lies the controller of all... He is the bridge that serves as the *boundary* to keep the different worlds apart."[19]

It's important to note that the corpus callosum develops as the individual develops, that it's not fully functional in childhood, and that it doesn't reach full maturity until the end of adolescence or early adulthood. Once again, if we employ the "ontogeny recapitulates phylogeny" model, we could see the brain evolving over many millennia to become less integrated, with more mutual hemispheric independence, just as the individual human brain, as a function of development in the first two decades of life, becomes less integrated, with more hemispheric independence. We could also see both the brain of our species evolving over millennia, and the brain of each individual developing over decades, adapting to their media environments (such as the challenges of literacy) by becoming more left hemispheric dominant for verbal thought. Thus, the "leftward shift hypothesis" would apply to both brain evolution in our species and brain development in the individual.

More specifically, in the case of schizophrenia, we can discern a reason for why the disorder has a relatively late typical age of onset, in late adolescence/early adulthood. If schizophrenia arises as a result of a malfunction of interhemispheric connectivity, and is specifically linked to a malfunction of the division or *mutual inhibition* of the dual hemispheric processing of verbal thought, which, by the end of adolescent brain development, must be completely divided, then we can understand the late onset of schizophrenia as a malfunction that coincides with the final stage of brain development involving hemispheric independence. The *"controller of all,"* the divider that keeps *"the different worlds apart,"* has stumbled in its final task, leaving the *"boundary"* open too wide, allowing the *"worlds"* to collide.

Crow concluded that "predisposition to schizophrenia is associated with inadequacy or delay in establishing dominance in one or the other hemisphere," and suggests that the breakdown in hemispheric integration is rooted in the gene that affects the lateralization of language in the left hemisphere.[20] Numerous anatomical and functional studies have revealed that language lateralization and cerebral dominance for language are reduced in schizophrenics, that language processing is more bilateral in schizophrenics, and that decreased language lateralization in schizophrenia correlates positively with the severity of hallucinations.[21]

In Crow's words: "…the nuclear symptoms of schizophrenia represent 'language at the end of its tether.'"[22] Language-based oral auditory hallucinations—the hallmark symptom of psychosis—are the unrecognized verbal thoughts of the disinhibited right hemisphere. Delusions arise both from the unrecognized voices themselves, and as a means of rationalizing the existence of these voices. For instance, the delusional schizophrenic may rationalize the voices by claiming that he's a prophet, that he hears the voice of God, or that aliens are telepathically communicating with him. The realization that the voices he hears are not "real" in the normative sense, forces him to question his own reality, to doubt his own senses, and to suspect that maleficent forces are conspiring to control his thoughts and perceptions—the fearful, foreboding, self-doubting, and distrustful suspicions that mark the essence of paranoia.

Other nuclear symptoms of schizophrenia, such as "thought broadcasting," "thought insertion," and "thought withdrawal," are so bizarre and idiosyncratic that, indeed, they only make sense *in light of* the theory that there is a very specific malfunction of verbal thought at play. In particular, the malfunction involves two simultaneous streams of consciousness that are mutually unaware of each other's existence, spilling over into each other.

The left hemisphere establishes mental dominance in thought by inhibiting the intrusion of right hemispheric consciousness into the left hemisphere's conscious train of thought. In schizophrenia, the breakdown of left hemispheric dominance results in the uncontrolled intrusion of right hemispheric verbal thoughts into the left hemisphere's stream of consciousness. What results is a virtual anarchy of the mind. Because the intrusions are uncontrolled, the left hemispheric stream of consciousness doesn't recognize the right hemispheric verbal thoughts as coming from the same mind as itself. The uncontrolled thought intrusions are perceived as alien, external psychic forces. This experience of self-alienation and split-mindedness is the essence of schizophrenia, and all other symptoms of psychosis proceed from this essential experience of internal disunity.

Of course, it's not adaptive for *all* right hemispheric thoughts to be inhibited *all* the time. A certain amount of right hemispheric influence is necessary for aspects of thought involving intuition, insight, creativity, and imagination. If, according to McGilchrist, the hemispheres each think about the world in different but complementary ways—the left hemisphere focusing on details while the right hemisphere taking in the big picture—then a stream of consciousness with no right hemispheric input at all would be quite maladaptive. In reference to the previous chapter, a left-only perspective would be "autistic." Similarly, a right-only perspective would excel at "getting the big picture," but would suffer from an inability to focus on details. (In subsequent chapters, I will argue that this form of cerebral disposition may be, in part, the cause of learning and behavioral problems such as attention deficit and dyslexia.)

In the case of schizophrenia, the problem isn't that the brain is lateralized too far to the left or too far to the right, but that there's seemingly no "dominant hemisphere" in control of inhibiting its other side, resulting in dual simultaneous streams of consciousness, always dueling it out, but with each side never attaining true dominance, as experimental studies in schizophrenics seem to illustrate:

Another distinctive characteristic that is often manifest in schizophrenic think-ing is a striking inconsistency or a tendency toward vacillating among alterna-tive responses to the world. One researcher describes the extreme variability of a given individual's responses—attributed to the tendency to keep changing his mind—as the main way in which various groups of schizophrenics differed from patients with affective illness across seven different tasks. On the object-sorting task schizophrenics will often show "endless hesitancy and vacillation between various aspects of the material," a tendency attributed to the patient's "inability to abstract one principle of the given material while he neglects the others." The schizophrenic often seems aware of a vast number of possibilities; but instead of focusing on only one, such as color or shape, it is as if he takes "all the possi-bilities into simultaneous consideration," thus leading to a competition among incongruous and incompatible modes of response. At times this may derive from a kind of "intellectual ambivalence"—what a patient of mine called a "coun-tervailing tendency" of the mind. One of Eugen Bleuler's patients (a man edu-cated in philosophy) described his experience in the following way: "When one expresses a thought, one always sees the counter-thought. This intensifies itself and becomes so rapid that one doesn't really know which was the first."[23]

In responses to the Rorschach test (an "inkblot" apperception test), schizophrenics and only schizophrenics display the "contamina-tion precept," in which "two objects or perspectives appear to be pres-ent simultaneously, as if overlaid on each other as in a photographic double exposure."[24] David Rapaport believed that the "frequent shifting among conceptual frames of reference" results in a lack of "automatic steering" in schizophrenic thinking.[25] Sass argues that this "perspectival shifting" may partially account for the slower reaction times in response selections that are very commonly found in schizophrenics.[26] "The schizophrenic ... seems more often to have a simultaneous awareness of several possibilities, frequently moving, or hesitating, among what are experienced, at least implicitly, as alternative worlds of orientation towards experience."[27] This "simultaneous awareness" of "alternative worlds" may, in part, explain both the psychotic experience of hallucina-tions, and the psychotic delusions confabulated to make sense of them. Sass believes that the confusion apparent in schizophrenic thought dis-order "stems from a kind of vertigo, a continual collapsing of one frame of reference into the next."[28]

Kurt Goldstein believed that schizophrenic cognitive perception suffers from "deficient figure-ground formation," resulting in an "inabil-ity to maintain adequate boundaries" between divergent thoughts and concepts. Goldstein's figure-ground metaphor is particularly intrigu-ing, if we momentarily take a very broad approach to the cerebral hemi-spheres, imagining the left hemisphere as the portal through which we experience the focal figure of attention, and the right hemisphere as the portal through which we experience the background or context in which the figure is embedded. If we can only focus on one thing at any given moment, our attention tends to stay fixed on the focal figure, the specific thing that stands out from the background, a figure which appears clearer and more distinct to us, as it is "in focus," as opposed to the ground, which remains unfocussed in the back ... indistinct.[29]

The key to adaptive cognitive perception would be for the brain to allow us to see both the figure and ground simultaneously, while giving us a clear point of focus on one or the other (usually the figure), so that what we perceive and think about at any given moment is one scenario with a focused figure and somewhat unfocussed ground, as opposed to simultaneously perceiving and thinking about *two* entirely different perspectives—one focused on the figure and the other on the ground—which would obviously result in chaos and confusion. In short, our sense of mental coherence and cognitive unity—our *sanity*—depends on our brain's ability to maintain cerebral dominance in one hemisphere, while allowing entry of the other hemisphere's thoughts into the dominant stream of consciousness in a controlled, unconscious, filtered way. It seems that in the case of schizophrenia, there is a gaping hole in that filter. But why?

Spectra within Spectra

Marian Annett, a renowned neurologist, espouses a "right shift theory," suggesting that there are different genes that determine cerebral hemispheric lateralization. Because her theory is based on studies of handedness, a "right shift" refers to a lateralizing shift of dominance towards the right hand, indicating a shift in cerebral dominance towards the left hemisphere (making it somewhat confusing for our purposes, as Annett's "right shift" in handedness corresponds with my "left shift" in cerebral hemispheric dominance). Annett's "RS+" gene would foster left hemispheric lateralization, and the "RS+" would foster right hemispheric lateralization. Annett believed that there may be a mutant variation of gene expression that would be "agnosic for left versus right," that is, a gene expression that does not distinguish between input from the left hemisphere and the right. This mutant gene expression would only be problematic when it affected both hemispheres. In her model, the calculations of risk for a genetic expression in which there was an agnosic gene affecting both hemispheres was estimated at about 1 percent, the same prevalence rate for schizophrenia in the general population.[30]

As a rule, patterns in nature fall along spectra of phenomena, rather than binary distinctions. *"Nature loves diversity."*[31] If we apply this principle to the variation of expression in the gene responsible for language lateralization, then we could imagine that the propensity for cerebral dominance in language created by this gene will express infinite varieties of cerebral dominance, which will nonetheless fall along a spectrum of expression. For the vast majority of people, language is lateralized in the left hemisphere, resulting in left hemispheric cerebral dominance. A normative expression of the cerebral dominance gene would place the dominant stream of consciousness in the left hemisphere, with varying but regular input from the right hemisphere, which is carefully filtered into the dominant stream of consciousness, so as not to upset the sense of conscious unity. Once again, cerebral dominance is *essential* in order to maintain a sense of cognitive unity. Hypothetically, this would result in a normative sense of consciousness, in which the individual has one singular train of thought, that generally follows a straight and linear path of thinking, but is occasionally diverted into tangential lines of thought, and even more occasionally, into whimsical flights of fancy.

We should note, however, that even in the normative individual, the gene for cerebral dominance would be expressed at different levels, depending on the situation and the individual's state of mind. When asleep and dreaming, for instance, left hemispheric dominance may be completely shut off, so that consciousness in the dream is experienced as a state of completely loose and un-linear associations, with no rhyme or reason dictating the direction of thought, no strict sense of reality or logic governing the experience. Jung's famous assertion, "Behold the dreamer, and you will see the mind of the psychotic," comes to mind.[32] However, as defined in the current model, the dream state is not psychotic, because dreams lack the cognitive anarchy of two streams of consciousness splashing into each other. Dreams merely represent a nonnormative experience of consciousness—the unfiltered stream of right hemispheric consciousness, rumbling away in the night, while the left stream slumbers.

On occasion, however, even the individual with "normative" consciousness may experience a state of cognitive disunity. The momentary disorientation of reality that we feel when we wake up in the middle of a dream could be due to the fleeting experience of duality, the unexpected intrusion of left hemispheric consciousness into the dream consciousness of the right hemisphere. For a moment, the two states of consciousness are experienced simultaneously, which feels uncanny and unsettling. The ancient Chinese parable comes to mind, of a man who was dreaming that he was a butterfly, and awoke with the conundrum: *"Now I do not know whether I was then a man dreaming I was a butterfly, or whether I am now a butterfly, dreaming I am a man."*[33]

Similarly, the wonder and terror experienced in the peak state of psychedelic hallucinatory drug experiences are glimpses at the psychosis of dual consciousness. Weaker hallucinatory drug experiences evoke the more subdued sense of diminished cerebral dominance, the change in the balance of consciousness from left hemispheric to right hemispheric, resulting in consciousness drifting from its focused state of mind into a more dreamy and unfocussed state, though without the jarring sense of duality that arises from a complete loss of cerebral dominance. In both schizophrenic and drug-induced psychoses, the sense of a unified self—the mirror of identity—is shattered, as uncontrolled, unfiltered, and unrecognized voices fill the head, seemingly monitoring and broadcasting our private thoughts, commenting on our behaviors, exposing unconscious desires, and making unwanted commands and insinuations. The shattering of the illusion of unity doesn't fracture only thought and speech, it fractures identity, it fractures one's sense of reality, one's relationship to the world and everything in it, one's phenomenological experience of "self."

Schizophrenic Thinking and Pollyannaism

There's a growing consensus among schizophrenia researchers to frame the disorder as primarily a disorder of thought, especially verbal thought, and to understand symptoms of schizophrenia as the product of schizophrenic thought disorder. Leonhard and Brugger (1998) found that participants on the schizophrenia spectrum were more likely to use right hemispheric semantic processes—to make loose associations that fostered creative analogies—than participants without schizophrenic traits. For instance, participants with "thought disorder" responded to indirect word associations, such as STRIPES and LION, more than nonthought disordered participants, who tended to respond only to direct word associations, such as STRIPES and TIGER. Looser associations represent a train of verbal thought that is less dominated by the "close focus" of the left hemisphere, which tends towards very tight associations between very clearly related stimuli.

Schizophrenics display significant deficits in both short term and long term verbal memory.[34] This specific function is very much entwined with inter-hemispheric transference between oral language (processed mainly in the left hemisphere), and private verbal thoughts (processed in both hemispheres). If there's a dysfunction in schizophrenia arising from hemispheric nondominance for verbal thought, then the deficits in verbal memory so reliably found among schizophrenics would be the perfect indication of such a cause for the disorder. Confusion regarding the storage, access, and interpretation of verbal memory, would result in many of the "positive" symptoms of schizophrenia. Oral auditory hallucinations, for example, could be the unwanted and uninhibited recalling of verbal memory from the right hemisphere. Delusional thinking could be related to partially recalled, and therefore only partially understood, memories or thoughts. Thought broadcasting, thought withdrawal, and thought insertion would all be related to the feeling that one's own memories and ideas were not under one's own control. Loose associations and thought derailment would also result from dysfunctional short term memory for verbal thought, as one would constantly be losing one's train of thought, forgetting what you were just thinking or talking about, without even realizing that your thoughts and speech sound loose and derailed to others.

Another reliable and interesting research finding is that schizophrenics do not display the universally occurring "Pollyanna principle" in tests of verbal memory.[35] (The Pollyanna principle is the tendency shown among virtually all people to have better memory for positive stimuli than negative stimuli. That is, we tend to remember the "good" more than the "bad.") Because verbal memory in particular and verbal thought in general are, for the vast majority of people, processed primarily in the left hemisphere, we can think of "Pollyannaism" as a trait of left hemispheric thinking. The left hemispheric approach to the environment is to focus on details, a narrowing of perception that, by its own nature, excludes and excises information from its own field of awareness. The complementary approach of the right hemisphere is to remain open to the big picture, to ingest wholly all of the information within its field of information, including the information discarded by the left hemisphere.

Now, if we define the content of our own focused awareness at any given moment, quite generally, as "consciousness," then the discarded content of our unfocussed awareness, could be labeled as "unconscious" content. In this configuration, we can see the Freudian dichotomy of "conscious/unconscious" awareness as a fairly good descriptor of the left/right dichotomy of hemispheric dominance for verbal thought. That is, thoughts that we are aware of are "conscious," thoughts that we are not aware of are "unconscious," and conscious thoughts are processed more in the left hemisphere, while unconscious thoughts are processed more in the right hemisphere.

In Freud's model, an extremely important aspect of consciousness is a cognitive "filter" that suppresses or represses unwanted negative unconscious thoughts or memories from "rising" into conscious awareness. This is, in essence, a psychoanalytic explanation of the Pollyanna principle. In configuring his model of ego defense mechanisms such as denial and repression, Freud asserted that thoughts that were potentially harmful to the ego were ignored by the conscious mind, though they still existed in the unconscious mind. For Freud, we "Pollyannaize" our experience of the world in order to retain a singular fixed perspective regarding ourselves—a singular "ego"—that is both defended and supported by our own positively biased selective memories.

The ego defense mechanisms in Freud's model employ an arsenal of cognitive tricks—denial, repression, rationalization, intellectualization, projection, deflection, etc.—that cover up the fact that most of the world we experience is filtered out of conscious awareness and stored away secretly in the vast storehouse of the unconscious mind. For Freud, the filter between conscious and unconscious awareness was absolutely necessary to defend the ego from a destructive level of "neurosis," which is an internal conflict between one's unconscious desires and one's need for social and personal restraint. In the current model, the filter between conscious and unconscious awareness is achieved by the cerebral dominance of the left hemisphere in verbal thought, which effectively silences the right hemisphere enough to maintain a singular voice of consciousness, thus defending the singular "ego," not only from negative reflective thoughts and associations, but from the destructive splitting of consciousness, which would result in the psychotic experience of having two egos, rather than one.

Research done on split-brain patients and stroke patients has revealed that the left hemisphere tends to take a more positive and optimistic outlook on anything that reflects on the self, actively focusing on positive details while actively ignoring or denying the negative. This outlook is opposed to that of the right hemisphere, which takes in the whole picture, both good and bad, without selectively focusing on the good and discarding the bad. For example, patients with right hemispheric strokes (resulting in a unilaterally left hemispheric mode of awareness), were found to be extremely prone to "anosognosia" (denial of having a disability), even when the disabilities to the left sides of their bodies, caused by their right hemispheric strokes, were extremely severe. Some patients who were completely paralyzed on the left side of their bodies categorically denied having any disability, despite the obviousness of their conditions. Patients with left hemispheric strokes, however, were not prone to anosognosia. "Denial," McGilchrist asserts, "is a left-hemisphere specialty."[36]

Absence of Pollyannaism in schizophrenics would seem to indicate a less dominant left hemisphere. It's presumed that the unusual levels of negative information that pass through the filter of awareness into consciousness for schizophrenics is related to many of the "negative" symptoms of schizophrenia, which resemble depression. (The links between higher levels of right hemispheric input into consciousness and depressed thought and mood are explored further in the subsequent chapter.) The "positive" symptoms of schizophrenia, symptoms of psychosis, would also relate to the absence of Pollyannaism, the function of which is to effectively filter out information that is negative, conflicting, or in any way damaging to the ego. When these bits of information are released from the "unconscious" hemisphere and invade our conscious thinking, the effect is more than merely confusing and disorienting. Since the actual content of the unconscious intrusions are generally negative towards the self—hurtful, derogatory, accusatory, spiteful, self-destructive, harsh, and critical—the psychotic intrusions are extremely damaging to the ego.

Thus, the schizophrenic is doubly tormented, not just by the existence of unwanted "voices," but even more so by the hurtful things about the self that these voices have to say. If "the truth hurts," then psychotic "truth" hurts doubly, because it speaks the hidden truths about the self that we normally hide away from everyone, including ourselves. The unwanted and unrestricted intrusions of ego-damaging information that cut to the quick because of their preternatural insight into the unconscious self, would also give rise to other schizophrenic symptoms, such as paranoia, delusions, and depression.

Madness, Genius and Eccentricity

If the spectrum of schizotypy relates to the spectrum of genetic expression for cerebral nondominance, then schizophrenia itself would represent the high end of the spectrum, the consequence of severe and profound cerebral nondominance. Mild cerebral nondominance, on the other hand, would convey benefits in cognitive flexibility, such as the ability to make unique associations and original intuitive leaps. Advantageous combinations of thinking styles, merging both hemispheric specializations, would arise, such as creative/analytical and imaginative/ meticulous. Concomitant disadvantages of moderate cerebral nondominance would be related to tangential or flawed thinking resulting from intermittent uncontrolled overflow or confluence of one stream of consciousness into the other. These disadvantages would present themselves as symptoms associated with the less severe disorders on the schizophrenia spectrum—schizotypal or paranoid personality disorder—including paranoia, mild delusions, peculiar or eccentric behavior, odd or magical beliefs, unusual perceptual experiences or mild hallucinations, and odd speech or thinking.[37]

One scenario in which the previous pattern could be potentially adaptive is in the case of creative artists, whose art depends on the unique perspective of dual consciousness. The artist in some cases may trade off the single-minded security of the sane for the dualistic voices and apparitions of the unbalanced visionary. Theories regarding the oft-observed "commonalities between madness and genius" can be seen throughout the psychological and philosophic literature, going back for centuries.[38] Aristotle observed, "No great genius was ever without some tincture of madness." Many empirical studies have shown the links between schizotypal loose associations and creativity in a variety of realms, especially in the attribute labeled "overinclusiveness"— the trait of seeing relations between things that most people perceive as being completely unrelated.[39]

Creativity is not so much about generating completely new ideas de novo, but rather about perceiving new and original connections between ideas that nobody ever considered before. While the "vertical" thinking of the left hemisphere, which is focused, linear, and sequential, is necessary for refining ideas that are already defined, the "lateral" thinking of the right hemisphere, which is more associative, circumferential, and serendipitous, is necessary for making heretofore unseen associations that give birth to original creative insights.

The works of great creative geniuses such as Leonardo da Vinci, Edgar Allan Poe, and Albert Einstein are marked by this interplay of both vertical and lateral thinking. In their work, we see the gradual building up of scientific or artistic styles or models, propelled intermittently by great leaps forward, stemming from incredibly creative and unique discoveries, that invariably originate from innovative perceptions of the relationships between things.

James Watson's model of the double helix strands of DNA came to him in a dream about a spiral staircase. Einstein came upon his theory of relativity while pondering in a daydream upon how he would experience gravity if he were free-falling from the roof of a house. Friedrich Kekulé saw the structure of the benzene ring in a dream, in which dancing atoms coalesced into a snake that coiled back onto itself to swallow its own tail. In all of these instances, the theories would not have been possible had not the theorists studied the respective issues for many years, and the theories would also not have been developed if the theorists hadn't followed up on their insights with diligent study for many years, but the moment of creative insight—the burst of intuitive inspiration that catapulted the models into an altogether different and higher dimension of theoretical understanding—was derived from these rather loose and far-out associations between unrelated objects and fields.

Creativity, at its moment of inception, is a qualitatively different mode of thinking than the normal everyday thinking of the average individual. We're left with the troubling conclusion that the odd and eccentric thinking indicative of the creative genius is indeed related on a neurological level with the loose associations and peculiar connections that are symptomatic of schizotypy.[40]

Here too may be another example of an evolutionary tradeoff. People in the mild-to-moderate range of the schizotypy spectrum may be gifted with creative insight, while those in the severe-to-profound range may be cursed with schizophrenia. The highly disadvantageous condition of schizophrenia remains in the gene pool and is propagated, due to the highly advantageous condition of heightened creativity that's experienced by those with a less extreme version of the same underlying genetic predisposition. Because creative insight isn't beneficial only to the individual who has it, but to all society, who gain the benefits of these insights, the genes that cause havoc among schizophrenics must remain in the gene pool, because of the great benefits to society that result from them.

On an historical level, if the psychotic confluence of consciousness is accepted by the individual and his society as a beneficial trait, such as a spiritual gift—as in prophets, oracles, witch doctors, shamans, etc.—then the symptoms of what we now call "psychosis," would be perceived by the individual and his culture as the auguries of the gods. Far from being shunned from society, the individual would be elevated. The voices that in our society cause paranoia and distress, and which need to be rationalized away via delusions, were in some cases in the distant past welcomed and understood as boons for the individual and his society—except, of course, when the voices were perceived as demonic, in which case the individual was also considered severely disturbed, possessed of a demon, and in dire need of exorcism.

Nevertheless, in the historical and cross-cultural acceptance and reverence of so-called prophets, shamans, and oracles, we could even see a potential evolutionary advantage for schizophrenia itself; an advantage which now no longer exists, at least not in modern post-literate civilizations. Thomas Szasz noted wryly: "If you talk to God, you are praying. If God talks to you, you have schizophrenia." In a similar vein, Julian Jaynes wrote: "The modern schizophrenic is an individual in search of a culture ... he is a mind bared to his environment, waiting on gods in a godless world."[41]

Literacy and Thought Disorder

Literacy invokes a literate train of thought. When reading or writing, the lines of ink on the page or screen are heard as a "continuous ribbon" of silent sound, running straight ahead on linear tracks of thought, towards a preconceived destination. It's the *linearity* invoked and required by literate thinking that conditions the left hemisphere's parietal lobe to think in long sequential trains of verbal thought. These trains of thought run so far and so fast into abstraction that they're quite easy to derail. In a brain that lacks clear cerebral hemispheric dominance, the long train of thought chugging towards its distal logical point in the left hemisphere, is quite easily derailed by unrestricted right hemispheric thoughts, that abruptly cut across the tracks of thought and derail the train.

Thought disorders are a number of related symptoms of abnormal verbal thought and speech, that, I argue, all stem from the nuclear symptom of thought "derailment." As a psychotic symptom, derailment is not purely a compound result of literacy and hemispheric nondominance. Literate thought does not exist in a vacuum. No mind is an island. Literate people grow up in a literate society where literacy, as the primary medium of academia, is engrained in formal schooling that lasts anywhere from 13 to 30 years. Long trains of linear sequential thought, linked together by logical connections and directed towards logical endpoints, are required modes of verbal thinking in school and in the society that creates these schools. Hence, derailment as a symptom is likely to be much more severe in a formally educated individual whose thinking process has been trained to think in long extended trains of thought. Furthermore, derailment as a symptom of abnormal behavior, can only exist in a society that expects everyone to think and speak in long linear trains of logical sequential thought. Literate society creates its own norms, thereby creating its own deviations from the norms, its own psychopathologies. This is true not only for psychotic symptoms such as derailment, but for every other deviation from the expectations of literate society, deviations that are labeled as pathologies, such as dyslexia, dysgraphia, dyscalculia, attention deficit, intellectual disability, and so on.

In a preliterate society, an illiterate person's thoughts will not be trained to stretch out into long sequential lines of logic, because the models for such thinking are not engrained in their mind as a product of formal education. Also, within that society, the thought and speech of the illiterate individual will not be expected to differ from the norms of thought and speech of everyone else, which will also necessarily be less linear. Hence, hemispheric nondominance in an illiterate person in a preliterate society will not result in severe derailment of thought. Furthermore, the derailment that would exist in such a person in such a society would not be perceived by both the individual or his society as being nearly as problematic or psychopathological, as derailment entails in a literate person in a literate society. The corollary of this argument is that schizophrenia as a disorder would have a positive correlation with literacy, and that both the severity and prevalence of schizophrenia would increase in tandem with the levels of literacy in society.

Schizophrenic speech tends to digress from linearity via "loose associations" into long irrelevant tangents. The schizophrenic does not intend to ramble. However, since his literate mind has been trained to think in long trains of thought, each uninhibited interruption from the right hemisphere will hijack the train of thought, redirecting it onto a different track, which by nature of the thinker's own thought process will be long, taking it far away from the original track of thought, a long digression from the original point.

The "incoherence" of schizophrenic speech is a product of the speaker's frequent digressions and the aforementioned loose associations, both arising from derailment. The "illogicality" of schizophrenic speech follows from the lack of linearity, as logic is based on linear sequential thinking, in which one thought logically builds upon and follows from the previous thought, and then logically follows into the next thought. When derailment occurs, the linear sequence is broken. The verbal thought and speech of schizophrenics is full of non sequiturs, making it seem entirely irrational and illogical. In severe cases, or in periods of "florid" psychosis, derailment occurs so often that no two words seem logically linked in any meaningful or linear way, resulting in the "word salad" of acute psychosis, or as Crow put it, "language at the end of its tether."

Literacy and Duality

The medium of literacy fosters the internalization of language into private verbal thought. A literate mind is more prone to "silent deliberation" or "pensive consideration," but there is no true silence within the mind of the thinker, whose thoughts are still heard as a "continuous ribbon of sound." Within the experience of verbal thought there's a dialectic, an inner dialogue, with both an internal speaker and an internal listener. When both the speaker and listener of verbal thought become aware of each other's existence, consciousness—our awareness of our own awareness—is born. It's no coincidence that consciousness itself is born out of duality, an internal dialogue, and that consciousness itself is dualistic, as it requires the self's acknowledgment of itself. Duality, in this sense, is a prerequisite for consciousness. Yet, at the same time, the mind must conjure the illusion of mental unity for the purpose of maintaining sanity. This fragile illusion, this veil of sanity, is lost in the absence of hemispheric dominance.

"Hallucinations," the red flag of psychosis, are the clearest symptom of psychotic duality. The "voices" of psychosis are the unrecognized verbal thoughts of the right hemisphere, the noisy un-cancelled neural feedback of a mistuned brain. "Paranoia," another nuclear symptom, arises as a natural corollary to hallucinations. If you cannot trust your own senses, if the origin and content of your own thoughts and perceptions are untrustworthy and suspect, if the sane straightforward world you once knew is now twisted and convoluted into a strange world of contradictory thoughts and experiences, if you're constantly forced to question the nature of your own reality, putting yourself in the position where you must conclude either that there are forces in the world conspiring against you or that you've completely lost your mind, then paranoia arises as a natural reaction. In R.D. Laing's words: "Insanity ... a perfectly rational adjustment to an insane world."[42]

"Delusions," yet another nuclear symptom, arise as another corollary to duality. If you find yourself forced to decide between two options—(1) You are insane; or (2) There are extraordinary forces at play that explain the abnormality of your reality—then the second option would clearly be preferable. As Freud explained, when forced to defend itself in the face of devastating ego-crushing information, the conscious mind will use any means necessary to defend, deny, repress, rationalize, intellectualize, justify, or in any other way delude itself into believing that it—the ego, the self—is sound and sane, and it's the world that's deluded and mad. Delusions in a deranged mind serve this ego defensive function.

The Haunted Unconscious

The main theme of McGilchrist's work is that as the left hemisphere of the brain trailblazes its way towards ever-higher abstraction, it becomes more dissociated from the right hemisphere, and more detached in general from the environment and from "phenomenal reality," or life as it's being lived. The left hemisphere is busy cloistering itself within the cerebral and conceptual life of the mind, a mind that, according to McGilchrist, has become more dualistic over the past few centuries, as the language-based consciousness of the left hemisphere becomes louder and more dominant, while the less verbal and more imagistic consciousness of the right hemisphere gets increasingly drowned out and silenced. The emergence of the "unconscious" in the 19th century as a relatively new idea may, in fact, actually point to the emergence of the unconscious as a new phenomenon.

If we imagine preliterate minds to be less fragmented—less divided by the abstract detachment of the left hemisphere, less disconnected by the illusion of unity that veils the input of the right hemisphere—then the unconscious arises as a consequence. If, in McLuhan's words, "The unconscious is a direct creation of print technology, the ever-mounting slag-heap of rejected awareness,"[43] then it would make sense for this "slag-heap" to emerge at the same time as the mass psychological effects of literacy on the population. So, at the same time that Freud was venturing into the "dark continent" of the unexplored, unconscious psyche, other scholars, such as Max Weber, were noting a distinct change in the way that people in the Western world were experiencing life, and also identifying the cause of the change: "The fate of our times is characterized by rationalization and intellectualization, and, above all, by the 'disenchantment of the world.'"[44]

As the left hemisphere intellectualizes and rationalizes its outlook on the world, its selective focus simultaneously denies, ignores, disregards, and discards all ideas and beliefs that fail to conform to the left hemisphere's rationalistic and intellectual point of view. Nevertheless, the right hemisphere, whose outlook is inclusive and holistic, is still aware of the ideas and beliefs discarded by its partner across the cerebrum, and it still remembers them, though its memories are not directly accessible to the dominant hemisphere's process of conscious awareness. So, at the same time that Weber's world, the Western world, was becoming "disenchanted," the world was also becoming haunted.

The late 19th and early 20th centuries saw the rise of the literary and cinematic genres of supernatural horror. While "ghost stories" have always existed, the tone of the ghost story dramatically shifted in the Victorian and Edwardian ages, due primarily to the change in which Western people experienced the world. Prior to the Enlightenment, it was an accepted truth among everybody that there was a spiritual dimension to existence, a soul in every body. As the soul is immortal and the body transient, belief in spirits and souls would also entail belief in disembodied spirits—ghosts. Hence, it requires no leap of the imagination to deduce that preliterate Europeans believed in ghosts, just as much as they believed in spirits, souls, angels, demons, and God.

It's significant to note that in contemporary preliterate societies, belief in the spiritual side of existence, and in the omnipresence of spirits, is still universal. We should also note that preliterate folk in modern Western societies—little children—also, as a rule, believe in spiritual or magical beings, such as the Tooth Fairy, the Easter Bunny, Santa Claus, as well as ghosts. Belief in the supernatural was never a conflicted issue in the Western mind until the "rationalized" and "intellectualized" mind of modern literate thinkers exorcised the demons of irrational thought from conscious awareness. Once exorcised, the demons of irrationality did not disappear. Instead, they were submerged into the subliminal awareness of the subconscious right hemisphere, only to rise again in the form of twin specters: horror and madness.

McGilchrist argues quite convincingly, citing copious neurological studies, that the seat of spiritual experience lies in the right hemisphere.[45] If so, then the ascent of atheism and agnosticism over the past few centuries is more than coincidentally synchronous with the rise of literacy. The left hemispheric shift in verbal thinking required of literacy, and the simultaneous detachment and dissociation of consciousness from right hemispheric input, caused a change in spiritual experience. Renowned theologian Karen Armstrong pointed out in her bestselling book *A History of God* (1993) that the term "atheist" didn't exist anywhere prior to the Renaissance, and even after the term was invented, its use prior to the Enlightenment was as a sort of religious insult, referring to anyone who transgressed religious norms or had divergent moral ideas. Karen Armstrong quotes a typical use of the word "atheist" in the late 16th century: "...the hypocrite is an Atheist; the loose wicked man is an open Atheist, the secure, bold and proud transgressor is an Atheist: he that will not be taught or reformed is an Atheist."[46] According to Armstrong, prior to the 19th century, "Nobody would have dreamed of calling *himself* an atheist."[47]

As literacy became the norm in post–Enlightenment Western society, "religiosity" continued to be an important part of life in Western society, because the rules and dogma of religious creeds—the theology of religion—are perfectly suited to the left hemisphere's intellectual perspective. At the same time, however, "spirituality," the actual spiritual experience of hearing, seeing, or feeling a spiritual presence—the *theophany* of spiritual life—began to diminish quite rapidly and suddenly. The time of the Reformation saw drastic changes within both Catholic and Protestant churches. There was a general redirection of religious focus onto the literal interpretation of scriptures, an amplification of the importance of theological doctrine, and a desperate need to enforce scrupulous religiosity via legal punishments, forced conversions and confessions, as well as communal witch hunts of "atheistic" transgressors.

The new singular focus on the "good book" as the central aspect of religious life indicates an ascension of the left hemispheric literate experience of God, and a descension of the right hemispheric experience of God, which is unrelated to scriptures, dogma, or theology, and is more about feeling and directly experiencing the spiritual presence of God. It is this shift in religious experience from the experiential/perceptual to the theological/cerebral that Weber is referring to when observing the "disenchantment of the world."[48]

As a result of the Western "disenchantment" of both gods and ghosts, the spiritual world—once embraced as an embodied part of the human world—was detached from conscious awareness. The realm of the spiritual, once an integrated and "natural" part of the human experience, became "super-natural"—dissociated from normal human experience—exiled into the haunted unconscious realm of the "unbelievable," the "irrational," the "unreal."

The protagonist of a classic Victorian or Edwardian ghost story is invariably a modern person, well-read and educated, who finds himself in the undesirable position of having to doubt the veracity of his own senses. The ghosts in a ghost story appear subliminally, with strange mysterious sounds ("things that go bump in the night"), barely audible whispers, hushed warnings, and fleeting glimpses of unseen otherworldly apparitions.

The sense of "spookiness" in a classic ghost story, the creepy feeling that Freud, in 1919, labeled as "uncanny," arises from the self-conscious paranoia of the protagonist, whose surreal sense perceptions lead him towards one of two conclusions, both of them horrifying. Either the things I think I'm seeing and hearing are "unreal," in the sense that they do not exist—hallucinations—or they're real, but "unworldly"—"undead" ghosts. If the former is true, then I've lost my mind.... I'm mad! If the latter is true, then I'm encountering a completely alien, menacing, paranormal presence. This state of paranoid self-doubt, accompanied by a heightened neurotic acuteness of the senses, a fearful perceptual vigilance towards the subliminal, and a questioning of the true nature of reality, is exactly the same psychotic paranoia felt by the schizophrenic.

Indeed the experience of the uncanny could be said to be the defining experience of schizophrenia as first described by Kraeplin and Bleuler—what is known in current psychiatric terminology as "delusional mood," in which the experienced world is bizarrely altered in a way that is hard to define, and appears vaguely sinister and threatening.—McGilchrist.[49]

The "horror" of ghost stories is essentially the same horror of the schizophrenic, who has perceived the "uncanny" in himself, the secret reality that should remain hidden. The feeling of the uncanny is completely related to the doubting of one's own reality, to paranoia, as the mind wrestles with the conflict created by the left hemisphere's rejection of the existence of all irrational experience, and the right hemisphere's unwelcome intrusion into that sterilized domain. To the left hemisphere, anything that can't be held firmly under the microscope of intellectual analysis, anything that is both unclear and un-clarifiable, anything that cannot be reliably and concretely "sensed," is therefore "non-sense," and must be discarded into the "slag-heap of rejected awareness." But what happens when the "slag" emerges out of its "heap" to confront the rejecter with reflections of its own discarded perceptions?

The haunted person is a very modern persona, a victim of their own duality. He or she is stuck in the "no man's land" of dual consciousness. Unable to believe their own eyes and ears, they constantly question their own sanity, balancing that doubt with the paranoid sense and delusional belief that their perceptions are real, which would therefore mean that they are sane, but the entire world, to their own horror, has become glaringly "unreal."

Hyperconscious Self-Reflection and Alienation

> *The world is too much with us; late and soon,*
> *Getting and spending, we lay waste our powers;—*
> *Little we see in Nature that is ours;*
> *We have given our hearts away, a sordid boon!*
>
>   —Wordsworth, "The World Is Too Much with Us" (1807)

The great achievement of oral language is our ability to "utter" our innermost thoughts, so that they may be shared and understood by others. The word "utter" is derived from the Old English word for "out," so an uttering is truly an "outering" of thought.[50] The great achievement of literacy is, by contrast, the "innering" of thought—the internalization of oral language—and the utilization of this function for private verbal thought. This relatively newfound ability of humans to distance themselves cognitively from their environments in order to think about their actions rather than reacting instinctively, is the defining feature of "Homo sapiens sapiens," the very wise ape…

> Oral cultures act and react at the same time. Phonetic culture endows men with the means of repressing their feelings and emotions when engaged in action. To act without reacting, without involvement, is the peculiar advantage of Western literate man.—McLuhan.[51]

The wisdom of humanity is revealed in our interaction with technology, which we use to master the world, but at the cost of becoming so neurologically intertwined with our technology that our thoughts are literally molded by it, often to our own detriment. The modern world of technological innovation arises from a modern species of thinkers that revere the technology of their own secular industry, rather than the magic of unworldly gods. Modern thought is trained via literacy to proceed visually along straight lines of black ink on white paper. This "neutral visual world" produces thinking that aspires to the visual ideal of clarity, thinking that's very fast and efficient, and proceeds along straight and logical lines of thought.[52] The words and thoughts of the schizophrenic seem "bizarre" to us, imbued with "magical thinking" and mystical connections, because the thought patterns are not fettered to the straight tracks of linear thinking. The interrupting thoughts from the largely illiterate right hemisphere are still yoked to oral language, still immersed in the auditory world of mysterious unseen connections and invisible mystical forces, the "magical world of the ear…."

> The interiorization of the technology of the phonetic alphabet translates man from the magical world of the ear to the neutral visual world.—McLuhan[53]

While literate thought provides us with cognitive distance from the world, a "neutral" stance of forced perspective and suspended judgment, it also provides distance from the self, as we reflect upon ourselves from a distanced, objective perspective, separating our intuitive self that exists in the moment, from our abstract sense of self that simultaneously observes, analyzes, criticizes, and otherwise reflects upon its own thoughts, feelings, and behaviors. Cognitive distantiation, the process of creating distance between our world and our interaction with our world, is furthered by the media and technology that created it. The more literate a society becomes, the more literate its people become, and the more distanced they become cognitively from the world, from each other, and from themselves. Modern technology allows us to master our environments, but in mastering them, we become estranged, "alienated," and "disenchanted" with our world, from each other, and from ourselves.[54]

With the automobile, we master the road, but in doing so, we become alienated from the land. No longer strolling upon it in the open air, we speed over it in sealed-off machines. With the tractor, we master the field, and we also become alienated from it. The vital connection between the land that provides food and the humans who live off the land, the connection between Mother Earth and her children, is lost; first when we step off the land and onto the tractor, and then again when we leave behind the tractor and the field for the city and the suburb.

There are a million other examples, all pointing to the same conclusion: that media in particular and technology in general enhance our lives by providing us with mastery of our thoughts and our environments, but mastery in-and-of-itself leads to distantiation from the primary object, whether that object is someone else, our self, or our world. At the current endpoint, our cognitive distance, our technology, and our media have enabled our species to understand and to communicate to everyone exactly how and why our own technology is killing the planet via the emission of greenhouse gases. Yet at the same time, we are so distanced, disconnected, and alienated from ourselves and from each other and from our world that we, as a species, cannot come together to adapt our technology in order to save our planet and ourselves. Like the premise of a dystopian sci-fi story, we've become "servo-mechanisms" to our own machines, enslaved by our own technology, which is killing us.

Inside the splintered mind of the schizophrenic, the same sense of alienation is at play. The schizophrenic, like all modern humans in post-industrialized societies, lives in a world from which he is disconnected…

> Today all the available sources of intuitive life—cultural tradition, the natural world, the body, religion and art—have been so conceptualized, devitalized and "deconstructed" (ironized) by the world of words, mechanic systems and theories constituted by the left hemisphere, that their power to help us see beyond the hermetic world that is has set up has been largely drained from them.—McLuhan[55]

The modern post-literate sense of alienation from the world and from oneself results in a tendency towards "hyperconscious self-reflection,"[56] a maddening neurotic state of mind that is both a cause and result of psychosis.

Most people think of schizophrenia as a disorder as ancient as humanity itself. Furthermore, there's a common presumption, especially from proponents of the psychoanalytic paradigm, that schizophrenia represents "a regression into a more primitive, unself-conscious, emotive realm of the body and the senses."[57] McGilchrist, among others, argues that schizophrenia in its modern form, which is severe and debilitating, is a product of the relatively modern industrial and post-industrial world:

... all the evidence suggests that schizophrenia is a relatively modern disease, quite possibly existent only since the eighteenth century or thereabouts, and that its principal psychopathological features have nothing to do with regression towards irrationality, lack of self-awareness, and a retreat into the infantile realm of emotion and the body, but entail the exact opposites: a sort of misplaced hyper-rationalism, a hyper-reflexive awareness, and a disengagement from emotion and embodied existence.—McGilchrist[58]

To be clear, the premise thus far is that while the genetic predeterminants of schizophrenia are indeed as old as humanity itself—originating in the neurological capacity for oral language and the subsequent potential for cerebral nondominance of verbal thought—the present-day expression of schizophrenia, which is debilitating and severe, is a relatively modern phenomenon; which I argue is a byproduct of literacy on both the individual and societal levels.

Although we can say that the potential for mass literacy began with Gutenberg's first printing press in the 15th century, the implementation of this potential didn't arise until the establishment of free public education in Western societies, beginning in the 17th century but not encompassing all of Western society until the early 20th century, thereby making the effects of mass literacy at the population level unapparent until quite recently, and even then, only in the Western world. So, in terms of a timeline, the argument that the modern form of schizophrenia is a relatively recent phenomenon, arising over the past few centuries, coalesces with the present argument, that schizophrenia is linked with literacy in individuals and mass literacy in societies.

McGilchrist's argument that schizophrenia is "an excessively detached, hyper-rational, reflexively self-aware, disembodied and alienated condition,"[59] presupposes in the schizophrenic a perspective of detached cognitive distance, a condition that stems from literate mindedness. The schizophrenic, according to McGilchrist, suffers from a duality of mind, such that "Phenomena that were previously uncomplicatedly experienced as part of a relatively unified consciousness now become alien."[60] McGilchrist doesn't inculpate literacy specifically in the schizophrenic experience of self-alienation, but rather, points to the general co-opting of conscious thought and perception by the left hemisphere since the ancient Greeks—a process of cognitive evolution in which literacy plays a primary, if not defining, role. Previously, I mentioned that one of the effects of literacy is to objectify thought, by equating heard words with visual objects on the page, that then become conceptual objects in the mind. When the subject of thought reflects upon itself, therefore, we begin to objectify our own minds:

Intuitions, no longer acted on unselfconsciously, no longer "transparent," no longer simply subsumed into action without the necessity of deliberation, became objects of consciousness, brought into the plane of attention, opaque, objectified. Where there had been previously no question of whether the workings of the mind were "mine," since the question would have no meaning—there being no cut off between the mind and the world around, no possibility of standing back from one's own thought processes to ascribe them to oneself or anyone or anything else—there was now a degree of detachment which enabled the question to arise, and led to the intuitive, less explicit, thought processes being objectified as voices (as they are in schizophrenia), viewed as coming from somewhere else ... the tendency in schizophrenia to bring into conscious awareness processes normally left unconscious and intuitive.—McGilchrist[61]

The "hyperconscious self-reflection" McGilchrist refers to is not a product of schizophrenia, it's a product of the objective detached perspective attained by modern humans via literacy. The particular problem in schizophrenia is the lack of hemispheric dominance that results in the confluence of the dual streams of consciousness. Only when the illusory veil of unity is split does the schizophrenic experience aspects of their own dual consciousness as unrecognized objects of thought, which are then scrutinized, analyzed, and deconstructed in the "hyper-self-conscious" style of the literate minded left hemisphere, in a desperate attempt towards self-understanding that, tragically, just causes more and more self-alienation, more and more self-objectification.

To compound the problem, the schizophrenic is not just an alien to himself, he is an alien to others in his society, as his thinking portrays neither the simplistic unity of a preliterate child's nor the complex logicality of the literate adult, but a cognitive mishmash of conflicting and clashing modes of thought, an ongoing train wreck of derailed ideas. Quoting psychologist Louis Sass, McGilchrist suggests that the habits of thought engaged in by philosophers, in which "objective" thought is turned inwardly via "self-conscious" observation, reveals an inner world that is "bizarre, alien, frightening—and curiously similar to the mental world of the schizophrenic...."

Sass explores the idea that "madness ... is the end-point of the trajectory [that] consciousness follows when it separates from the body and the passions, and from the social and practical world, and turns in upon itself." For Sass ... abstraction and alienation ... detachment from body, world and community, can produce a type of seeing and experiencing which is, in a literal sense, pathological.[62]

Sass's term "hyperconsciousness," from his book *Madness and Modernism* (1994), refers to a modern state of mind, a sensibility that I argue is fostered by literacy, and which in some cases, leads to psychopathology. In the case of schizophrenia, hyperconsciousness is only pathological when it's exacerbated by hemispheric nondominance, as the combination of the two conditions merge to create what Chris Firth identified as the "core abnormality" in schizophrenia: "an awareness of automatic processes which are normally carried out below the level of consciousness."[63] In other cases, such as anxiety and depression, hyperconsciousness in-and-of-itself becomes the root of pathology (discussed in the next chapter).

Reading is a hyperconscious process. When reading anything more sophisticated than a grocery list or dinner recipe, anything with "literary depth," the mind of the reader must assume an interpretive stance, in which meaning is extracted from the text, in order to reveal the "subtext." We must "read into things" to understand anything beyond the surface level of the written word. The underlying meaning of the text is revealed not simply by reading the words, but by deconstructing and reading *beyond* the words, revealing broader concepts, ideas, and theories. The schizophrenic, in his hyperconscious state of detachment and objectification, winds up "reading into" his environment, reading into others, and reading into himself, as if he were reading a book. His paranoia is revealed in his constant deconstructionism. He's always reading into things—imagining secret connections where there are none, creating layers of plot and symbolism where there is only simple action and setting, concocting malicious conspiracies where there is only the blank slate of phenomenal experience—reading and interpreting meaning into the simple statements of others, as if they were the dialogue of a dense prose text rather than the speech of real people.

In the paranoia of the schizophrenic, deconstructed reality is dissolved in the acid of hyperconscious analysis. The focus turns from the apparent surface of things, to what could be interpreted as lying hidden beneath the surface, to the symbolic underlying meaning of things. To quote Nietzsche's interpretation of the state of the modern world in his day: "More and more, the symbolic replaces that which exists."[64]

Westernization

> *The print-made split between head and heart is the trauma which affects Europe from Machiavelli till the present.*
>
> —McLuhan[65]

If the condition of cerebral nondominance for verbal thought is in part genetically determined, then it's likely to have existed in the human species since the advent of oral language in the Paleolithic age.

However, the condition itself is not necessarily a disorder. I've argued that schizophrenia as we know it is a product of both the neurological predisposition towards cerebral nondominance, and a media environment that evokes the symptoms of psychosis. In particular, when literacy becomes engrained within the fabric of a society to the point where everybody in the society is forced to become literate, schizophrenia as a disorder is much more likely to arise. Literacy changes the way we think, both as individuals and as a society. Research on the epidemiology of schizophrenia—longitudinally, since such records have been kept, and cross-culturally, across the world—has demonstrated that schizophrenia occurs more in Western countries, that it's more severe in Western countries, and that the rates of diagnosis have been steadily increasing in Western countries over the past two centuries.

> In England schizophrenia was rare indeed, if it existed at all, before the 18th Century, but increased dramatically in prevalence with industrialization. Similar trends can be observed in Ireland, Italy, the United States, and elsewhere. However, even at the end of the 19th Century schizophrenia appears to have been relatively rare compared with the first half of the 20th Century, when it steeply increased…. What is beyond reasonable doubt, however, since it has been established by repeated research over at least half a century, is that schizophrenia increased *pari passu* with industrialization; that the form in which schizophrenia exists is more severe and has a clearly worse outcome in Western countries; and that, as recent research confirms, prevalence by country increases in proportion to the degree that the country is "developed," which in practice means Westernised.—McGilchrist[66]

According to studies by the World Health Organization (WHO), schizophrenics in developing countries experience far less severe symptoms than schizophrenics in developed (Western) countries, with higher rates of recovery, lower rates of relapse, shorter periods of active psychosis, and much better prognoses.[67] Indeed, if the WHO used the contemporary modes of clinical assessment found in the current edition of the *Diagnostic Statistical Manual of Mental Disorders* (DSM-V), then the majority of diagnoses of schizophrenia made in Third World countries would have indicated that the patients were merely on the schizophrenia spectrum, and they would be diagnosed with less chronic and severe disorders, such as schizophreniform disorder or schizotypal personality disorder, rather than full-blown schizophrenia.[68] Assays of African mental health demographics in the mid–20th century found specifically that: "In regard to schizophrenia, delusional systemization in **nonliterate** Africans is relatively lacking, and accordingly, the categories described as paranoia, 'paraphrenic,' and 'paranoid' are seldom seen."[69]

According to Sass, "what the WHO studies suggest … is that the more persistent and ... more prototypical forms of this illness ... may well be more common in the more modern and developed socio-cultural settings ... where the allied forces of modernization, Westernization, and industrialization ... have a significant degree of influence." Furthermore, Sass points out that the WHO study surveyed diagnostic rates in both developed and developing countries, but not in truly *undeveloped* or "primitive" societies, which have rarely been studied at all in reference to modern psychiatric diagnoses. In short, we don't really know if true schizophrenia is common in preliterate societies, because those studies have not been done, and if they were done, they would be difficult to assess, as preliterate individuals tend to have spiritual beliefs and practices that would blur the line between thinking that's sane, rational and logical, and thinking that's insane, irrational, illogical and, in a word, "schizophrenic."

Sass quotes anecdotal evidence from anthropologists such as Sir Andrew Halliday, who noted in 1828, "We seldom meet with insanity among the native savage tribes of men; not one of our African travelers remark having seen a single madman." Similarly, Curt Seligman wrote in a 1929 article that he could find "no evidence of the occurrence of mental derangement" among the preliterate New Guinea highlanders. George Devereux wrote in 1939 that the rarity or absence of schizophrenia among primitive societies is a "point on which all students of comparative society and of anthropology agree," and he noted that schizophrenia does seem to appear quite quickly once a society has become Westernized.

Later empirical studies in New Guinea found that the rates of schizophrenia in the coastal districts—which are much more modern and Westernized than the inland districts—were "five to ten (or even twenty) times higher than in the more isolated highland areas." Similar studies have revealed lower rates of schizophrenia in non–Westernized groups, and also that even in Western societies such as America, schizophrenia is less prevalent in rural areas as opposed to suburbs and cities. Sass concludes that the "most clear-cut cases of schizophrenia—those characterized by the core symptoms of chronicity and social withdrawal, by flat and inappropriate affect, by Schneiderian First Rank Symptoms, and by unusual and abstract styles of thinking—may well be less common in cultural settings where traditional or premodern forms of social organization prevail." Historical evidence (or lack of such evidence), suggests that "schizophrenic illnesses did not even appear, at least in any significant quantity, before the end of the eighteenth century or the beginning of the nineteenth ... just after the most intense period of change toward industrialization in Europe." Sass argues that the cross-cultural and historical evidence combine to indicate that "modern Western civilization does seem to have a statistical association with schizophrenia, or at least with its severely chronic or autistic forms."[70]

Summing up, it seems that the well-known statistic stating the worldwide prevalence of schizophrenia at 1 percent is misleading, as the numbers in third world countries are much lower, and—perhaps more significantly—the form of schizophrenia found in non–Westernized countries is much less severe, much less chronic, and—for lack of a better word—much less *psychotic* than the very severe and chronic form of schizophrenia that we're familiar with in the West. I personally believe that the 1 percent statistic indicates a universal human vulnerability to the disorder, but that the form and course of schizophrenia are molded by the culture and media environment of the individual.

Specifically, in light of the findings above, I'm suggesting a causal relationship between literacy and psychosis, as literacy in Western countries has for centuries been far more entrenched than in developing countries. The long range effects of literacy—industrialization, urbanization, and fragmentation—have triggered changes in Western society that have created a modern environment and culture that further evoke the onset of schizophrenia. Moreover, the modern media environments created by electronic media and digital media have additional evocative effects on the spectrum of schizotypal thought and behavior in the modern world.

Fragmentation, Intellectualization and Alienation

Just as a tree is the product of both the acorn and the soil it grows in, so too is every psychological disorder an offspring of two parents: the genetic clay of its origin, and the nurturing loam of its environment. The genetic origin of schizophrenia, I suggest, is a genetic variation for cerebral dominance of language, expressed as a predisposition towards nondominance. This neurological predisposition, however, is not inherently disordered or flawed. Like an ambidextrous baseball player, the condition of cerebral nondominance could, in the right environment, be quite advantageous, as it would reflect a mind that is well-balanced between the hemispheres, and capable of integrating in the same thought process, both the deep-focused, detail oriented, analytical sensibility of the left hemisphere, and the holistic gestalt perspective of the right hemisphere. The condition of cerebral nondominance only becomes pathological when it exists in an environment that is hostile towards it. The modern world, especially in the West, is an environment that is hostile towards cerebral nondominance, an environment that breeds "an excessively detached, hyper-rational, reflexively self-aware, disembodied and alienated condition."[71]

Engrained literacy, the primary product of schooling, creates a distinctly powerful internal voice of verbal thought. The literate mind takes on the linear and sequential form of the medium of literacy, engaging in private verbal thought that speeds along linear tracks towards highly abstract, decontextualized, theoretical concepts. The dominant left hemisphere detaches itself so far from the phenomenal world of lived reality that it creates its own walled-off "kingdom of mind," separate and disconnected from both the outside world and the inside world of right hemispheric thought. It is at this point of detachment that the duality of mind is created, in which the hemispheres think and operate together, but also separately, with the left hemispheric voice of consciousness functioning with complete obliviousness towards the existence of a second sense of consciousness in the opposite hemisphere.

It's my argument that the preliterate mind is not nearly as dualistic as the literate mind, because the voice of consciousness in the preliterate mind is less detached, less abstract, less disconnected from both the natural environment, and from the input of the right hemisphere. Schizophrenia expresses itself more severely in the literate mind, not only because literacy amplifies the volume of the conscious "voice" inside our heads, but because only in the literate mind is consciousness so severely separated and split into the opposing hemispheres as to create dual consciousness. Schizophrenia, the split-mind, can only exist in a mind in which the cognitive split between the hemispheres is so great that the disinhibited revelation of one hemisphere's thoughts and words by the opposing hemisphere is experienced as a completely alien and foreign intruder. Only in a mind of dual consciousness can a person become a "stranger to himself."

Intellectualization, the brainchild of mass literacy, is born out of the scientific, skeptical, reason-based perspective of academia. In applying the scientific method to our environment, intellectual humans mastered their environment to levels of technical wizardry that go well beyond the dreams of our preliterate ancestors. Nevertheless, the same hyper-intellectual mindset that gave us computers and satellites forces us to examine and comprehend every aspect of our world within the same skeptical reason-based mindset. Concepts that have no scientific basis, ideas that have no foundation in rational thought, beliefs that cannot be proven to exist via physical measurements or intellectual calculation, are exiled and abandoned by the intellectual mind. In doing so, the Western world increasingly becomes a "disenchanted" land, bereft of gods and goddesses, spiritless, soulless, alive but unanimated, existent yet hollow of meaning.

The disenchanted world is particularly perilous to the mind that's opened to dual consciousness. Prior to Weber's "disenchantment," spiritual experiences were normative and generally positive. Ghosts were merely the disembodied spirits of our dearly departed friends and loved ones, paying us a visit, or comforting us in times of need. Angels were God's messengers, reminding us of His presence and involvement on the earthly plane. Even a demon, when properly understood and correctly exorcised, was just another member of the natural spiritual order. But in a disenchanted world, the uninhibited intrusions of right hemispheric input, rather than being understood as "normal" experiences of the ever-present spiritual dimension, become terrifying apparitions and disturbing voices arising from "nowhere," as the disenchanted world has no place for the spiritual. While small children, whose preliterate minds are not yet formatted to logicality, and whose minds are not yet expected to be rational, are allowed to indulge in these "strange openings," adults are not. As Aldous Huxley lamented:

> Strange openings and theophanies are granted to quite small children, who are often profoundly and permanently affected by these experiences. We have no reason to suppose that what happens now to persons with small vocabularies did not happen in remote antiquity, in the modern world ... the child tends to grow out of his direct awareness of the one Ground of things; for the habit of analytical thought is fatal to the intuitions of integral thinking, whether on the "psychic" or the spiritual level.[72]

The modern adult schizophrenic, living in a post-literate intellectual society, is put in a "double bind"[73] situation: to either doubt his own sanity, or to doubt the nature of his reality. Both responses, it turns out, result in behaviors that are diagnostically psychotic.

The modern world promotes a fragmentary rather than cohesive mode of existence, resulting in the individual's sense of alienation from his community, family, home, and other sources of stable identity-building cohesion. This results ultimately in a sense of alienation from oneself, which, for somebody with a schizophrenic disposition, is quite treacherous. There is incontrovertible evidence that rates of schizophrenia are directly and positively related to urbanization, with a conservative estimate of causation calculated as a factor of two.[74]: A person living in or close to a city is at least *twice* as likely to become schizophrenic as a person living in the country. On the broadest level, city life is very much disconnected from nature. Rather than living within nature, city dwellers are often cut off from much of nature. They're always inside—but even when outside, they're always surrounded by buildings, immersed in unnatural electric light—with nature as an impediment to the actions of life, rather than the vessel for all living beings.

Alienation from nature is in a very real sense alienation from oneself, as humans are natural beings. If, as most people believe, there's an aspect of humanity that yearns to be connected with nature, like a baby yearns for connection with its mother, then that aspect is fragmented in urban life. *An indoor life is disconnected from both the outer world and the inner self.* Though this sense of alienation from nature affects nearly everyone in industrial and post-industrial societies, the effects are most devastating on the schizophrenic, whose sense of alienation from reality, and whose fragmented sense of conscious self, are already dangerously intense.

The heightened mobility of industrial and post-industrial societies cause fragmentation. In agricultural societies, people tend to grow up in small farming communities and stay in those communities their whole lives. Many people live in the same farmhouse with their extended families for their entire lives, while some marry off, only to join a nearby family, and live in that nearby farmhouse for the rest of their lives. This multigenerational connection to family, to home, to community, to church, to nation, and to the land, all served to ground people in deep, meaningful interpersonal connections with other people, with specific places, and to specific institutions.

The mobilization offered by the planes, trains, and automobiles of modern society, coupled with the freedom of vocation attained via higher education, has created a species of mobile people who are free to pick up and move anywhere, whenever they want to. Though this rootlessness frees the individual from the smothering ties that bind, it also excises the individual of a sense of rootedness or belongingness to any one place. Deep meaningful connections with people and places are lost, replaced by sterile, anonymous, interchangeable apartment complexes that offer convenient lodgings but no sense of "home," with meaningful interpersonal connections replaced by vacant superficial posts on social media, and limitless Facebook "friends" who offer no real connection to anyone.

The freedom of mobility is a curse to the person who needs grounding and a sense of belonging and connection in order to feel stable and secure within his own identity, in order to feel "whole" or unified inside. Portable, mobile individuals risk cutting the ties that bind them not only to others and to home, but to their own unified sense of personal identity. The mobile stranger in a strange land is likely to become estranged from himself.

Though there are many at factors at play, it's plausible that the timing of schizophrenia onset, in late adolescence and early adulthood, is significant not just because it coincides with the maturation of brain development, the synaptic "pruning" of neurological connections, and the consolidation of the affects of literacy on conscious thought—but also because this is a time when many young people in modern society leave home for the first time—in order to study at a faraway college or to embark on a new career path, off alone in perhaps the bright lights of the big city. For many young people, the overpowering sense of social isolation that they experience for the first time when they're disconnected from family, friends, and home, that sense of solitude and alienation experienced in the "lonely crowd" of the university campus or the cold hard city, can result in the stark sense of alienation and disconnection from the self experienced by schizophrenics.

Career is a cornerstone of personal identity. For the vast majority of human history, people didn't get to choose what work they did. In prehistoric times, everyone was a hunter or gatherer. Following the Agricultural Revolution, nearly everyone was a farmer or rancher. As civilization progressed, however, opportunities for specialization in alternate careers arose. People became blacksmiths, carpenters, butchers, bakers, etc. Following the Industrial Revolution and the breakdown of agricultural society in the West, public education opened up new fields of work to entire populations whose parents may have been uneducated factory workers, and whose ancestors had been farmers for many generations.

Careers in the modern world are highly specialized, requiring many years of specialized education. It should be noted, however, that the foundation stone of education—literacy—is a trained "specialist" skill in-and-of-itself.[75] It takes many years to learn literacy. Though a variety of subjects are taught in school, the medium for that content is invariably literacy, so while the interchangeable school subjects—history, science, social science, etc.—comprise the *content* of learning, the *medium* for learning remains constant: Literacy. McLuhan's adage, "the medium is the message," applies here more than anywhere, for the most drastic effects that education has on the brain are not achieved through educational content, but through the continuous and constant focus on the specialized medium of education, the proverbial "three R's" of education: reading, 'riting, and 'rithmetic. In other words, Literacy. (Mathematics, as will be discussed in greater depth in later chapters, is merely another form of literacy, in which the phonetic alphabetic code is replaced with a logico-mathematic code of numerals and logical operations.)

My point, long in the making, is that work in the modern world has become extremely specialized, and the prerequisite for work, i.e., education, has also become elongated and, at its tail end, highly specialized. If we understand specialization as yet another aspect of fragmentation, we could discern yet another way in which modern society has become more fragmenting—more "schizophrenogenic"—more likely to evoke schizophrenia.

Consider the lot of pre-industrial farmers, working on the old traditional family farm. They work the land that their parents worked, and their parents' parents before them, going back countless generations. They share the work—husband and wife, brothers and sisters, daughters and sons, uncles, aunts and cousins—all working together. With the fruit of their labors and the sweat of their brows, they feed and sustain the entire family, and community as well. The farmer reaps the same grain he sowed, grinds the grain into flour, and sees it baked into his daily bread. Everything that needs to be done is done by him and his family. One day the farmer plows behind the mule, the next day he's a painter painting the barn, the next day he's a shearer of sheep, the following day mending a fence, and so on. The family farmers are nonspecialists, which strengthens their personal connections to every aspect of farm life, to every part of the farm itself, and to every animal and family member living on the farm with them.

Compare this farmer to the modern office worker. He or she sits all day staring at a screen, watching letters and digits go by. If they share their work with others, they're still virtual strangers, many of them only existing in the virtual netherland of digital and telephonic communication. Neither the workers nor their coworkers claim ownership or any personal relation to their common enterprise. If necessary, they could empty their desk into a single box and find the exact same job somewhere else. They own nothing that they work on, and have no familial or personal connection to their labor. They do the same thing every day, their skills specialized so explicitly to their specific task that they could hardly do anything else.

Though the office workers support themselves and their family, the many transmutations by which their work in the office translates into digital numbers added automatically to their bank account, are largely unknown to them. They feed themselves and their family with processed food made many miles away by strangers, paying for it with electronic digits drawn invisibly from a plastic card. Is there any sense of meaningful identity and personal connection that these Kafkaesque workers gain from their career? Their skills and his deeds are so fragmented and disassociated from nature and from themselves, that a psychotic sense of self-doubt and alienation would be altogether expected of someone in their schizophrenogenic situation.

Fragmentation, Electronification and Digitization

For the past million years, at each stage of communication evolution, our media have become more fragmented. When mimetic communication and toolmaking evolved as crucial adaptations in humans more than a million years ago, the need to establish cerebral dominance emerged. A gene (or genes) moderating the trait for cerebral dominance for either hemisphere along a spectrum of expression, included a variation of expression resulting in cerebral nondominance. So, while we could presume that, according to the current theory, there were Stone Age humans who did not have a dominant cerebral hemisphere for handedness and mimetic communication, we should not presume that these ancient humans were schizophrenic. The environment they lived in—more specifically, the *media* environment they lived in—would not have evoked schizophrenic symptoms. It goes without saying that a creature who has no language cannot hear voices or form delusions to rationalize those voices, nor can they speak in loose associations, and so forth. If schizophrenia is a disorder of language and verbal thought, it can only exist in post-lingual humans. "Psychosis has never been observed outside of our own species."[76]

Mimesis, as a form of communication, is contextual. The person communicating is usually within the same context of what they're expressing, such as when I point to an animal, or mimetically demonstrate how to make a fire. The person communicating is also in the same context as the person they're communicating with, making it a very personal form of communication. A person must be right there in front of you to express something mimetically. Finally, the signs used in mimesis are direct analogical representations of what's being expressed. A mimetic sign for "apple" directly represents an apple, without any further levels of symbolization or encoding taking place between the person expressing the sign, and the person receiving it. The sign for apple is therefore a "whole" message. It isn't fragmented or broken down in any way. Mimesis is a fairly concrete, nonabstract means of communication.

Oral language, on the other hand, is largely noncontextual, as a word could be used to refer to something completely abstract, to something that may have existed in the past or may exist in the future, or to something that couldn't exist. Though abstract, oral language is intensely personal, as a person must speak to you face-to-face (or within earshot), and there's a large degree of personal emotion and identity expressed in the voice while speaking. Furthermore, much is expressed nonverbally in an oral language exchange, via gestures, facial expressions, tone of voice, etc. Oral language subsumes mimesis as a vital part of its means of expression. Also, like mimetic signs, spoken words are direct analogical representations. The spoken word "apple," heard by the listener, is understood as the object "apple" without any further symbolization or encoding. Spoken words are whole, un-fragmented messages.

Compared to previous media, literacy is remarkably noncontextual, as the abstract written word could refer to anything at any time in any place, while the writer need not even be around for their writing to be expressed—the writer may even be dead—making literacy a relatively depersonalized medium. Written words are not direct analogical representations. When reading or writing a word, we take the sound of the word, break it down to its smallest auditory components (phonemes), and using the code of the phonetic alphabet, create a re-representation of the sound of the word using visual symbols (letters). Literacy, as a medium, is much more fragmented than previous media, as the process of literacy deconstructs the analog of the spoken word, fragments it into its most basic phonetic elements, and then reassembles it using a visual code.

Print standardized the medium of literacy. Because printed material is much cheaper and made much faster than handwritten manuscripts, the print medium is even more decontextualized, as inexpensive books, pamphlets, leaflets, and newspapers can travel around the world, and are relatively unconstrained by the limits of time and space. Compared to the spoken word, or even the handwritten letter or script, typographic print is quite impersonal, as the standardization of the printed letters and the mechanization of the printing process strip the personal element from the message. Just as a Hallmark birthday card is far less personal than a handmade card, print literature is far less personal than handwritten scriptures. In the print medium, there's no trace of any personal physical interaction between the writer and the reader.

There's also another level of representation and fragmentation added on in the print process, as the written word of the author must be broken down by the printer into typographic blocks, standardizing the appearance of the author's written words, both in appearance, and also in grammar, spelling, word choice, and any other editorial revisions seen fit by the publisher or printer. The print medium has also increased the volume of literary material made available to the reading public. As the first mass medium, print democratized literacy, creating the mass public—entire societies of literate people—which in turn created even more literate societies, as well as societies that are highly engaged in the exceedingly intellectual, abstract, and fragmented endeavors of reading and writing literary material. At this point, at around the 18th century, when free public education began to create entire populations of literate people in Western society, we see the emergence of schizophrenia in the historical literature.

Electronic media decontextualize and fragment the message even more. Films of deserts and jungles are experienced by viewers in dark windowless theaters. Silent films, a new mass medium in the early 20th century, presented characters that looked real but lacked voices. These unvoiced personas must have resonated in the minds of schizophrenics, as they too often feel "unvoiced," as if the words of their verbal thoughts were stolen by some malicious force, directly from their minds. Radios and telephones project disembodied voices that could also feed delusions about thought transmission and interception, as well as self-doubt about hearing voices.

It was a popular belief for much of the 20th century that silver fillings in teeth could act as antennae for radio broadcasts, resulting in the sound of external voices or music being heard in one's head. Many people reported experiencing this phenomenon. In fact, though it's technically possible for this to happen, it's so exceedingly *unlikely* that its actual real world occurrence would be extremely rare. So most of the people who reported this experience were probably delusional—not at the level of full-blown psychosis, but at a much broader level of the schizotypal spectrum, a level where hallucinations occur at a more subliminal level. Proof of the delusional basis of these reports also stems from the unusual nature of the experiences themselves. For instance, typical reports claimed that the listener heard either constant music or constant voices, but never any advertisements, station identification announcements, static, weather reports, or any of the other standard content of radio broadcasts. It seems that the mere suggestion that a wireless electronic signal could be picked up by a tooth filling resulted in mass auditory hallucinations. Psychosis, in the modern electronic world, lurks very close beneath the surface of everyday life.

The invisible, omnipresent, pervasive machinations of electronic media seem to supply some of the core delusional language of schizophrenia: "mind control," "thought broadcasting," "satellite tracking," "global conspiracy," "mind hacking," "thought transmission," etc. The chicken-or-the-egg question of origin is raised here: Does electronic media reflect certain qualities of psychosis, or is psychosis—in some way or in some part—evoked by electronic media? For instance, nobody—schizophrenic or otherwise—ever claimed that their private verbal thoughts were being broadcast, transmitted, or intercepted, before radio and telephones were invented. Prior to electronic media, schizophrenic delusions regarding hallucinations and thought interference typically had parapsychological, magical, or spiritual bases. The schizophrenics believed that the voices were coming from angels or God, or that their minds were being read telepathically by a witch or magician, or a sorcerer or mesmerist was inserting thoughts into their heads.

The 20th and 21st century versions of these hallucinations and delusions, based on the technology of electronic media, have not only a more modern sound but a more sinister tone. Since radio and telephone function at the macro-system level of society, the origin of the mind control technology being directed at the individual would clearly be either the government, or some powerful corporate entity, giving psychotic paranoia its peculiar conspiratorial tone. The fact that the modern world is, in fact, packed to the brim with electronic signals and messages being broadcast across the globe, passing through our bodies and brains constantly, is a notion that could evoke paranoia in anyone.

Paranoia in-and-of-itself owes much to the modern technology of electronic media. Prior to electronic media, any suspicion that one is being watched or monitored by malicious forces would have to based on the sensed presence of actual physical observers, or on the sensed presence of magical or spiritual observers. In the modern world, however, video and audio surveillance is ubiquitous. Satellites can track and observe our movements anywhere and everywhere on the planet. Even as I write this sentence, I can't be 100 percent certain that some nefarious institution isn't surreptitiously using the video camera and microphone on my laptop to spy on me. Or they may be using the internet connection on my laptop to furtively transmit my written thoughts.

The NSA and Verizon and Facebook and other omniscient government agencies and global corporations track, trace, and store our phone calls, posts, and text messages. Ad companies and media corporations monitor our internet clicks and viewing habits for targeted advertisement. Ratings agencies gauge our media preferences in order to predict and suggest what we may want to view. Hackers hack into our personal emails and computer files.

Given all of this monitoring, surveillance, and theft of personal information and identity, even the most trusting individual must give pause to how every data point reflecting our personal thoughts and behaviors is gathered and measured by unseen observers. If paranoia didn't exist before the electronic and digital ages, it would certainly have been created by them. And though schizophrenia predates electronic and digital media, it's very clear that one of the primary symptoms of the disorder—paranoia—has been given its distinct flavor and its extreme posture by the advents of new media that have the sinister power to peer deeply into the most hidden recesses of our personal lives. If the computing device is an extension of our mind, an extension of private thought, then the walls of the "kingdom of mind" that once guarded our sacredly private and personal sense of identities, have been breached. In a world where privacy as a concept is rapidly becoming obsolete, it's a wonder we're not all paranoid schizophrenics.

The 20th century introduced the world to notions of disembodiment and alienation that simply did not exist before. The disembodied voices of singers in the opera house were heard by listeners via radio or the phonograph in the privacy of their own living rooms. The everyday life of the sitcom family was viewed everyday by real families on TV, though the sitcom family—a collection of unrelated actors on some Hollywood soundstage reciting lines written by television writers—is in no way connected to the actual families they pretend to portray. The technology of electronic media seems to accelerate the process of fragmenting and decontextualizing the content they transmit. Yet, in other ways, electronic media are more personal and less fragmented than previous media.

The voice on the telephone, though disembodied, is still more personal than a letter (especially a printed letter). The phone call is also more contextual, as it happens in real time, with both speaker and listener mutually interacting in the same moment. Though the method of transmission itself is more fragmentary—telegraphic and telephonic messages are broken down into electronic signals, as are radio and TV broadcasts, while film breaks down live action into 24 separate photographic frames per second—the actual content expressed via electronic media appear to the user as much more personal and animated than print content. An actor in a film or TV show, though decontextualized, appears to his audience as a whole person, speaking words that could be directly heard, making movements and mimetic gestures that could be directly seen, and expressing emotion that could be directly appreciated by the audience, despite the fact that the actual images and sounds are merely ethereal projections of descrambled electronic signals.

Most radio and some TV is broadcast in real time, so that the performers and their audience share in the same moment of expression. There are many forms of electronic media that have many different effects on society and the minds within it. Some electronic media heighten the sense of depersonalization and fragmentation experienced by people, while others decrease those senses. This issue is picked up again throughout this book.

The Digital Stranger

Forever I shall be a stranger to myself.

—Albert Camus (1942)

On the surface, digital media are clearly the most fragmenting of all media. Digital media, by definition, function by "digitalizing" the content being sent, deconstructing every expression into a series of binary digits, 0 or 1. Binary digital code is the most fragmentary code possible, reducing content to the most elemental fragments of information, with 0 and 1 representing positive or negative, just as a nod or a shake of the head, representing "yes" or "no," represent the most elemental form of human communication. Nevertheless, the effect of digital media, quite ironically, is often one of defragmentation, or more simply, one of integration. FaceTime on an iPhone is face-to-face real time communication with both spoken words and facial gestures.

FaceTime, as well as Skype and Zoom and all other video-telephonic media, provide an integrated communication experience that is much more personal, contextualized, and direct than a phone call or even a handwritten letter. Nevertheless, the ease of use and instantaneity of digital media, rather than having an integrative effect on society, seems to create more fragmentation.

Though FaceTime and Skype exist, most people prefer to text or email most of their messages, opting for the quicker, easier, faceless, voiceless, far less personal media. While social media sites such as Twitter and Facebook offer instant multimedia communication with countless users, the laser-fast pace of digital media and the overabundance of digital media content circumscribe the use of social media messages into brief trite statements that could be "liked" or "disliked," "shared" or "posted" within an instant of being seen. Real communication, which is often complicated and time-consuming, is not only impeded by digital media, it's functionally obsolesced.

Though I know I cannot express my complete thoughts on a subject via a text, Instagram, Facebook post, or tweet, I also know that nobody in this digitalized world of instant everything has the time, patience, or inclination to sit down and discuss the topic fully, so the topic goes undiscussed. In depth editorials have given way to the 10 second sound byte. Even the current president addresses the nation in 140 character tweets, compressing national policy into cryptic tweeted outbursts that create more confusion than understanding. Intellectual conversations have devolved into the aphoristic post or retweet. Visits to and from grandma have been replaced with photo posts on Facebook. Even the semi-communal act of the family gathering around the television to watch a pretend family interact, has fragmented into each member of the family sitting separately, engaged in their own separate media ... isolated together in the same house.

Though it may be too early to determine its effect on schizophrenia, I would argue that the fragmented, depersonalized, alienating aspects of society that certainly do have an effect on the levels of schizotypy experienced within it, are being amplified by the digitization of media in the modern world. Despite the claims that digital media in general and social media in particular are designed to connect people and make them feel closer, all of the evidence seems to indicate the opposite: that digital media, in all its forms, increases our tendencies towards social isolation, heightens our sense of alienation within our environments, depersonalizes our interactions with others, and has an overall effect of increased fragmentation on our identities.[77] The fragmented culture created by post-industrial digital society projects the objective mechanistic viewpoint of the left hemisphere outwardly, fashioning a society and a landscape that is entirely unnatural and even destructive to nature, as well as alienating to the individual.

In *Madness and Modernism,* Louis Sass argued that the schizophrenic experiences "an 'unworlding' of the world: a loss of the sense of the overarching context that gives coherence to the world, which becomes fragmented and lacking in meaning."[78] According to Sass, schizophrenia isn't just a condition of many people in the modern world, it's a condition of the modern world itself. Since the stone ages, media of communication necessarily fragmented our expressions in order for the messages to be communicated and accessible. As our ability to communicate has increased, the fragmentation of the communication process has increased in tandem, right through to the modern digital age, in which fragmentation seems to have reached its logical endpoint. The modern world of digital media provides us with a mirror that reflects our limitless expressions of ideas, images, and identity. But with infinite vastness and instantaneous speed, we lose the warm feel of personal contact, the secure rootedness of context, and the wholeness of complete expression.

There's a cinematic trope of an actor, after committing an unconscionable crime, pausing to gaze at his reflection in the mirror. He lingers for a moment, as if he doesn't recognize the man in the reflection, and then he does, and he realizes that he doesn't know himself. He smashes the mirror, as if to destroy the man reflected within it, but in doing so, he creates a crack in the glass, resulting in the optical illusion of a split man in the mirror. The inner duality has been "outered" and split. He has become a stranger to himself.

• FIVE •

Anxious Depression

THE CONSEQUENCES OF CONSCIOUSNESS

The growing consciousness is a danger and a disease.
        —Friedrich Nietzsche (*The Gay Science,* 1862)

I swear to you gentlemen, that to be overly conscious is a sickness, a real, thorough sickness.
        —Fyodor Dostoevsky (*Notes from Underground,* 1864)

Under the categories of "mood disorders" and "anxiety disorders," the DSM-V lists three primary types: Depressive Disorders, Anxiety Disorders, and Bipolar Disorders. "Major Depressive Disorder" (MDD) is the primary DSM diagnostic category for depression, marked by the experience of "depressive episodes." There are some sub-categories of depression, such as "dysthymia," a less severe but more chronic form of depression, and a new addition to the club, "premenstrual dysphoric disorder"; but for the most part, when people refer to "clinical depression," they're referring to MDD, a malady that will affect over 18 percent of American adults, with similar prevalence rates seen throughout the Western world.[1]

The DSM category of anxiety disorders currently has several sub-categories, such as "Separation Anxiety Disorder" and "Social Anxiety Disorder," as well as other disorders that are marked by anxious symptoms, but are so common that they've become entitled to their own categories, such as "Obsessive Compulsive Disorder" and "Posttraumatic Stress Disorder." Nevertheless, just as MDD is the primary diagnostic category for depression, "Generalized Anxiety Disorder" is considered the primary diagnostic category for anxiety. This disorder is marked by the experience of intense anxiety that's relatively chronic and not limited to just one type of stressor, such as school, public speaking, or various specific fears or "phobias." The symptoms of the disorder are often referred to rather whimsically as "free-floating anxiety," though those who suffer from GAD would certainly not describe their own anxiousness with the fanciful terms "free" and "floating." Anxiety disorders are "the most common mental disorders" in America. Nearly a third of all Americans will experience clinical levels of anxiety in their lifetimes, and more than 6 percent of all Americans will experience the symptoms of GAD.[2]

Bipolar Disorder is a mood disorder marked by the alternating experience of both depressive and manic episodes. If mood is visualized on a spectrum with mania at the high end pole of the mood spectrum and depression at the low end pole, then Unipolar Disorder represents being stuck at just one pole, and Bipolar Disorder represents an alternating cycle of mood that goes to the extreme of each pole. The terminology here seems somewhat pointless, because there's no such thing as a person who is always manic, as the human brain and body simply cannot function at that level of hyperactivity indefinitely. Hence, unipolar disorder is just another term for depression. (The term "Unipolar," in this light, makes little sense and has no real purpose, as it was only invented as a taxonomical counterpart to Bipolar.) There are a couple of sub-categories of bipolar, such as "Cyclothymic Disorder," a less severe but more chronic form of bipolar, and "Bipolar II Disorder," in which the sufferer experiences major depressive episodes and "hypomanic" episodes (less severe mania than in regular bipolar).

In any case, the primary diagnostic category for bipolar disorders is regular Bipolar, officially referred to as "Bipolar I Disorder." Prior to 1980, the disorder was referred to as "Manic Depression," which I feel is a better term, as it adequately describes the experience of the disorder as an alternating rotation between mania and depression. The DSM-III, however, changed the name in 1980, in order to avoid the stigma that had become attached to the name "manic depression," and also to apply a more clinical, scientific title to the disorder. The psychiatric industry often changes the names of disorders for the reasons listed above, but I suspect that the industry itself and the readers of its literary product, the DSM, have fallen under the spell of the "nominalist fallacy," the false belief that providing a newer or more specific name for a phenomenon denotes a better understanding of it. This fallacious reasoning is why a layperson interested in the disorder at hand will need to consult a dictionary if they want to know what "Bipolar" and "Unipolar" are, while the older terms, "Manic Depression" and "Depression," were self-explanatory.

This chapter introduces my construct of "Anxious Depression," pairing generalized anxiety and major depression, conceptualizing both conditions as two sides of the same coin—the coin at hand being the consequences of consciousness—or more specifically, too much consciousness, otherwise referred to as "hyper-reflective consciousness," or more simply, "hyperconsciousness." By framing anxiety and depression as differing symptoms of the same underlying problem, I answer the relatively old and extremely important question, "Why do anxiety and depression typically co-occur?" It's well known that MDD and GAD are so commonly co-morbidly diagnosed that psychiatrists and therapists generally assume that if their patient has one disorder, they also have the other.[3] It doesn't help that the typical modern treatment for both disorders—SSRI drugs—is the same, which means that when psychopharmacological treatment is effective (or when its placebo effect is effective), it seems to be addressing the root cause of both anxiety and depression. Another "coincidence" is the fact that women are twice as likely as men to be diagnosed with both depression and anxiety.[4]

So, if two disorders almost always co-occur, if they have similar onsets (adolescence/early adulthood), similar treatment models, similar epidemiological patterns, and largely overlapping symptoms, then why are they considered different disorders, rather than differing symptom patterns of the same disorder? The answer, I believe, is that anxiety and depression feel so different that we intuitively assume that they must be different phenomena altogether. However, we also know that sometimes the symptoms of a disorder can be expressed in ways that are so different, that they seem completely opposite, yet upon close observation, we see that all of the symptoms are actually the expression of the same underlying condition.

Bipolar disorder (referred to throughout the remainder of this chapter with the antiquated but more descriptive term "manic depression") provides the perfect example. Mania and depression seem like opposite moods, but when we see that these mood episodes alternate in such a way that one mood episode not only precedes the other, but actually precipitates it, then we understand that mania and depression are two sides of the same coin, and are caused by the same underlying pathology. My argument in this chapter is that anxiety and depression are, indeed, two sides of the same coin, much like mania and depression. However, whereas the "coin" in question for manic depression is mood, the "coin" for anxious depression is conscious thought.

Before proceeding, it's crucial to remember that mental disorders are complex phenomena with many interacting factors. There is the emotional element to mental disorder, which affects our mood, our feelings, our emotional reaction, and so forth. There's also the physiological element to mental disorder—how our bodies experience and express the disorder—observed in symptoms such as lethargy, nausea, headaches, etc. There's the biological element: the genes, organs, neuro-transmitters, neurological connections, and other biological factors involved. And finally, there's the cognitive element to mental disorder—what we think about and how we think about it. Mental disorders are so complicated because every one results from and is an expression of a combination of all of these elements, with each element being infinitely complex in-and-of-itself, and with each of these infinitely complex elements interacting with the others to make the conditions even more complicated and difficult to figure out.

As I have neither the ability nor the inclination to explain mental disorders in the light of all of these elements and factors, I have limited my explanations to the cognitive dimension, as my focus in this book is the way that media shape and influence thought. As for the disorders referred to thus far in this chapter, both anxiety and depression are discussed at length, but only in reference to their cognitive symptoms, and primarily in reference to my argument that anxiety and depression are essentially two different patterns of thought disorder, both arising from a similar state of hyperconsciousness. As for manic depression, while I believe that the cognitive symptoms associated with bipolar depressive mood episodes are similar to the cognitive symptoms of regular depression, I also believe that the disorder as a whole is precipitated by the neurological dysregulation of emotional mood and physical activity, which is almost certainly caused by biological factors, or more precisely, neurological factors deep within the brain. Hence, manic depression itself will not be discussed in this chapter, other than my use of manic depression as an analogy for my construct of anxious depression.

The Pendulum Metaphor

Consider the simple movement of a pendulum as it swings from side to side. When the ball is pulled towards the left side, it will move leftwards, but when the leftward force ceases, the ball not only swings back to the center, it's driven by the momentum of its own swing towards the right side of the pendulum. Once the rightward momentum ceases, the ball swings back towards the left, and then back to the right, and so on. Once set in motion—regardless of the direction—the ball of the pendulum will continue to swing from side to side until it runs out of momentum. Now, imagine for a moment that your stream of consciousness is like the ball on the pendulum. A leftward swing, now, represents a cognitive movement of conscious thought towards the left hemisphere. If the brain of the imaginary person in this metaphor is one in which consciousness is not strongly skewed towards either hemisphere, that means that consciousness in this person will tend to be pulled towards the middle, like the ball on the pendulum, which is always being pulled by gravity down to the middle. However, just as the ball on the pendulum, when pulled leftward and then released, will swing past the middle and, driven by its own momentum, swing towards the right—consciousness, in this metaphor, will likewise swing leftwards when drawn to the left—and it will then swing rightwards, past the middle, driven by its own momentum. I don't want to overuse or extend this very simple metaphor too far, but I do believe that at a very simplistic level, the metaphor provides an apt model for my construct of "anxious depression." To clarify, I'll re-employ the analogy between anxious depression and manic depression.

Manic depression is a condition in which one's emotional mood swings back and forth between the two poles of manic episodes and depressive episodes. While depressive episodes are relatively normative—everyone gets depressed now and again—manic episodes are relatively abnormal. Hence, it would make sense to assume that something out of the ordinary in the brain of the manic depressive pulls that person's mood aberrantly towards the extreme of mania. The experience of mania, however, is extremely fatiguing. Euphoric mood, hyperactivity, racing thoughts and other manic symptoms drain the body and brain of energy, making manic episodes temporary affairs. But what happens when the manic individual is inevitably drained of his manic energy? The end of a manic episode brings with it feelings of physical exhaustion and mental fatigue, feelings of sadness and disappointment that the excitement has ended, feelings of shame or regret for misdeeds done during the manic flight, feelings of hopelessness and helplessness in regards to controlling one's own mood, feelings of worthlessness and inferiority that arise from the knowledge of one's own mental abnormalities...

In short, the extreme high of the manic episode and the problematic behaviors that accompany it, set the stage for a physiological and emotional crash. When the mania ends, the manic depressive's mood goes into freefall, a rapid mood swing that descends past normality and continues to swing—propelled by its own downward momentum—down to the abysmal lows of depression; just like the ball on the pendulum, once the force driving it to one side is spent, will swing back in the other direction, past the middle and all the way to the other side. Thus, in this model, depression in manic depression is not so much a product of something causing depressiveness in the brain but the mood hangover that naturally follows a manic bender. Just as everything that goes up must come down, every episode of mania must eventually descend, typically in the form of a crash, all the way down to the depths of depression.

The mood swings of manic depression, in which mania precipitates depression, are similar in theory to the cognitive swings in my construct of "anxious depression," in which anxious thoughts precipitate depressive thoughts. The general idea is that anxious thoughts are evoked by a sense of uncertainty regarding the future. In my model, anxious thinking is marked by consciousness lateralized in the left hemisphere of the brain. (The reasons why anxiety is left hemispheric and depression right hemispheric are explained below.) Because the left hemisphere tends to "perseverate" (to remain fixatedly focused on a stimulus for extended periods of time), the person engaged in perseverative anxious thought will eventually become mentally and physically exhausted, because the deep focus required of this kind of thought tires the brain, and the physiological arousal caused by the stress and fear evoked by these thoughts are physically draining. Mental and physical exhaustion precipitate a cognitive crash, in which consciousness swings from left to right hemisphere, and the thoughts switch from anxious presentiments about the future to depressing ruminations about the immediate or distant past.

It's been said that anxiety is a future-oriented emotional experience, while depression is past-oriented. I agree with most of that statement. Anxiety, certainly, is future-oriented: worrying and stressing about the unknown and unpredictable things that may come to pass. Depression can be past-oriented, but it depends on how you conceptualize the past and the present. Since depression can be related to a feeling of disappointment with oneself or one's situation in the present, we could say that depression is also a present-oriented emotion. However, since the present does not exist per se at any given moment, every reflection on the present becomes a reflection on the immediate past. Despite these splitting of semantic hairs, I think we may safely say that both anxiety and depression represent ways of thinking that aren't focused simply on the present moment or on the present space but somewhat abstractly on potential future fallings or on recalled past failures.

More significantly, both anxiety and depression are born of verbal thought and self-consciousness—the hyperconscious rumination on one's own thoughts that encapsulates both our fears of a possible future that will make us feel bad, and our thoughts of regret and despair regarding our immediate or distant past, that make us feel sad. As discussed in Chapter Two, if we did not have private verbal thought, we could not mentally maintain an abstract ongoing personal narrative of our own lives, which stretches back into our remembered and reconstructed past, and stretches forward into an imagined, and often dreaded, hypothetical future. Thus, we may say that both anxious and depressive thoughts would be impossible to experience without the medium of verbal thought—consciousness. If this is so, then by extension, we can say that the hyper-implementation of verbal thought—hyperconsciousness—will result in increased anxious and depressive thought, what I've named: "anxious depression."

Who's likely to suffer from anxious depression?

Consider the shape of a standard population distribution, otherwise referred to as a "bell-shaped curve" or a "spectrum." In the standard distribution, the curve rises steeply upwards in the middle, indicating that the vast majority of the population falls within a couple of standard deviations from the center of the distribution. If we apply the standard distribution model to the hemispheric lateralization of conscious thought in the brain, we could imagine the left side of the distribution representing the population whose brains have consciousness lateralized in the left hemisphere, and vice versa for the right side. Using this model, we can say that most people are not excessively lateralized towards either the right or the left hemisphere. Rather, most people fall somewhere in the middle. Therefore, if "anxious depression" is caused by the perpetual swinging of conscious thought from left to right hemispheres, going side to side continually as on a pendulum, then the people who are most likely to experience anxious depression are the people who are in the middle of the distribution. That is to say, according to my theory, that the majority of people in a society afflicted by hyperconsciousness will also experience anxious depression.

In short, anxious depression is not so much a disorder, but a normative state of being for people in modern society. Anxious depression is the price we pay for having sophisticated brains that can predict the future and interpret the past using private verbal thought. Anxious depression is the cognitive rent we pay for the private kingdoms of minds in our heads. Anxious depression is the consequence of consciousness.

It's well known that women are diagnosed with both anxiety and depression more than men. According to the National Center for Health Statistics, between the years of 2005 and 2008, nearly a quarter of all American women were on antidepressants, with similar rates for anti-anxiety medications.[5] "The onset of anxiety and depressive disorders peaks during adolescence and early adulthood, with females being at significantly greater risk than males. Women have twice the lifetime rates of depression and most anxiety disorders."[6] There are psychosocial reasons for this gender difference, such as the notion that men, traditionally, have been expected by their cultures and societies to be "strong and silent" in the face of anxious and depressive thoughts, while women have had no such constraints, making the expression of anxious depression (if not the experience of it), more noticeable and therefore more identifiable and more diagnosable in women.

Beyond this psychosocial factor, there's also the well-known neurological phenomenon that women's brains are generally less lateralized than male brains.[7] Within the model being drawn out in this chapter, a generally less lateralized brain in women would presumably result in a higher incidence of anxious depression, as a brain that isn't particularly lateralized for conscious thought would be more conducive to the left/right back and forth of anxious/depressive thoughts. The good news for women is that a less lateralized brain would also, in my model, be less conducive to disorders resulting from left hemispheric hyperactivity and/or right hemispheric hypoactivity, as in the case of autism, which has a much higher incidence in males, with a male to female diagnostic ratio of 4:1.[8]

How Melancholia Became Anxiety and Depression

In his book *How Everyone Became Depressed: The Rise and Fall of the Nervous Breakdown* (2013), psychiatrist and psychiatric historian Edward Shorter explains that for most of the history of medicine and psychiatry, anxiety and depression were not considered discrete disorders in-and-of-themselves, but rather, they were considered common symptoms of one broader underlying condition. Well more than 2000 years ago, Hippocrates stated that "If fear or despair continues for a long time, such a thing is melancholia."[9] This statement presupposes that "melancholia" is the underlying condition that reveals itself in symptoms of both anxiety ("fear") and depression ("despair"). Melancholia (along with synonymous conditions) was the diagnosis given to people with those symptoms for the next two millennia.

With the lack of a standardized taxonomy of mental disorders such as the DSM, psychiatrists in the 19th century and first half of the 20th century came up with various alternate titles for melancholia, such as neurasthenia, neurotic depression, depressive neurosis, anxious melancholy, neurotic anxiety, and mixed anxiety-depression. All of these different titles shared a common set of symptoms, that included anxiety, depression, obsessive thoughts, fatigue, and other somatic complaints. Psychiatrists and laymen alike in the 19th and early 20th centuries considered anxiety and depression to be symptoms of the same underlying condition. Even Emil Kraepelin, the psychiatrist famous for dichotomizing unitary psychosis into two different categories of psychotic disorder, considered anxiety and depression to be two symptoms of the same underlying condition: "a union of dysphoria with inner tension."[10] In the first half of the 20th century, doctors and their patients often referred to symptoms of anxiety and depression with the very broad and general term "nerves," so that someone suffering from anxious and depressive symptoms was said to have a "bad case of nerves," and if the individual's nerves got so bad that he or she couldn't function, it was called a "nervous breakdown."

The psychoanalysts of the early 20th century created the diagnosis of "depressive neurosis" to denote the "commonest of the neuroses," a condition of combined anxious and depressive symptoms, which became "the workhouse of everyday psychoanalytic practice."[11] Between the early 1920s and the late 1970s, the similarly termed diagnosis of "mixed anxiety-depression" was the primary condition being treated by psychiatrists. Shorter noted: "...empirically it was obvious that most depressions were accompanied by anxiety—and vice versa ... mixed anxiety-depression is by far the commonest presentation of either anxiety or depression."[12] It wasn't until 1980 that anxiety and depression were formally separated by the *DSM-III* into two separate categories of mood disorders. The question is, why do so?

Shorter makes a strong argument that the decision to dichotomize mixed anxiety-depression was not based on a change in the clinical population—who have always and will always experience anxious depression concurrently—it was based on a change in the dominant treatment model. The long wake of Freud's influence on psychiatry began before the 1920s and peaked in the 1940s, but began to wane in the 1950s in favor of the new psycho-pharmaceuticals that were available. Over the next few decades, the medical/psycho-pharmaceutical model gradually but steadily displaced the psychoanalytic model as the dominant psychiatric paradigm, so that by 1980, traditional psychoanalysts had become passé, and psychiatrists who had a prescription handy for any psychological problem were, and still are, all the rave. It was outside pressure from the pharmaceutical industry, Shorter argues, that created the need for separate diagnoses.

> Until *DSM-III* in 1980, the supposed difference between anxiety and depression lived on mainly in the world of pharmaceutical advertising, where diseases were found to fit the compounds on hand, rather than the other way around. The benzodiazepines, launched in 1960 with Librium, are actually quite suitable agents for mixed anxiety-depression. But they would be spun either toward anxiety or depression, depending on the needs of commerce. The Upjohn Company, for example, wanted to introduce its benzodiazepine alprazolam (Xanax) in 1981 as

an antidepressant and was blocked from doing so only by the absence of an inpatient study. So they ended up with a marketing hit for panic disorder! Big bucks were riding on the question of whether anxiety was a separate disease: If separate, different agents would be needed to treat it. If the same, the patient could be spared one prescription. The entire issue became degraded by commercial considerations…. It is difficult to put it this way but I cannot think of any other way to say it: The fact that they separated depression and anxiety into two entirely different disease basins shows that they did not know what they were doing…. In the decades ahead, depression and anxiety would in academic disease classification be seen as separate diseases requiring separate treatments.[13]

Adaptive and Maladaptive Anxiety

Anxiety is a normative experience. The phenomenon is rooted in the more basic emotion of fear, our body's and our mind's natural reaction to perceived danger in our environment. Following the DSM, diagnosticians differentiate between fear and anxiety as follows: "*Fear* is the emotional response to real or perceived imminent threat, whereas *anxiety* is anticipation of future threat."[14] Julian Jaynes referred to anxiety quite succinctly as "the knowledge of our own fear,"[15] even though we may oftentimes be clueless about what exactly we're afraid of.

Imagine being a chimpanzee living in the jungle. You're knuckle-walking along, minding your own business, when you hear what sounds like a growl. Immediately, your heart rate leaps, your breath quickens, your sweat glands kick in and your skin moistens, your senses turn up to high alert. The body is instantly prepared for fight or flight. Images of tigers and lions appear in your head, as your imagination conjures the possible origin of the alarming sound; the brain is instantly prepared for discovering and encountering the perceived threat. Feelings of trepidation and apprehension suddenly dominate your mood. The mind is emotionally set to the condition of danger. You investigate your surroundings, and you find an old chimp friend lying asleep in the bushes, his snores creating the sound that you momentarily mistook as a growl. Immediately, all the symptoms of fear fade away, and in a moment, you're walking along again, worry-free and without a care in the world. The chimp experiences fear in the moment of perceived danger, but not anxiety before or afterwards, because without the process of internal verbal thought, it cannot compose a cohesive and detailed private personal narrative that stretches back into his remembered past, and reaches forward into various hypothetical imagined futures.

Internal verbal thought creates an "inner mind-space"[16] of conscious rumination that's generally filled with our own narrative voice, which makes sense of the environment and our place in the environment by telling us a story about ourselves. In order for us to tell a story, we must be able to conceive of a timeline in which things happen to us ... a past, present, and future. Most animals probably cannot deliberately access specific events from their pasts without an external association, because the substance of the past—memories—are inaccessible without a sophisticated retrieval system for memories. Linguistic thought is that retrieval system. Most animals do have memories, they just can't consciously access these memories, because they're not "conscious" (in the way humans are) and they don't have the cognitive tools to deliberately recall and access memories. Imagine a huge library full of books. The books themselves are relatively useless unless there's some sort of cataloging system that uses categories and labels to access the books based on their title, author, subject, or content. An animal's memory system is like a library without a catalog. Memories come to them like flashes of images in a dream, but they're evoked either by unconscious association or by direct contact with a stimulus that evokes an unconscious association, not by conscious retrieval. Hence, the waking state of an animal, at least in terms of its experience of memory, is probably very much like the dreaming state of humans while we're asleep. Associations of memories float by in their minds, but they don't think about the memories or deliberately access the memories. Humans, however, deliberately recall certain memories and consciously think about them as we narrate our own stories to ourselves. Hence, the inner mind-space of conscious narrative thought creates a sense of past, present, and future in humans that doesn't exist in animals who lack verbal narrative thought. Without the ability to tell a story about itself in linear narrative form, the animal is always in the present—the here and now—as it has no conscious or deliberate cognitive access to its past, no concept of a linear timeline in reference to itself. So, while it can experience memories that are recalled unconsciously via association, it cannot navigate back and forth in its own narrative timeline deliberately, because it cannot conceive of a timeline to begin with. Therefore, the animal without verbal narrative thought cannot conceive of either a hypothetical future or a reconstructed past— and this is the crucial point in terms of anxious depression.

Now, imagine you're you, a modern human, walking without a care down the street of a modern urban jungle. Suddenly you hear a clanking sound emanating from a dark alley. Immediately, your heart rate leaps, your breath quickens, your skin moistens, your senses turn up to high alert—the body is instantly prepared for fight or flight. Images of muggers and rapists appear in your head, as your imagination conjures the possible origin of the alarming sound. The brain is instantly prepared for discovering and encountering the perceived threat. Feelings of trepidation and apprehension suddenly dominate your mood as the mind is emotionally set to the condition of danger. You cautiously investigate the dark alleyway, and you find an old alley-cat rummaging in a garbage can, creating the sound that you momentarily mistook for an attacker. Immediately, the symptoms of fear fade, and in a moment, you're walking along again—but not necessarily worry-free and without a care in the world.

You are now hyperconscious of the potential danger in your environment and can reflect on the fearful experience of your recent past, and ruminate on the possible dangers in your immediate or distant future. What if you really were attacked? What about that time ten years ago when you were almost attacked? What about the friend you had that was once attacked? What about all those media reports about people being attacked every day? What about that dark alley up ahead ... might there be a real attacker (and not just a cat), up the block a ways? The hyperconscious You experiences not only fear in the moment of perceived danger, but anxiety *following* the moment of perceived danger. Furthermore, because anxiety is evoked by imagined danger rather than real or even perceived danger, anxiety can persist indefinitely, and can be evoked at any time by nearly any thing. We can be anxious about possibly losing our job in a few years, or about having enough money to retire in thirty years, or about how we're going to die, which could be in fifty years or in fifty minutes... We can even be anxious about things that may not actually exist, such as ghosts, demons, aliens, etc.

With all the above, we may conclude that anxiety is a distinctly *human* phenomenon derived from fear, but functionally autonomous of its root in fear, as it arises from the cognitive domain of imagined future danger, as opposed to imminent perceived danger. Furthermore, since our ability to ruminate about the future is made possible by consciousness, we may also conclude that anxiety is caused by consciousness of potential danger, rather than actual danger, hence anxiety is manufactured by consciousness itself. Anxiety disorder—a condition of chronic intense anxiety that's unrelated to any real danger or threat—can therefore be considered a product of too much consciousness (hyperconsciousness), especially hyperconscious rumination about the future.

There are other aspects about the modern human condition that seem to manufacture the pathological state of chronic anxiety, as opposed to the normative state of momentary fear. As children, we're taught to worry about our performance in a range of activities, especially academics, in order to secure a successful future. That is, we train children to stress out about tests and schoolwork so that, driven by anxiety, they study harder and longer, so that they get good grades in school, so they can go to a good college, so they can get a good job. At no point in that process do we tell kids to stop stressing out: to the contrary, the pressure to excel in academics and other areas increases as kids get older. So, if the "danger" that evokes fear is the possibility of becoming an unemployed, unemployable, penniless, homeless ne'er-do-well, the anxiety evoked by this imaginary fear begins in childhood and continues throughout adulthood, with the anxiety only becoming stronger and more chronic, as we grow into adulthood and take on not only more personal obligations and responsibilities, but the tremendously stressful obligations of adult parents, who have to worry and stress about not only their own careers and welfare, but the welfare of their young children, their elderly parents, and their other dependents.

In sum, whereas a nonconscious chimp only worries when there's a clear and present danger in his environment, a modern conscious human is trained from childhood to worry about potential "dangers" in the forms of academic and vocational requirements and assessments, as well as a constant list of things to worry about that never go away. So, while consciousness allows us to master our environments by giving us the ability to foresee potential challenges and obstacles in the future, it also condemns our minds to the cerebral prison sentence of *constantly* thinking about future challenges, causing us to *constantly* consider future pitfalls and obstacles, causing us to exist in a *constant* state of chronic anxiety, which is tantamount on physical, emotional, and cognitive levels to living in a *constant* state of fear.

The irony here is that consciousness has allowed us to master our environments to a point where the most frequently experienced immediate natural dangers—predators, starvation, serious injury—have been eradicated or largely mitigated; yet at the same time that our environment is the safest its ever been in the history of humankind, humans themselves are living in an unprecedented, extreme, and chronic state of fear of their environment. *Consciousness giveth, and it taketh away...*

To all of this, I might add that our media environment is constantly evoking fearful responses by bombarding us with fearsome images and stories of terrifying terrorists, attackers, and the myriad of physical and metaphysical dangers that both exist and potentially exist. The news media are well aware that "fear sells" almost as well as "sex sells," so they profit from the fact that their consumers are equipped with brains that make them constantly mindful of dangers in their environment (regardless of whether these dangers are real or imagined). The irony is that the same brains that made our species so fierce and dominant, also predispose us to a chronic state of anxiety and fear. We've become a dominant yet ironically fearful species, living in constant fear of imagined potential dangers, and at the same time, constantly adding to our fears by immersing ourselves in a self-created media environment saturated with fearful images and stories.

By manufacturing fear in our cut-throat assessment-driven academic and vocational environments, we realize—as Winston Churchill realized during World War II—that our greatest fear is of fear itself. That is, one of the main things that modern people worry about is the fact that they and their children worry too much. Meta-anxiety, anxiety about having anxiety, worrying about worrying too much, adds to the positive feedback loop of our fear-saturated environment, which keeps us constantly anxious and chronically stressed. Although I continue to examine our modern environment—especially our modern media environments—for the things that manufacture chronic anxiety in all of us, I should note that we must not presume there was a happy vanished time, way back when in the good old days, when people lived happy, stress-free, anxiety-free lives. Yes, I do think that our modern world creates more anxiety than in previous generations, and yes I do think that modern hyperconscious people are more anxious than pre-modern, preliterate people, but I don't presume that anxiety is a new phenomenon in the evolution of our species.

There's a common misunderstanding about the evolutionary process and the phenomenon of "happiness," in which people assume that a species such as ours adapts to our environment, and when a member of that species becomes perfectly adapted to his environment, he will be completely happy, as if the endpoint of evolution is a continuous nirvana-like state of peaceful, blissful grace. The problem with this line of thinking is that evolution is a never-ending process, so it has no "endpoint" or goal, and also, evolution as a process is completely unconcerned with "happiness," as the phenomenon of happiness is more-or-less irrelevant to the evolutionary pressures of sexual reproduction and survival.

If anything, a state of perpetual bliss would be evolutionarily maladaptive, as it would lead to complacency, laziness, and self-destructive profligacy. To the contrary, a state of chronic dissatisfaction with one's self and one's environment is actually a more adaptive evolutionary strategy, as chronic dissatisfaction—like a carrot on a stick—creates constant motivation for the individual to always work harder to improve himself and master his environment. Chronic dissatisfaction, in this sense, would be experienced as feelings of generalized anxiety (worrying about the potential for future happiness), and mild depression (sadness about the lack of happiness in one's distant or immediate past).

So, it may be that our evolutionary process has dealt us cards that predispose our minds towards anxious and depressing thought patterns that make us unhappy. Obviously, it would be maladaptive for people to be too unhappy all the time, as severe anxiety and depression are debilitating disorders that reduce productivity, reproduction, and adaptiveness, and may also lead to suicide and other self-destructive behaviors that anxious depressed people engage in, such as self-medicating with drugs and alcohol, overeating, media binging, etc. Once again, we must conceptualize these traits as they're distributed throughout the population, by applying the standard distribution model. If we place the hazily defined human trait of "unhappiness" caused by hyperconscious rumination on a standard distribution, then the majority of the population would fall out in the middle of the spectrum, which would represent mild-to-moderate unhappiness (or mild-to-moderate "anxious depression") in most people. Hence, in this model, most modern people are mildly to moderately unhappy ("anxiously depressed") a lot of the time, but relatively few people are severely unhappy almost all of the time, and relatively few people are extremely happy almost all of the time.

The lucky people on the low end of the spectrum will be blessed with very little anxious depression (although this trait could backfire, because without anxious depressive feelings pressuring us to better ourselves and our lives, we face the risk of complacency, which may reduce adaptivity and productivity). Anxiety, when channeled and sublimated well, has the benefit of making us more productive, more competitive, and more achievement-oriented. These traits make us more successful, but they also make us chronically dissatisfied and unhappy. Thus, the road to success is paved with anxiety. Anxiety is also perpetual, because "success" is fleeting in a conscious mindset that's always looking towards the future. When present success is perceived as a mere building block towards even greater future success, happiness or satisfaction is only experienced as a temporary fleeting moment, a brief reduction of stress in the present, followed by another wave of future-oriented anxiety. What is happiness, then? Since happiness is fleeting and anxious depression chronic, happiness for most of us is simply "what we feel the moment before we want more happiness."[17] The unlucky people at the high end of the spectrum are the people who suffer from more chronic and severe anxious depression, the people who find it hard, if not impossible, to experience even fleeting moments of happiness.

Anxiety to the Left of Me, Depression to the Right

McGilchrist noted that, in its capacity as the side of the brain that engages in deep focus, "The left hemisphere has difficulty disengaging."[18] The left hemisphere is monologistic—it focuses on one thing—and stays focused. This perseveration on stimuli is obviously quite useful for problem solving, but perseveration becomes a problem in-and-of-itself when the subject of perseveration becomes oneself, in which case perseveration on the "problem" of one's own existence becomes hyper-conscious self-reflection on conscious thoughts that evoke anxiety or depression.

Part of the problem has to do with the nature of consciousness itself. We may consider consciousness the "boss" of cognition, because we can consciously decide to do things or to not do things—even when those decisions are counter-intuitive and counter-instinctive—and we can even consciously decide what to think about. However, because consciousness is the boss, there's nobody to boss around consciousness itself. We cannot consciously turn off our own consciousness. We can manually override it with drugs or a swift blow to the head, but that merely delivers a temporary state of unconsciousness. Most of us cannot consciously decide to be nonconscious. Hence, a condition like anxious depression, which is caused by hyperconsciousness, cannot be cured simply by avoiding or eliminating conscious thought, because except for people who have the time, ability, and inclination to spend a majority of their waking lives in a state of ego-less, thoughtless, conscious-less, transcendental zen meditation, we are all subject to the perseverative and unstoppable rumination of consciousness.

As discussed earlier, the left hemisphere tends to discard information that doesn't conform to the worldview it prefers to perceive. This excluded information—the ash heap of discarded consciousness—is not eradicated, but silently stored in the right hemisphere, which explains the role of the right hemisphere as the librarian of negative memories, and it also explains its penchant for melancholy. Fixation on one's past, especially on those aspects of the past that evoke feelings of shame, guilt, or melancholic wistfulness for days gone by, will naturally result in depressed mood. If anxiety could be considered the knowledge of one's own fear, then depression could be considered the knowledge of one's own shame—encompassing feelings of guilt, inferiority, bereavement, and low self-esteem—resulting from any sort of shortcoming or failure. When consciousness is fixated on past failures and losses, it loses its ability to think forward, resulting in a paralysis of volition, an inability to proceed forward.

In depression, we see someone who is conscious of what they want to achieve, but unable to garner the volition required to move towards achievement. Whereas our preverbal hominid ancestors simply acted on their thoughts without significant forethought or afterthought, modern humans with conscious verbal thought ruminate over their thoughts endlessly, creating a gap between thought and volition. Depressed people may be stuck in this gap, able to understand what they want to do and even desiring to do it, but unable to actually proceed. This model of depression has been called the "rumination theory," the idea being that people who ruminate hyperconsciously on their own negative thoughts and feelings are more likely to be depressed. Empirical studies have demonstrated that people who ruminate are more likely to be depressed,[19] but—unlike my model—the empirical studies don't explain where rumination comes from, or why it exists in the first place.

Rumination can be described as a morbid fascination and meditation on one's own faults and foibles. The depressed person criticizes and berates himself for every defect, resulting in the self-doubt and self-loathing that interrupt volition. Interrupted volition, in turn, results in inactivity and the incompletion of goals, which then results in more self-consciousness, more self-criticism, more self-doubting and self-loathing, and so on...

McGilchrist has suggested that "the left hemisphere's raison d'etre is to narrow things down to a certainty, the right hemisphere's is to open them up to possibility."[20] The left hemisphere is always seeking certainty. In its role as the "problem solver," the left hemisphere is always seeking problems and trying to solve them. This modus operandi is perfectly suited for manual tasks and intellectual problems, but the "real world" often gives us problems that cannot be solved, problems without solutions, or problems that only devolve into other problems, and so are never completely resolved. The left hemisphere, in these situations, rather than letting go of the problem, will focus even harder in its desperate mission to resolve problems with solutions that provide absolute certainty. Obsessive-Compulsive Disorder (OCD) is an anxiety disorder that seems to function by associating certain anxiety-provoking worries, such as the fear of germs, with related anxiety-relieving behaviors, such as compulsive hand washing. Each obsession evokes a problem in the mind that must be solved, and each associated compulsion temporarily resolves the problem, thus relieving the anxiety, but only until the next obsessive thought comes around.

Anxiety can be conceptualized as the embodied need for certainty. It's a need that will perseverate indefinitely. One popular cognitive model of anxiety is the "intolerance of uncertainty theory," which posits that anxiety arises from a desperate and unyielding need for certainty, and which is supported by research that shows that "uncertainty intolerance" is strongly correlated with anxiety. My model not only assumes that anxiety is aroused and exacerbated by uncertainty intolerance, but it even explains where uncertainty tolerance originates, and how it operates in the mind.

Meta-anxiety, worrying about worrying, arises from not knowing why you feel anxious or depressed, and wondering whether there's something wrong with you physically, mentally, or spiritually. All this meta-worrying and stress result in even more severe feelings of anxious depression ... a positive feedback loop. Furthermore, feelings of guilt, shame, and worthlessness arise when you wonder why you can't just get over your depression, why you can't just pull yourself up by your bootstraps and face the day with a stiff upper lip, why you can't just be happy and satisfied like other people ... deepening the already existing feelings of anxious depression.

Ineffective Therapies: The Emperor's New and Old Clothes

A plethora of empirical studies have demonstrated that antidepressants such as the SSRI Prozac have a very powerful placebo effect, and that when the substantial placebo effect is subtracted from the main effect of the drugs themselves, there's very little effect left. That is, SSRIs are somewhat effective in treating depression and anxiety, but this effectiveness in most cases is due almost entirely to the placebo effect, and not the drug itself.[21] It's been argued that one of the main reasons why antidepressants such as the SSRI Prozac are so frequently effective is because the "chemical imbalance hypothesis" of anxiety and depression effectively dispels both the uncertainty of the origin of the disorder, and the feelings of guilt and shame that accompany it. The term "demystification" applies to the feeling of relief a patient experiences when an unexplained condition is finally explained and a course of treatment prescribed. Oftentimes the relief of stress is so great following demystification that the patient will experience a reduction or even elimination of symptoms, even if the prescribed treatment is known to be ineffective beyond the placebo effect.

When patients suffering from anxious depression are prescribed an SSRI, they are told that the cause of their anxiety/depression is a chemical imbalance; specifically, a shortage in the neural presence of the neurotransmitter serotonin. Immediately, all of the feelings of uncertainty—*Why am I this way? Why won't these feelings go away? Why can't I just will myself to feel better?*—are demystified and dispelled. Simultaneously, the feelings of guilt and shame for having the disorder are also dispelled. A person infected with a virus doesn't feel guilty for being sick, they just take their medication and feel better. Similarly, in keeping with the chemical imbalance hypothesis, a person suffering from clinical depression should not feel guilty for having a biological condition resulting from a deficiency of serotonin. They just take their Prozac and feel better. The demystifying psychological catharsis provided by the chemical imbalance hypothesis exorcises the patient's shame and self-judgments, relieving them from crippling and stressful feelings of uncertainty and guilt, resulting in a powerful placebo effect of diminished depression and anxiety. This is doubtlessly coupled with a traditional placebo effect, in which the patient feels better simply because he has faith in his doctor and he believes quite strongly that the medication will help him ("mind over matter").

The idea that the efficacy of modern antidepressants is capacitated in large part by these placebo effects is supported by studies in which the artificial depletion of serotonin did *not* cause depressive symptoms in patients, thus debunking the notion that serotonin deficiency has a direct causative effect on depression.[22] Dr. Irving Kirsch, associate director of the Program in Placebo Studies at the Harvard Medical School and author of the book *The Emperor's New Drugs: Exploding the Antidepressant Myth* (2011), provides incontrovertible evidence via meta-analyses of hundreds of clinical studies that antidepressants, for people suffering mild to moderate depression (that is, for the vast majority of people diagnosed with depression and prescribed medication), have *no significant clinical effect* beyond the placebo effect. He concludes: "It now seems beyond question that the traditional account of depression as a chemical imbalance in the brain is simply wrong."[23]

Most researchers in the field agree with Kirsch's judgment, but practitioners are still prescribing antidepressants by the barrelful to patients diagnosed with either depression, anxiety, or both, primarily because the placebo effect is quite powerful, so even though the clinical effect of antidepressants is insignificant for most people taking the medication, the drugs nevertheless seem to work—they just work because of the placebo effect, not because the drugs themselves rectify any "chemical imbalances" in the brain, because the "chemical balance" theory in-and-of-itself is simply incorrect. Despite these issues, "antidepressant medications are now the most commonly prescribed class of drugs, ahead of drugs for high blood pressure, high cholesterol, asthma, or headaches."[24]

The dubious effectiveness of antidepressant and anti-anxiety medications is mirrored in the dubious effectiveness of the traditional "talk therapies": psychoanalysis and psychotherapy. While many patients/clients strongly believe that talk therapy is helpful in their lives, self-reports indicate that over the course of therapy, anxiety and depression are not significantly reduced.[25] That is, the clients say that they benefit from the support of therapy, and that therapy provides them with tools to help them cope with stress and sadness, but their anxious depressive thoughts persist. Therapy seems to work by helping patients/clients deal with anxious and depressing feelings and thoughts. Like medication, therefore, therapy treats the symptoms of anxious depression, but doesn't address the root cause.

It was Freud who pioneered the field of talk therapy under the premise that neurosis (aka anxious depression), can be resolved if unconscious issues were made conscious. Like a demon or vampire who dissolves into a wisp of smoke when exposed to daylight, unconscious fears and doubts will also vanish once exposed to the light of conscious understanding. With all due respect to the Master, the theory I'm putting forth here is diametrically opposed to Freud's. My argument is that neurosis/anxious depression is actually *caused* by consciousness. It therefore follows that consciously focusing on these conscious neurotic thoughts—hyperconsciousness—will not only be ineffective in eliminating the thoughts themselves, it will cause them to persist. To a certain extent, we may even say that talk therapy is a form of hyperconsciousness, which may explain the adverse psychological effects of talk therapy, which appear in a significant minority of clients.[26] It would also explain why psychotherapy, unlike physical therapy, never has an endpoint. Unlike the body, which physically recovers from injury with time, proper exercise, and treatment, the mind will not mentally "recover" from the anxious depressive effects of hyperconsciousness, if the treatment is in large part hyperconsciousness as well.

In short, the reason why talk therapies, while helpful in many ways, are so notoriously ineffective at reducing anxious depressive thoughts, is because the medium of talk therapy itself—language—is the medium of anxious depression. Trying to cure or treat anxious depression with words is like trying to douse a fire with gasoline. To put it more prosaically, language is a medium of deep self-reflection, because it's the medium our mind uses for private verbal reflective thought, so it suits psychotherapy/psychoanalysis quite well, as the goal of these therapies is increased self-awareness and self-reflectiveness—to make the unconscious become conscious via the process of hyperconscious self-reflection. It has been my argument in this chapter, however, that hyperconscious self-reflection is the *cause* of anxious depression, rather than the cure. Once again, McLuhan's adage—"the medium is the message"—gets to the heart of the issue. If somebody wishes to be less anxiously depressed, he or she will seek out a therapist to talk about the content of their anxious and depressive thoughts, without for a moment realizing that the psychological effect of the *content* of their thoughts— the specific fears, stressors, or depressors—are relatively inconsequential in regard to their mental condition, compared to the overarching effect of the *medium* of thought itself—language. In a follow-up book, I plan to offer a suggestion for relieving anxious depression by channeling thought and behavior into different, nonlinguistic media of expression.[27]

The irony of 20th century applied psychology is that the "emperor's old clothes"—the Master's "talking cure"—was displaced in the latter half of the century by the "emperor's new clothes"—psychopharmacological medication—while both treatment models seem to be equally ineffective at eliminating the primary cause of psychological suffering among people seeking treatment for anxious depression.

The Optimist and the Pessimist Within

The left hemisphere perceives its environment as a landscape filled with potential problems. In its capacity as problem-solver, the left hemisphere will predict potential future problems and perseverate on the need to remediate these hypothetical problems, continuing in this process until it's certain about its future. In its desperation, the left hemisphere will create the delusion of certainty, based on its own self-made beliefs regarding the future that have the veneer of certainty, even though, of course, one can never truly know what will happen in the future. If the delusion of certainty is unapparent, or if circumstances in life dispel the delusion, the resultant feelings of uncertainty and insecurity, the desperate search for certainty—and the fear of never finding it—provide the essence of anxiety.

The right hemisphere, on the other hand, will contemplate the possibilities of life, basing its reasoning on the remembered experiences of the remote past as well as the immediate past (i.e., the "present"). If the illusion of possibility is dashed by prior experiences in the past, or if the "reality" perceived in the present is disillusioning, then the sense of impossibility—the "real-I-zation"—that one's dreams are truly out of reach, will naturally lead to a sense of hopelessness about one's self, and a sense of helplessness about one's situation, providing the essence of depression.

Although it's too simplistic to say that the left hemisphere in an optimist and the right hemisphere a pessimist, there's a good deal of evidence to support this argument, at least metaphorically, as a general dichotomy in the way that the hemispheres attend to the world and the individual's place within it. McGilchrist argues, "The right hemisphere is also more realistic about how it stands in relation to the world at large, less grandiose, more self-aware, than the left hemisphere. The left hemisphere is ever optimistic, but unrealistic about its shortcomings."[28] The left hemisphere's specialty is a narrow focus that operates by excising information that it deems irrelevant to the specific task at hand, lending itself towards a tendency for "pollyannaism"—neglecting negative information while focusing only on the positive. That modus operandi is a set-up for unbridled optimism. The right hemisphere's specialty is a broad focus that grounds our cognition and perception in the real world, making the right hemisphere's job that of a "bridle" or controller, keeping the left hemisphere grounded in the real world. Hence, we may consider the right hemisphere more of a realist as compared to its optimistic twin, and realism—looking at one's self and one's situation realistically as opposed to optimistically—is, by default, a pessimistic viewpoint. How is this so? I'll provide an example.

I've been a fulltime college professor for nearly 20 years. Part of my job is to advise students regarding their academic and vocational career goals. Occasionally, I'll speak with a student who expresses a desire to earn a Ph.D. in clinical psychology, and the problem is, I truly believe that this student does not have the academic strengths needed to get into a doctoral program in clinical psychology, much less complete said program and work in the field. So what should I do? Should I advise the student that he does not have a realistic chance at accomplishing his dream (my true assessment), or do I tell the student that—though it will be a great challenge—he should pursue his dream, regardless of the apparent impossibilities involved. While advising the latter may seem imprudently optimistic, advising the former may seem hopelessly pessimistic, even though the former advice is actually just a realistic assessment of the student's capabilities, based on my own evaluations of the student's academic performance as his professor and advisor. Hence, in this world of delusion, where we spend most of our mental time fantasizing about possible futures filled with success and good fortune, a realistic viewpoint, in contrast, will always seem hopelessly pessimistic. In other words, a pessimist is just a realist in practice.

McGilchrist summarizes the empirical evidence of the associations between the right hemisphere, pessimism, and depression, as follows:

Although relatively speaking the right hemisphere takes a more pessimistic view of the self, it is also more realistic about it. There is evidence that (a) those who are somewhat depressed are more realistic, including in self-evaluation... (b) depression is (often) a condition of relative hemisphere asymmetry, favouring the right hemisphere. Even schizophrenics have more insight into their condition in proportion to the degree that they have depressive symptoms. The evidence is that this is not because insight makes you depressed, but because being depressed gives you insight.[29]

The left hemisphere's inherent optimism is thwarted when it sees its own optimistic predilections in the light of uncertainty, transfiguring the positive excitement of anticipation into the negative apprehension of dread and anxiety. The right hemisphere's inherent realism, in turn, is easily experienced as pessimism, because in a kingdom of dreamers, romantics, and fantasists, the realist is just a gloomy wet blanket. In short, the left hemisphere tends to be optimistic, but also anxious, especially when its optimistic forecasts don't line up with the apparent dark clouds in sight. The right hemisphere tends to be realistic/pessimistic, but also depressive, especially when the real world and one's place in it seem to preclude the possibilities of an improved existence. That is, realism is often perceived as pessimism, and pessimism, even when correct (or *especially* when it's correct), is depressing.

When the twin hemispheres are working well together, they balance each other off. The left side's optimism keeps us motivated and striving towards what we perceive are achievable goals, while the right side's realism keeps us grounded in the real world, so we don't get too carried away by our own unbridled optimism. When the twin hemispheres aren't working well together, they create a positive feedback loop of anxious and depressive thoughts. The left hemisphere, in its eternal and overly-optimistic quest for perfection and certainty, will perseverate indefinitely on the apparent uncertainties and imperfections in its life. The psychological and physical stress of this chronic anxiety takes its toll, leading to emotional exhaustion and precipitating a pendular shift of both thought and mood to the right hemisphere, where the left hemisphere's aspirations for certain perfection now, in the dim light of realistic perception, seem hopelessly out of reach. This self-conscious "pessimism," this self-doubt in one's abilities to achieve one's goals and dreams—no matter how unrealistic those goals and dreams may be—provide the slippery slope of self-loathing and negativity that lead downward into a sinking pit of depression.

As was his wont, Freud provided an overly-complicated psychoanalytic model of depression. According to Freud, we all carry around an internal mental image of our imagined perfect selves, which he labeled our "ego ideal." When we feel or know that we're not living up to that ideal, we feel a sense of mourning for that ego loss, and that "imagined loss" of our own self-concept is experienced as depression.[30] The idea here is that we all live in a mental world that contains a virtual reality of our own selves. That idealized virtual self—the "ego ideal"—is used as a model with which to compare our real selves.

When projected into the future, the ego ideal is likely to make us feel anxious, because our left hemisphere will detect the discrepancies between our real self and our ideal self, and it will interpret these discrepancies as problems that must be solved post haste, and if they cannot be solved immediately, or ever, the residual stress and restless energy will be felt as anxiety. When reflecting on the present and past, the ego ideal is likely to make us feel depressed, as per Freud's interpretation, because the understanding that we are not the person we wish to be, and that we never were and will likely never be that person—this depressing *real-I-zation*—will be felt as a sense of mourning and loss for the perfect me that never was, and never will be.

The Brain's "Default Mode Network"

In a seminal paper published in 2001, neurologist Marcus Raichle noted that the "resting state" of the brain used in brain imaging studies—the state of the brain before and after the participant is given a specific task to perform—is actually just as active if not more so than the "active state" of the brain when it's performing a given task.[31] He labeled this paradoxical "resting" state as the brain's "default mode," because the term "resting" was inappropriate due to the high level of brain activity. In follow-up studies, Buckner et al. (2008) noted that "A common observation in brain imaging research is that a specific set of brain regions— referred to as the default network—is engaged when individuals are left to think to themselves undisturbed."[32]

The "default mode network" is so named because the state seems to be the default mode of the brain when it's not otherwise occupied with a specific task, and also because the default mode utilizes multiple neuro-systems from across different brain regions. It's a coordinated "network" of brain systems. They discovered that "the default network is active when individuals are engaged in internally focused tasks including autobiographical memory retrieval, envisioning the future, and conceiving the perspectives of others—what William James (1890) called the 'stream of consciousness...' the mental processes that make up fantasy, imagination, daydreams, and thought."[33]

The default mode is a state of rumination, usually about oneself, and often involved with imagining how other people think of us—"social comparison." Because the default mode is typically self-reflective, "some neuroscientists call it 'the me network.'"[34] Buckner et al. theorized that "the adaptive function" of the default mode is "to provide a 'life simulator'—a set of interacting subsystems that can use past experiences to explore and anticipate social and event scenarios." Buckner et al.'s construct of the default mode is essentially the same thing as hyper-self-conscious rumination, which I've inculpated as the root of anxious depression. The fact that the default mode is a network that involves systems from all different parts of the brain, supports my construct of anxious depression as a product of thought that relies on both hemispheres—access to memories from the past as well as perspectives on the self from other people's imagined points of view (right hemisphere)—as well as calculated projections of the future (left hemisphere).

In another seminal paper entitled "A Wandering Mind Is an Unhappy Mind," Killingsworth and Gilbert (2010) demonstrated that when people are engaged in the default mode (which they also referred to as "mind wandering" and as "stimulus independent thought"), people were significantly "less happy" than when they were not "mind wandering." Killingsworth and Gilbert concluded that "a human mind is a wandering mind, and a wandering mind is an unhappy mind. The ability to think about what is not happening is a cognitive achievement that comes at an emotional cost." The achievement in this case is hyper-consciousness, and the cost is anxious depression.

In his book on psychedelic research and therapy, *How to Change Your Mind...* (2018), Michael Pollan, in reference to the default mode, argues: "The price of the sense of an individual identity is a sense of separation from others and nature. Self reflection can lead to great intellectual and artistic achievement but also to destructive forms of self-regard and many types of unhappiness."[35] Pollan cites fMRI brain imaging studies of subjects on psilocybin (the psychedelic chemical in "magic mushrooms"), noting that the drug seems to quiet or partially deactivate the default mode, and "when activity in the default mode network falls off precipitously, the ego temporarily vanishes, and the usual boundaries we experience between self and world, subject and object, all melt away."[36] Pollan cites the neurological research on psilocybin to conclude that when the brain is on the drug, the default mode network is partially or temporarily deactivated, and "the brain appears to become less specialized and more globally interconnected, with considerably more intercourse, or 'cross talk,' among its various neighborhoods."[37] He supports the view that the deactivation of the default mode is the factor that causes significant and long-lasting reductions in anxiety and depression for people who have been treated with psilocybin. If one's default mode of consciousness has become a cognitive rut of anxious and depressive rumination, a never-ending stream of conscious neurosis punctuated with the inevitable "pity party," then the temporary escape from that rut can also serve a much larger and permanent purpose.

How do you know if your own default mode of consciousness is maladaptive, when all that you perceive and conceive is filtered through that same mode of consciousness? The only way is to perceive and conceive for a while in an altered state of consciousness—especially if the focus of that altered state is to be reflective about one's own mind and behavior. The promise of psychedelic therapy is that it may allow people to reflect upon and even reset their default mode. The current interest in psychedelic therapy is spurred by a general awareness of the ineffectiveness of both talk therapy and pharmacotherapy in the treatment of anxiety/depression (notwithstanding the psychosocial benefits of talk therapy, and the placebo effect of medications).

The Tyranny of the Anxious

In an earlier chapter, I explained how the process of learning to read had the effect of amplifying the internal voice of consciousness, strengthening it via the force of repetition, associating it with thought, as well as conditioning it to think narratively. While it would be incorrect to say that preliterate children and people in preliterate cultures do not hear their own internal conscious voices, it's safe to say that literacy evokes and then establishes the primacy of this internal voice within the domain of private thought. In childhood, we acquire literacy by reading stories about others. The narrator of those stories is heard within our own minds. In a short time, that internal narrator breaks free from the bonds of the page and dives into its own stories about itself.

In its role as the internal narrator, the voice of consciousness looks backward for backstory and looks forward for narrative devices such as surprising plot twists, drama, conflict, victory, defeat, and resolution. And it's precisely this tendency to disregard the present in favor of digging up the past and fretting about the future that predisposes us towards anxious depression. The argument, then, is that consciousness is a byproduct of oral language, and that hyperconsciousness is a byproduct of literacy. Anxious depression, therefore, is not caused by consciousness per se but by the ruminative and perseverative harping of hyperconsciousness.

If anxious depression is caused by hyperconsciousness, then we would expect to find the consequences of hyperconsciousness intensified among literate people in literate societies; and that's exactly what happened in the 20th century. The last century saw dramatic rises in both literacy rates and diagnostic rates of mental disorders reflecting symptoms of anxious depression. This correlation, I argue, is not coincidental, but causative. The good news, then, may be exactly what educators and administrators have been apoplectic about for decades: declining literacy rates in America in the 21st century.

In his book *The Shallows: What the Internet Is Doing to Our Brains* (2010), Nicholas Carr makes the point that few people would be willing to disagree with ... that electronic and digital media are increasingly displacing print media as the dominant medium for information: "Of the four major categories of personal media, print is now the least used, lagging well behind television, computers and radio...."[38] While the vast majority of modern schoolchildren do acquire "basic literacy" in school, because of high dropout rates language barriers among immigrant students, learning disorders, and a general lack of interest or motivation for extracurricular reading (aka "aliteracy") many children never reach the level of proficiency expected of them by our own educational standards for literacy. They remain at the basic or "below basic" level of literacy proficiency, meaning they can read signs and very short messages and passages of text, but cannot engage in more in-depth reading.

While these children grow up to be adults who can get by in our increasingly post-literate and aliterate society, they would be unable to get or hold down a job that requires higher levels of literacy proficiency, making them "functionally illiterate."[39] However, if children are reading less in favor of other nonliteracy based media, then we may be raising a generation of people who are less pre-disposed towards anxious depression than their parents. That is, a movement away from literacy might cause a decrease in anxious depression, as the internal narrator of hyperconscious rumination is born out of the reading of literature. I would like to come to this extremely optimistic conclusion, but I can't. There are a number of reasons why I see anxious depression increasing in the next generation rather than decreasing.

First of all, it seems probable that the aspects of literacy that would have the most profound effects on anxious depression are the amplification of the voice of consciousness, the automatic formatting of private thoughts into words (private verbal thought), and the adoption of a narrative style of self-reflective thought. These aspects of literacy occur at the acquisition phase of literacy development, which means that for most of us, by the time we learn to read at a basic elementary level of proficiency, most of the damage, in terms of hyperconsciousness and anxious depression, has already been done.

Another reason for increasing rates of anxious depression among younger generations, despite decreasing literacy, is alluded to above. Everyone in the field of education is concerned about the declining rates of literacy proficiency in American schools. In a field where the written word is considered fundamental and most essential, declining literacy is perceived not only as a present failure of the school system, but a direct cause of the future vocational failure of these less literate school children themselves. Teachers, administrators, and parents are stressing out big time about declining literacy and increasing aliteracy among modern people in general, and among modern children in particular. The education industry, in its sociocultural role as the bastion of literacy, has equated school success with future career success. And so, since literacy is the primary product offered by the education industry, literacy is thus placed at the same level of priority as survival.

The stressful reactions of teachers and parents and everyone else involved is an expression of panic over the future survivability of the children. This panic is funneled directly into our children, because even though the adults have caused the problem by introducing new media that will naturally displace older media, we expect the children to fix the problem by becoming even more literate, even as we saturate them in a media environment that is antithetic to traditional literacy. The result is that schools have become a place of stress, tension, and fear for children, as well as their parents and teachers. Everybody feels like they're being graded all the time, and they're right. As literacy inevitably declines, gradually becoming displaced and obsolesced by newer media of information, the primary product of schools is now stress. If schools cannot succeed as a manufacturer of increasingly literate students, they will resort to being manufacturers of increasingly anxious young people.

At the macrosystem level, if anxiety is driven by a need for control, then the people with an acute psychosocial need to control themselves, others, and situations, will tend to rise to positions of power and control, becoming our bosses, managers, instructors, etc. Meanwhile, the more laid back folks avoid those positions of power, precisely because those positions are both anxiety-evoking and anxiety-ridden. The effect of this upward psychosocial drift of the control-hungry people in society to positions of power and authority, when this occurs at the level of the entire population or culture, is a social structure where the most anxious people are in charge of everything and everyone, stressing everybody out about everything, so that high stress and high anxiety become the new norm, and everyone has to play along, because the expectations for stress and anxiety come down from the top, in a tyranny of the anxious.

One more reason why declining literacy will not necessarily result in a decline in anxious depression is that much of the newer media that displace the written word as the primary medium of information create even more anxiety than the written word. If anxiety stems from a perceived need to react to a potentially hostile environment, then an environment perceived as unstable, unpredictable, or uncontrollable, will naturally make us feel insecure and fearful. The media environment we live in now is such an environment. An environment that is in constant flux due to ever-upgrading new media technology inhibits our ability to adapt, so instead of feeling comfortable within our environments, we feel anxious, as McLuhan observed over a half-century ago: "It is plain today that change is not only the constant in our society but that adjustment to change is quite impossible. We have no time to adjust and must substitute, instead, understanding of the process of change."[40] The modern media environment evokes anxiety, not only by its constantly altering presence, but also by its demands for "commitment and participation" in the digital field of social interaction, as McLuhan again prophesied over a half-century ago:

> This is the Age of Anxiety for the reason of the electric implosion that compels commitment and participation, quite regardless of any "point of view." The partial and specialized character of the viewpoint, however noble, will not serve at all in the electric age.... If the 19th Century was the age of the editorial chair, ours is the century of the psychiatrist's couch.[41]

Digital media in particular seem to manufacture anxiety and depression in ways that are much more powerful and direct than literacy. Whereas older media such as the written word, movies, and television, offered passive engagement without participation, digital media is inherently interactive. However, unlike physical interaction, digital interaction never completely resolves itself, never completes its action, but rather is perpetually engaged in re-action. A digital post evokes a response, and that response evokes another response, and another and another and another... Unlike a printed book, magazine, or newspaper that has a last page, digital homescreens for news and social media typically have an "infinite scroll" function, which loads content continuously as the user scrolls down the page, so the page never ends. The news feeds, the tweets, the snaps, the posts, the comments—they never stop. The never-ending cycle of reaction never satisfactorily finds resolution, as it never formally resolves into a settling of all disputes, or a restful unworried disengagement. There will always be another tweet, another text, another post, another annoying selfie to comment upon, another anxiety-provoking news feed to look at.

These anxiety-evoking effects of the media are compounded by the similar effects of the media content, which in many cases consist of dismaying reports of global warming, associated natural catastrophes, impending plagues, horrifying acts of terrorism, and shocking acts of political corruption. Because fear sells, it's constantly being sold to us in the form of "news," but unlike a newspaper or an old-fashioned TV, digital news comes to us 24/7 without respite, an incessant barrage of terrifying, horrific, unnerving fear. By extending consciousness into the digital world and, via the internet, linking it with infinite information, digital media allows us to linger and ruminate indefinitely on the fears of our future, as well as the failures of the present/past.

People of my generation learned in school that if we studied long and worked hard, we could master our environments and find those elusive, mythical places called "success" and "happiness." No one told us that within our lifetimes, the rules of the game would change, as the medium of the game itself morphed from paper books, letters, and articles to digital screens displaying electronic information. Less than a century ago, our media environment was largely dominated by print media. As that environment steadily and quickly dissolves into the mercurial and ethereal landscape of electronic and digital media, we exchange the security and dependability of knowledge acquired from books and newspapers, for the speed, convenience, and variety of ever-changing information gleaned from a scrolling screen that is constantly changing and never-ending. Once again, McLuhan foresaw this transition over a half-century ago: "Inner direction towards remote goals is inseparable from print culture.... The fact that no such culture is compatible with electronic simultaneity is what has involved Western man in new anxiety for a century."[42]

I have little doubt that digital social media platforms such as Facebook, Twitter, Snapchat, Instagram and the like, are the primary culprit in establishing new generations of anxiously depressed media consumers. The hyperconscious mind is always doubting itself and its host (its body and identity). How am I to know if I'm a success or a failure? How do I know if I deserve to be happy, or if I need to work much harder to become the kind of person who's deserving of the self-complacent state of happiness? The only way to know is via "social comparison," the act of comparing our lives, bodies, and identities with the lives, bodies, and identities of others. Social comparison is the standard method we use to measure our psychosocial selves.

The problem with social comparison is that it invariably leads to dissatisfaction with yourself, because there will always be someone prettier, taller, richer, cooler, or in some way better than you are. Social comparison is a game you can't win, because it will always make you feel like a loser. The danger of digital social media is that it provides a media environment filled with infinite images and portraits of infinite people doing infinite things. The average person can never compare favorably to the profiles of all those people, in large part because people rarely if ever post negative images or information about themselves. "Fa[k] ebook" and other social media are fantasy worlds projected by consumers, consisting of fantasies of how they would like to be perceived, with all the un-fantastic bits censored out. The danger of these platforms is that people compare their own real lives with the fake lives on the Fakebook pages of others, causing them to feel inferior, self conscious, anxious, and depressed, because everybody on Fakebook seems to be much better off than they are. One cannot even adopt the passive tactic of nonengagement made famous in the movie *War Games* (1983)— "the only winning move is not to play"—because if one refuses to engage in social media, one runs the risk of being called "asocial," "antisocial," "unfriendly" or even "autistic."

The effect of digital and social media on our sense of identities is explored in depth in Chapter Seven. For now, it's time to move beyond anxious depression, in order to focus on the primary manufacturer of anxiety in our society: School...

• Six •

Disordered Learning
and Neurological Intolerance

That we continue to prescribe drugs to our children in such massive numbers is appalling.

There are no historical precedents for a society perpetrating such a travesty on its offspring.

—Joseph Chilton Pearce (2004)[1]

It is more difficult to provide uniqueness and diversity than it is to impose the uniform patterns of mass education; but it is such uniqueness and diversity that can be fostered under electric conditions as never before.

—Marshall McLuhan (1964)[2]

More than four billion people in the world wear glasses, primarily because of myopia, a medical condition precipitated in most cases by the ocular strain required for reading.[3] If literacy has clear and present physical consequences, such as the permanent degradation of our vision, then we shouldn't be surprised to "see" that there are equally clear and present psychological consequences. There's no argument that "learning disabilities" such as dyslexia (aka reading disorder) and dysgraphia (aka writing disorder) would not exist if reading and writing were not required to be mastered by nearly every child in the post-industrial world. *Learning disorders do not exist in preliterate societies.* These disorders, and all the pain and strain experienced by affected schoolchildren, as well as their parents and teachers, can be considered direct consequences of literacy. Similar learning disabilities such as dyscalculia (aka mathematics disorder) can be considered an extension of the same consequences, as mathematics, in its elementary form (arithmetic), is essentially a form of literacy (I explain this idea later in this chapter).[4]

One further extension of the consequences of literacy includes the specific type of attention required by the mind of a child to focus on literacy-based tasks for extended periods of time. Children whose minds aren't adept at this specific type of highly focused attention are labeled "ADHD" (Attention Deficit Hyperactivity Disorder). Cumulatively, these direct and dire consequences of literacy—dyslexia, dysgraphia, dyscalculia, and ADHD—affect nearly a third of schoolchildren worldwide, with most of these children co-morbidly diagnosed with two, three, or even all four of the disorders mentioned above.[5]

ADHD

> *Of course Johnny must read. He must follow the lines of print. He must roll that hoop down the walk. He must roll his eyes in lineal, sequential fashion. We have only to proceed to engraft the old right-handedness on his new left-handedness in order to win our point. But in the meantime we shall have lost his attention, and he may be subdued, but he will be utterly confused.*
>
> —Marshall McLuhan (1959)

Attention deficit hyperactivity disorder is the most prevalent psychiatric disorder among schoolchildren in America, affecting nearly 10 percent of all children (and 13 percent of all boys).[6] Most of these six million children—some of them as young as two years old—are taking some form of prescribed medication for their attention issues. While ADHD is diagnosed in other countries and also treated with medication in other countries, America claims the extremely dubious honor of having both the highest diagnostic rates of ADHD, and the highest medication rates for children diagnosed with ADHD. Perhaps even more troubling than these grave statistics is the fact that everyone, especially psychiatrists, knows that ADHD is for the most part a childhood issue, but not because the attention of ADHD kids suddenly balloons once they hit adulthood—ADHD is a childhood issue because it's evoked by the specific media environment that children are forced, often unwillingly, to adapt to. Once children leave the literacy-based media environment of the classroom, once they're free to play and to focus their attention in ways that are more congruent with their particular ways of thinking, the symptoms of attention deficit, for the most part, either simply go away or become manageable to the point where no true dysfunction is apparent.

Similarly, once children grow up and move into work environments where they have more control over the way they focus their attention, their childhood symptoms of inattention simply go away. This case example provided by psychiatrist Richard Friedman in a 2014 article in the *New York Times* illustrates my point:

> A patient of mine, a 28-year-old man, was having a lot of trouble at his desk job in an advertising firm. Having to sit at a desk for long hours and focus his attention on one task was nearly impossible. He would multitask, listening to music and texting, while "working" to prevent activities from becoming routine. Eventually he quit his job and threw himself into a start-up company, which has him on the road in constantly changing environments. He is much happier and—little surprise—has lost his symptoms of A.D.H.D. My patient "treated" his A.D.H.D simply by changing the conditions of his work environment from one that was highly routine to one that was varied and unpredictable. All of a sudden, his greatest liabilities—his impatience, short attention span and restlessness—became assets.[7]

In his article, Dr. Friedman posits an evolutionary model of attention, which assumes that neurodiversity in attention is extremely important for the adaptability of our species:

> Consider that humans evolved over millions of years as nomadic hunter-gatherers. It was not until we invented agriculture, about 10,000 years ago, that we settled down and started living more sedentary—and boring—lives. As hunters, we had to adapt to an ever-changing environment where the dangers were as unpredictable as our next meal. In such a context, having a rapidly shifting but intense attention span and a taste for novelty would have proved highly advantageous in locating and securing rewards—like a mate and a nice chunk of mastodon. In short, having the profile of what we now call A.D.H.D. would have made you a Paleolithic success story.... Recent neuroscience research shows that people with A.D.H.D. are actually hard-wired for novelty-seeking—a trait that had, until relatively recently, a distinct evolutionary advantage.... In short, people with A.D.H.D. may not have a disease, so much as a set of behavioral traits that don't match the expectations of our contemporary culture.[8]

While Friedman acknowledges that "Some of the rising prevalence of A.D.H.D. is doubtless driven by the pharmaceutical industry, whose profitable drugs are the mainstay of treatment," he believes that the highly contrasting media environments that exist for the child inside and outside of the classroom play a major role as well:

> ... the increasingly stark contrast between the regimented and demanding school environment and the highly stimulating digital world, where young people spend their time outside school ... would seem even duller to a novelty-seeking kid living in the early 21st century than in previous decades, and the comparatively boring school environment might accentuate students' inattentive behavior, making their teachers more likely to see it and driving up the number of diagnoses.[9]

Returning to the brain and the "leftward shift" model, the classroom is an environment created to teach literacy, an environment that promotes the shift in hemispheric dominance for attending leftwards, towards the hemisphere that specializes in deep focused sequential tasks. The classroom environment is unconducive to learning for many (if not most) children for many reasons—reasons that are addressed in this chapter one by one...

Decontextualized Learning

Information is alienated experience.

—Jaron Lanier[10]

All things have a context. Learning about something within its context helps us to understand the whole thing in relation to the things around it. For example, if one wants to learn about the life of a lion, the ideal way to study this would be to observe the lion in its natural habitat, where you can see it hunt, mate, fight for dominance, etc. Studying a lion by observing it in the zoo is less ideal, because the zoo is not the lion's natural habitat ... the lion has been decontextualized from its home in the jungle and stationed for observation in its cell in the zoo. Therefore, as a product of its decontextualization, the zoo lion doesn't give you a very good idea of what the life of a lion is really like. Studying a lion by reading about it in a textbook in a classroom is least ideal, because the information is completely decontextualized. Both the subject of the lion and the subject's context, the lion's habitat, are decontextualized and represented abstractly in the book. The child is not learning directly about anything.

Lions are of course not part of ordinary schools, so they must be decontextualized for the sake of safe and convenient study. Decontextualizing something also makes it easier to study it in detail, because you can isolate, freeze, and zoom into specific details in ways that you can't do with real subjects existing in real time within their real contexts. Nevertheless, decontextualized learning will always offer only a partial restricted view of a subject. Subjects usually need to be recontextualized in order to be fully understood.

More significantly for the present discussion, if a media environment such as a classroom functions via a process of decontextualization, there will be many students whose minds are not predisposed towards that sort of learning. What about the students who learn better when things are learned within their context? What about students whose minds seek to grasp an understanding of a whole subject, in which each topic is perceived as an interactive component of the whole, rather than as an isolated unit of decontextualized information? These students, whose brains are likely to be less lateralized towards left hemispheric dominance, are also likely to be labeled "ADHD," simply because their mode of attending is divergent from the norm.

In short, an analytical and deconstructive mindset favors decontextualized learning, while a holistic and gestalt mindset favors learning about subjects within their contexts. Ideally, a balance between both learning styles would encourage learning and thinking in both ways. Unfortunately, schools—because of their reliance on literacy as their primary mode of media engagement—mainly provide only one type of learning, the decontextualized type.

The Classroom: A Toxic Media Environment

> *The classroom is now a place of detention, not attention.*
> *Attention is elsewhere.*
>
> —Marshall McLuhan[11]

The world we live in now—the digital media environment—provides stimuli in ways that are much more engaging than the way that stimuli are presented in the classroom. The problem of the "distracted" or "inattentive" child is currently dealt with primarily by adjusting the attention of the child biochemically using drugs, even though it seems quite clear that the problem lies in the media environment of the classroom, and in the huge discrepancy between the classroom media environment, and the media environment that children are immersed in outside of the classroom. McLuhan noted this extremely important discrepancy over a half-century ago, well before digital media became mainstream, when television was the most recent innovation in media technology:

> The TV child finds it difficult if not impossible to adjust to the fragmented visual goals of our education system after having had all his senses involved by the electric media; he craves in-depth involvement, not linear detachment and uniform sequential patterns. But suddenly and without preparation, he is snatched from the cool, inclusive womb of television and exposed—within a vast bureaucratic structure of courses and credits—to the hot medium of print. His natural instinct, conditioned by the electric media, is to bring all his senses to bear on the book he's instructed to read, and print resolutely rejects that approach, demanding an isolated visual attitude to learning rather than the *Gestalt* approach of the unified sensorium. The reading postures of children in elementary school are a pathetic testimonial to the effects of television: children of the TV generation separate book from eye by an average distance of four and a half inches, attempting psychomimetically to bring to the printed page the

all-inclusive sensory experience of TV. They are becoming Cyclops, desperately seeking to wallow in the book as they do in the TV screen.[12]

Boredom in the classroom is considered a given, but why? From a media psychology perspective, boredom in the consumer is an indication that either the medium or the medium's content isn't stimulating enough. If I were a programming director at a TV station and I found out that my viewers were tuning out because they were bored, I would immediately get to work changing either the content of my programming, or adjusting aspects of the medium itself to make it more stimulating. I wouldn't attempt to alter the brain chemistry of my viewers in order to get them to sit still and keep watching the boring media.... I'd change the media.

Obviously, the government or the forces-that-be would never allow me to introduce powerful psychoactive substances into the delicate brains of my young viewers, simply because they find my media boring. If so, then why does the government or the forces-that-be allow, and often insist, that millions of schoolchildren be drugged in order for them to sit still and be quiet while they're exposed to media that bore the hell out of them? While there are many targets to point the finger at—pharmaceutical companies who profit from selling drugs, psychiatrists who profit by writing prescriptions for drugs, school administrators, counselors, and teachers who recommend and often insist that their students take drugs in order for their classrooms to function efficiently, parents who follow the advice of the "experts" and make their children take drugs in order for their children to conform to the behavioral norms of the classroom—but in the long run, I truly believe that all of the people mentioned above have the best interests of the children in their hearts, they just don't know of any other viable options.

I have vivid memories of being so bored in school as a child that I created entire fantasy worlds in my mind, replete with characters and settings and far out plots. McLuhan compared the boredom of a schoolchild to certain forms of hypnosis and torture. Hypnosis, and some forms of meditation as well, occur as a function of narrowing your sense perceptions down to *one* point of focus—"a steady assault on one sense, like a tribal drumbeat"[13]—resulting in a trancelike state of cognitive simplicity. Mental torture, on the other hand, can be achieved via confinement in a room where *all* senses are unstimulated, like in solitary confinement. "Modern torturers in Chile break down prisoners by putting them in cells where everything—walls, furniture, utensils, window covers—is painted white."[14]

The classroom of my own childhood seemed just as sterile as the Chilean torture chamber, evoking a profound sense of boredom that at first seemed like torture, until it softened into a hypnotic inward focus, leading to the freedom of mind that I could only experience within. But is it really necessary to force children to sit in a torture chamber called the "classroom" for hour upon hour, day upon day, year upon year, just so they could learn? There seems to be a culturally shared and accepted fact that school is torture for most kids, but that's ok because it's always been that way. It was torture for me when I was a kid, and now it's torture for my kids. It's like a form of sociocultural hazing that everyone must go through. But why? Can't we create a school environment where learning is interesting and engaging rather than understimulating and boring? Can't we educate our kids without torturing them or forcing them to retreat into the stupor of a self-hypnotic state of detachment?

When we put a child in a media environment called a "classroom," and that child shows the classic symptoms of boredom—fidgeting, disengaging, getting distracted, seeking stimulation, etc.—we presume that the problem is not in the media environment at all, but in the child's brain. The current etiological theory of ADHD is the "Understimulation Theory"—which posits that ADHD is caused by a chemical imbalance resulting in understimulation of the brain's perceptual processes. This theory was created and advanced by backwards science, as a way of explaining and thereby rationalizing the fact that psycho-stimulants seem to increase attention in kids with ADHD.

The fact of the matter is, any psycho-stimulant, whether it's Ritalin, caffeine, amphetamine, or cocaine, will increase arousal and thereby increase focus and attention. When I wake up in the morning, I'm still mostly asleep. I'm understimulated, under-aroused. I cannot focus or pay attention to anything until I've ingested a powerful psychostimulant, the caffeine in my morning cup of coffee. I know perfectly well why I experience such a severe state of attention-deficit when I wake up. It's because I'm addicted to caffeine, and I'm going through caffeine withdrawal. The more significant question is, why do people diagnosed with ADHD experience similar severe states of attention-deficit in certain situations?

The current medical model of ADHD presumes that symptoms of inattention are caused by a chemical imbalance, resulting in a deficit in the presence of the neurotransmitter dopamine in the brain. The only evidence behind the underarousal theory is the fact that, when given psychostimulants that increase the presence of dopamine in the brain, children with noted attention deficit exhibit demonstrably increased focal attention for as long as the drugs are in effect. However, we all know that psychostimulants increase arousal, thereby enhancing attention. That's what they do! Just like my morning cup of coffee. Yes, Ritalin has a more pronounced effect on attention in children diagnosed with ADHD than in children without the diagnosis, but that doesn't prove the validity of the disorder, or of the treatment.

Psychostimulants increase attentiveness in everyone. The more inattentive you are, the more pronounced the effect will be. So while the underarousal theory gives some level of rationalization for the medication of millions of children with powerful drugs in order to make them pay attention the way we want them to, it doesn't even come close to answering the real question, which remains: "Why do people diagnosed with ADHD seem to be more inattentive than others in certain situations?"

Answering this question by positing a "chemical imbalance" in the brain of millions of children is at best unhelpful and at worse extremely damaging. The brain does one thing: It adapts to our environment. Every neuron and every process in the brain is ultimately functioning towards the never ending goal of ecological adaptation. If a child's brain is truly understimulated, the obvious reason is that there isn't enough stimulation in the environment. That is, the media in which the stimulation is being provided are insufficient to sustain the child's attention. Placing the fault for the problem inside the child's brain rather than in the media environment surrounding the brain is, again, wrong.

Chemicals in the brain are merely responding to their environment. Mediating inattentiveness in schoolchildren by changing the balance of chemicals in their brains is like mediating restlessness in your dog by giving him a sedative. If the dog is restless, it's because he needs more exercise. Sedating the dog mediates the restlessness, but only temporarily. Similarly, giving a child Ritalin does seem to increase attentiveness, but only temporarily. The next day, or even later on in the same day, he'll need more Ritalin, because the issue of inattentiveness wasn't resolved, only the behavioral symptoms were temporarily treated. This is why we usually see significant behavioral changes after administering Ritalin—the child is less fidgety, less active, less disruptive—but actual learning does not necessarily improve significantly over the long term. The sedated dog is not getting the exercise he needs, he's just not acting like he needs exercise. Similarly, the drugged child is not focusing in a way that really enhances learning, he's just not acting like he's understimulated and inattentive, and thus he's less disruptive in the classroom, and less of a problem for the teacher.

The drug is a tool, a powerful tool, and its main use is to modify the behavior of the child by altering his brain chemistry, in order for the child to conform to the cultural norms of the classroom environment— to be quiet and docile and undisruptive. The drugged child is likely to become psychologically and neurologically dependent on this drug. The obvious reason for the child's perceived deficits—deficient or inefficient stimulation in his environment—is overlooked. Why? Because it's far easier to change the mind and behavior of a five-year-old child with a simple pill than to change the structure and operation of a 500-year-old institution that has not significantly altered its approach to teaching since its inception.

If we think of the standard education model as an institution devoted primarily to the mastery of literacy in languages and math, with the various subject matters providing the content for the mastery of the medium, then we can easily see that the standard education model in today's world has become obsolete, and ill-equipped to prepare modern students for the new world of digitality. For the most part, the children and adolescents of today learn to master digital media outside of the classroom, while time inside the classroom is devoted to obsolete learning methods.

The old "one-size-fits-all" model of education, in particular, seems a relic of a bygone age. The old model puts too much emphasis on only two media of thought—linguistic and logico-mathematical—to the near exclusion of the musical, the artistic, the naturalistic, the bodily-kinesthetic, etc. The old model is intolerant towards minds that are not well-formatted for linguistic and logico-mathematical modes of communication. This intolerance of neurological diversity is the reason why such a large percentage of modern students are treated as disabled and labeled with psychopathologies such as ADHD, dyslexia, and other behavioral, language, and learning disorders. The old model depends almost entirely on passive, unimodal, decontextualized, and obsolete modes of engagement, such as listening quietly to lectures, memorizing facts and mathematical procedures by rote, and repetitively calculating numbers by hand.

In the digital world, learning needs to reflect modern modes of engagement that are interactive rather than passive, multimodal rather than unimodal, and focused on finding, using, and integrating the limitless information that is now instantly accessible, rather than on needlessly memorizing information and procedures and regurgitating them on tests, for the sole purpose of demonstrating effort in schoolwork. The assessment driven world of academia is consumed by a constant need to prove and reaffirm that students are busy learning, so we give them busywork to prove it. The teachers are then consumed with the busywork of inventing new tests and assignments and then administering and grading them. The principals and other administrators have their hands full with busywork too, making sure that everyone else's busywork is in proper order.

The same system extends through colleges and universities and beyond. But with all of us so consumed in busywork all the time, we forget that the true effects of the education system on thought and learning are not achieved through the content of education (busywork), but through the medium (literacy). "The medium is the message." If an education system is based on literacy, it will manifest itself in literary form—busywork—and it will evaluate itself only according to the measures of its own standards. Creative yodeling is typically not a significant advantage for a student in the public education system, because it cannot be translated into a high mark on a standardized test, nor does it lend itself to literary exposition, so it can't be used for busywork. But in a nonliteracy-based media environment, such as the digital environment fostered by streaming video sharing platforms like YouTube, creative yodeling would be much more popular and successful as media content, and would certainly gain more views and likes than a page of small black coded symbols slowly scrolling downwards and from left to right against a white background.

The world our children are inheriting is changing at the speed of light, because that's the speed of information when it's traveling via electric signal. Rather than preparing them for this new world, we sequester them in tabernacles of obsolescing media, and stupefy them with overloads of information that are not remembered beyond the test date, because information is only retained in the ever-efficient brain when it serves some practical purpose, and once you've passed the test, in most cases, the information has no more value, especially in a digital world, where virtually all information is instantly accessible. The ancient academies prized literary information so highly because the ancient scrolls were so rare, and each scroll represented countless hours of labor by scholars and scribes.

There was no greater tragedy in antiquity than the burning of the library at Alexandria by fire. But now that we live in a world where information, in the form of electronic digital signals, is literally swarming through every inch of our physical and psychological environments, we can finally admit that information, in-and-of-itself, is useless. Unless we put something to use, it's use-less. Our current education focuses on stuffing information into children's heads, and then testing them to see if they remember it. If the information is not put to any practical use other than being regurgitated for the test, then once the test is over, the highly efficient brain will soon forget the useless information.

When I was a child, I "learned" (i.e., memorized) the names and inauguration dates of each of the first ten U.S. presidents, and each of the ten most recent U.S. presidents. I forgot just about all of that information almost immediately after taking the test. So what was the point of memorizing the information? As far as I can tell, the content of the learning (names and dates) was relatively inconsequential. This I know, because I've lived many years since then, and have *never* needed to use *any* of that information. So if the content of school learning (information) is relatively inconsequential (especially in the age of instantly accessible infinite information) then we must admit that the useless information is merely serving as the content of a medium (literacy) and the content's entire raison d'être is to be used as exercise in literacy-based tasks, so that the medium of literacy is mastered. In short, the curriculum of academia is media content, and it's only purpose is to serve as practice for mastering the medium of literacy, which means that it doesn't really matter what we make Johnny read and what we make Susie write, just as long as we get them to read and write.

Information in school is gained primarily by reading, and its recollection is tested by written assignments and examinations. These literary tasks, the heart and soul of academia, are obsolete in a world where information must be accessed quickly and used interactively as a means to producing something beyond a literary re-representation of the information itself. *Information in the digital world is a means to an end, not an end in itself.* Learning by repetition and memorization is obsolete in the age of instant access to all information. Learning math by memorizing times tables and repeating calculation after calculation by hand is obsolete in a world where all calculations done outside of the classroom are processed by machines.

The products of the digital age—computers and calculators—perform the function of storing information and making calculations quite efficiently. Digital age students need to learn how to apply intellectual and mathematical concepts, rather than wasting time and energy imitating the functions of computers and calculators. Students are people, not machines. Digital age students need to learn how to gather and organize information in order to discern and express new patterns of thought, rather than wasting mental energy memorizing facts that will soon be forgotten, and that are accessible instantly with just a swipe on a phone.

If Education as a field emerged as a response to the demands of literacy and the need to create new generations of literate citizens, then Education must now accept the fact that digital media have subsumed literacy, and that the demands of a digital society require a new approach to education, an approach that reflects a digital sensibility towards information and learning...

> The outer environment is a great big teaching machine charged with messages, whereas the inner environment of the schoolroom is paltry, feeble, specialist, classified data, like looking up words in a dictionary.—Marshall McLuhan[15]

Most importantly, Education must accept neurological diversity as a fact, and it must stop trying to force square pegs into round holes...

Literacy and Education: A Brief and Brutal History

> In ordinary human past, there'd been more in knowledge and information available inside the classroom condition than outside. With this spectacular reversal of this condition, it would seem to be possible that the business of the school has also reversed, that the business of the school is no longer instruction but discovery. And the business of the teaching establishment is to train perception upon the outer environment instead of merely stenciling information upon the brain pans of children inside the environment.
>
> —Marshall McLuhan[16]

Literacy has its roots in the development of the first phonetic alphabets in the Near East about 4,000 years ago. For several thousand years, literacy was an extremely specialized skill mastered only by a few scribes, clerics, and scholars. In agricultural societies where nearly everyone labored in the fields or engaged in some form of ranching, craft, or manual labor, mass literacy was unnecessary. Only after the Industrial Revolution in the late 18th century did the need for a population of literate citizens arise. Public education arose to meet this need in the Western world in the 19th century, but it didn't reach the point where the majority of children went to school until well into the 20th century. Therefore, the democratization of literacy via public education—*mass literacy*—has only been around for a little over a century, and that only in the post-industrial world.

Prior to the 20th century, the vast majority of the world's population was illiterate. By the mid–20th century, it was estimated that more than half of the world's population was literate. By the end of the 20th century, about three-quarters of the world's population was literate. The numbers now seem to be increasing at the rate of about 5 percent a decade.[17] Since literacy is a highly specialized skill that takes years and years of training to master, the project of educating billions of people a year in literacy requires a form of industrialized mass education that resembles, in practice, the industrialization processes of modern societies that heralded the need for mass education in the first place.

Mass education (aka "public education") was born as a byproduct of the Industrial Revolution. Print technology, the first true industrial system of mass manufacturing standardized products, and also the first mass medium, created the shared information network necessary for inventors and engineers and entrepreneurs to recreate the Western world from an agricultural society into an industrial one. The new industrial world needed workers. Farmers and their families, who could no longer compete with industrialized agriculture, left their ancestral farms to work in industry. Children, who had always worked on farms with their families, were now put to work in factories.

The horrific conditions of industrial child labor were appalling. Furthermore, children were now taking away desperately needed industrial jobs from adult men who had to support their families. Western governments, aware of the horrors of factory labor for children, and also aware of growing socio-political tensions caused by mass poverty and unemployment, realized that their new industrial societies needed to breed a new generation of workers, people who could not only operate industrial machines, but repair and build new ones. This new industrial world also needed people who could specialize in certain fields: engineers, electricians, doctors, lawyers, accountants, etc. In short, print technology, the first industry and the first mass medium, created a demand for more people who could read and write. This industrial demand for literate industrialists would be supplied by yet another industry: Education.

In his bestselling book *The Perfectionists: How Precision Engineers Created the Modern World* (2018), Simon Winchester explains how the standardization of precision instruments and industrial parts made mass industrialization feasible, thus remolding the shape of the world in the image of industry. Industrialization and standardization of products go hand-in-hand. In an industrial environment, innumerable basic things like faucet heads and lighting fixtures need to be made according to precise standard measures, so that most mechanical things have interchangeable parts. Mass production on a large scale is only achievable when the machinery is assembled with standard precision parts that are interchangeable. When everything is made to the same precise measurements, the wheels of industry keep moving, unhindered by broken parts, because all industrial parts and products were interchangeable and thus easily replaced.

When Education arose in the wake of the Industrial Age, the same template was applied to this new industry, whose job was to mass produce multitudes of literate people for the industrial world. The brains of these people were assumed to be essentially the same in reference to learning. That is, all people have brains that learn in the same way, therefore, all people can be taught in the same way. In this way, the industrial process was applied to the education process, creating a standardizable system of manufacturing literate people, whose cognitive functions were all presumed to be precisely the same. The minds of all students and all future workers were meant to be standard, interchangeable, and easily replaceable. The Education industry applied a standardized curriculum, standardizing the same methods and materials for all students, presuming that the brains of all students were a "tabula rasa," or blank slate, for learning, just like a sheet of paper is a blank page for printed material. This presumption, we now realize, couldn't be more wrong. The brain is not a blank slate at all!

Human brains are born "hardwired" for many faculties, and they're quite divergent in the variety and array of those "wirings." No two brains are exactly the same, even in identical twins. Brains are also constantly adapting to their environments in real time, via the establishment and management of neural connections, and through epigenetic adaptations in the expression of genetic traits. The mistaken presumption that all brains are the same (standard), and thus all children's learning should be the same (standard), gave birth to the standardized curriculum (aka the "push-down curriculum"), which utilizes standardized teaching methods, and standard assessments via standardized testing.

Winchester makes the point very early in his book that precision is only feasible in certain materials, like metal. Organic materials like wood are no good in terms of true industrial-grade precision, because wood breathes—it's alive—and always adapting to its environment. Precision is only possible in nonorganic materials that are insensitive enough to their environment, in that they stay exactly the same regardless of subtle changes in their surroundings. The brain, though very complex, is not a precision instrument, *precisely because it's incredibly sensitive to its environment*, and is constantly changing. In handling organic brains as if they were standardizable products, the Education industry created an industrial byproduct in the form of a large subset of students who could not conform to the rigid curriculum. For many decades, these students tended to drop out early and earn a living without the benefit of a standard education.

In his well-known book *In the Mind's Eye: Creative Visual Thinkers, Gifted Dyslexics, and the Rise of Visual Technologies* (2009), Thomas West provides many stories of people who could barely function at school, dropped out, and went on to become major successes in a diverse array of fields. However, as the post-industrial world itself became more standardized, it became less feasible for even the brightest young people to find gainful employment without some level of formal education. When dropping out no longer became a viable option for the students whose natural ways of attending didn't fit the standard mold, they stayed and suffered. Most of them were sent to "special" schools or "special" classes to be taught the standard curriculum, but in a "special" way.

The latter decades of the 20th century saw rapid change in the treatment of children who required "special education" services. New laws passed by the Supreme Court mandated that students must be included in the general classroom if at all possible, rather than excluded and sent off to "special classes" or "special schools." Happening concurrently was the pharmaceutical revolution in psychiatry, which shifted treatment models for everyone—including children—from psychotherapeutic and cognitive-behavioral therapies to psychopharmacological medication. Now, many of the "special" students who formerly would've been in special ed. classes or special ed. schools, were now subdued biochemically in order to exist in the standard classroom while not being disruptive to others. This is the standard treatment.

In the short but brutal history of education, it was accepted that teachers could and should beat their students with paddles, whips, and rods, in order to force them to learn the curriculum, and in order to force them to conform to the behavioral norms of the classroom. To a large extent, these brutal tactics have fallen out of use, not so much because they were cruel, but because they were inefficient in subduing the brain into complete conformity. The paddle, the whip, and the rod afflicted the body directly, but only indirectly affected the child's mind, and even less so his brain. The new weapons of psychological conformity are much more efficient, and in their own insidious ways, more brutal. A drug such as Ritalin doesn't cause physical pain, but it causes psychological dependency, physical side effects, and worst of all, a crushing blow to the child's self esteem, who must accept the fact that his brain is "abnormal," and that his ways of learning and thinking are, in certain ways, "deficient."

Specialism versus Generalism

> *The more information one has to evaluate, the less one knows.*
> *Specialism cannot exist at the speed of light.*
>
> —McLuhan & Powers[18]

Our brains evolved over millions of years in the capacity of hunters and gatherers and, more recently, over the past 12,000 years or so, as farmers and ranchers. The occupations of hunter/gatherer and farmer/rancher are generalist occupations. A hunter/gatherer is an opportunist who hustles for a living, following anything that may lead him to food, whether it's animal prey, fruit on the trees, berries on the bushes, roots in the ground, fish in the stream—whatever's around. Similarly, on the farm, a man may work in the fields in the morning, and then find himself a carpenter in the afternoon—mending a fence or building a shed—and then become a cooper at dusk, constructing a barrel for the apples in his orchard. On Monday he's a rancher breaking in a horse, on Tuesday he's a shepherd shearing his sheep, on Wednesday he's a butcher at work on a pig, on Thursday a veterinarian for a birthing cow, on Friday a hunter of deer, on Saturday a fisher of fish, on Sunday a mechanic repairing a cart, and every evening he's a musician and storyteller for his kids. The farm matron, even more so, is a mistress of many jobs. All of these tasks are vocational, not incidental. Catching a fish so that your family could eat fish for dinner rather than just vegetables and grains isn't a hobby, it's a job. Similarly, the housewife who nurses and cares for the baby, cooks every meal from scratch, sews clothing, spins thread, cleans the house, washes the clothes, pickles vegetables, jams fruit, bakes bread and cake is fulfilling a generalist occupation. Since the dawn of humanity, we've been learning to master our environments as generalists—jacks-of-all trades—dilettantes who can adapt our knowledge and skills to every task at hand.

Now, in the post-industrial world, we go to school to learn how to become specialists. Literacy is the embodiment of specialist work. Unlike hunting or farming, literacy is not a task that can be learned on the job by observing someone else and then working on it yourself with minimal direct instruction. Literacy, a specialist task, takes years and years of direct instruction. It takes years of intense focus on specific details—letters, grammatical rules, punctuation—until the specialist literate person emerges. The same is true for math and other specialist domains. The modern world, shaped and invented by the very recent focus of humans on literacy and education, has become a world in which we're expected to master our environments as specialists. If a modern man's car is broken, he takes it to a mechanic—he doesn't dare to try fix it himself. If his fence falls down, he calls a carpenter. If his pipe bursts he calls a plumber. For a dark house he calls an electrician, for a cold house he calls a furnace repairman, a hot house requires an air conditioning repairman, and so on. We live in a world of specialists now, a world created by literacy, because literacy demands and therefore engenders education, and education specializes in creating specialists of every kind...

> As is the biblical story of the Tower of Babel, the architects will no longer know how to speak to the engineers; the stonemasons will no longer understand the carpenters; the laborers will no longer be able to call the water carriers. Excessive specialization seems to bear the seeds of its own destruction.[19]—Thomas West

The primary tool of literacy, the book, is only useful if it specializes in a specific subject. A book about everything would be useless. When we go to school, we begin by learning to read books. The function of school is to teach us the specialist craft of book-reading, along with the associated specializations of writing and mathematics. We learn the fundamental "elements" of education—the three "R's." The old word for elementary school, "grammar school," encapsulates the notion even better. We begin by learning the medium of literacy itself, the basic grammar of letters and words, as well as numbers and calculations. Once we understand the basic grammar of the medium, we specialize by dividing our attention into specific subjects: History, Science, Social Studies, etc. At first the different subjects are divided by specific periods with specific textbooks within the same classroom, but eventually, the process of specialization requires separate classrooms with specialized teachers in each subject. The high school degree is a specialist degree in literacy, the content areas—history, science, social studies, etc.—are incidental. The only thing high school truly qualifies anyone for nowadays is the pursuit of a more specialist degree in college.

Higher education, in turn, presents another universe of specialties. Every class presents a specific topic for study (e.g., media psychology), every professor is specialized in his own field (my specialization, for example, is developmental psychology, with a focus on media), every specialized professor teaches in his own department (e.g., psychology), every department resides in its own specialized division (e.g., social sciences), and every division is in its own school (e.g., arts and sciences). Each college student must select a major, which typically means that when they graduate, they are ready to "commence" even further specialization in graduate school, where they will attain the degree that certifies their mastery in an area so specific that only people with those specialist certifications are allowed to practice that particular specialization. The course of continuously more specialized education culminating in a very specific profession follows the analog of literacy. Each individual, like a book, becomes a storehouse of specialist information and specialist abilities.

After following the road of literacy and specialism for 500 years, we're now presented with a new medium. The digital medium is a generalist medium. It shakes the very foundation of education as we know it, because it belies the notion that each individual must specialize his attention and understanding. When information is instantaneously and universally accessible, we no longer need specialization, as long as each individual generalist is capable of accessing and then applying the information at hand. Given a good enough YouTube instructional video and a 3D printer that can manufacture parts and tools, I can fix my own car, making the specialist trade of the auto mechanic obsolete. The same principle stands for plumbing, carpentry, air conditioner repair, surgery—*anything.*

Digital media, with its ability to stream audio-visual demonstration, belies the need for literacy itself, and recreates a world where intuitive and adaptive generalists can master their environments without dependence on an endless series of specialists. The old book, made of paper and ink, must specialize—it cannot be about everything. The new "book," composed of interactive and infinite electronic digital information that's instantly updated and accessible in real time, is composed of an ethereal fabric that enables it to transcend specialization. Indeed, what is Google, if not a book about everything?

The 500-year-old tradition of specialist education must now reinvent itself. This is not an option, it *will* happen, because the dominant cultural medium of information has already begun to transform itself. The question is not *if* the transformation in education will happen, but *how.* The invention of the printed book, by its own existence, precipitated the ever-increasing need for books, precipitating the invention of schools to teach the mastery of printed books, and the ever-increasing need for more schooling to master the specialist skills and trades that, of course, were created by the proliferation of education and literacy. The changes in the mind required for literacy and cognitive specialization to take hold are not universal (which is why so many people struggle with school in general and book learning in particular).

The leftward shift in human brain lateralization is just a temporary adaptation to the specialist medium of literacy. As the dominant media change, the brain will re-adapt, likely by shifting rightwards, as the digital media tend to be more generalistic, more holistic, more multisensory, and more multimodal than prior media. Minds in general will probably become less specialized. How could they not, when the brain that has evolved for millions of years to adapt to a generalist context, has only been confronted with a specialist context for a mere century? The resulting backlash of generalist minds being thrust into a specialist context is seen in the designation of new behavioral disorders and cognitive pathologies—ADHD, dyslexia, dysgraphia, dyscalculia—specific disorders that exist only within the context of specialist training in literacy. However worrisome these disorders may be, they must be understood within the context in which they occur (education), and within the world in which they are evoked (the world of specialism).

The shift from specialism to generalism, the neurological shift from left to right, will probably occur from top down pressure. That is, rather than Education encouraging students to take a more gestalt approach to learning, the world outside the classroom will change first, and it will demand a new type of learner, a new kind of thinker. This is happening now. Once the demand for more holistic thinkers outstrips the supply being produced by our education system, it's likely that our education system will begin to change, not due to foresight of the effects of changing media, but due to the practicality of the education industry needing to keep up with its supply of workers who have the ability to perform and compete in the brave new world of digital generalism. In a 1972 lecture entitled "The End of the Work Ethic," McLuhan declared: "The job as specialism, as a fixed position in an organization chart, will not hold up against the simultaneous jostling and the interfacing of simultaneous information. What is taking the place of the job is role-playing."[20]

It seems likely that the education industry as a whole may begin to return to an educational system that preceded it by millennia. Before classrooms, children learned by doing. For crafts that required a lot of doing to learn by experience—crafts such as that of the blacksmith—apprenticeships provided the primary medium of education and vocational training. Learning in these situations avoids the issues mentioned above in relation to specialization and standardization, because learning as an apprentice is contextualized, and the learning itself is experiential rather than abstract, multisensory and multimodal rather than a focus on just one sense (such as vision in literacy), and one modality (such as the book).

While the future of Education is speculative, the present state of Education is manifest. A system that declares nearly a third of its members to be "disordered" because they cannot adapt to the system, must be, in actuality, a disordered system in itself. But as we enter into a new phase of our system, we have the opportunity to take off our blinders so that we understand that a properly operating system doesn't run by designating a third of its members as dysfunctional. To the contrary, a properly operating system recognizes functionality in all of its members, and it also recognizes mass dysfunction in its members as a symptom of its own inherent dysfunction. Only this recognition will allow us to create a new system that is free of "disorder."

Age Segregation and Specialism vs. Age Integration and Generalism

Education has created an "age segregated culture,"[21] in which children learn, adults work, and the elderly retire and engage in leisure activities. Prior to the advent of public education (and in countries where public education is still not provided), children, adults, and the elderly all worked together (usually on a farm or ranch), and they all learned from each other, and they all engaged in leisure activities together as well (though people in traditional agrarian societies, admittedly, have little time for leisure). When the family farm was obsolesced by industrial agriculture, families moved to the city where everybody— including the children and the elderly—went to work in industry. As industrial labor was ill-suited for both the very young and the very old, child labor laws and the system of education were set up for children, and eventually, retirement laws and social security benefits were set up for the old, turning age integrated cultures into age segregated cultures.

Age segregation and specialism go hand-in-hand. The young are expected to specialize their learning in a specific field by late adolescence (choosing a college major), so they can further specialize in a specific field of labor as adults. In the adult world of work, all labor is becoming increasingly specialized. While I work in my office, a landscaper mows my lawn, as a teacher teaches my children, a mechanic fixes my car, a baker bakes my bread, restaurant and food corporation chefs cook my food, doctors tend to my body, dentists to my teeth, and so on. All these different forms of labor are segregated and relegated to specialists. However, the advent of digital technology may reverse this trend, as digitality is a generalist medium, opening the door to generalist workers. If my work revolves around information, there's really no need for me to go to the office, I could just work at home on my computer—a situation that frees me up to mow my own lawn, bake my own bread, cook my own meals, fix my own car, paint my own house, and even, to a certain extent, tend to my own body and teeth.

Applying the generalist model to school, we can just as easily say that if schoolwork is primarily about information, then most if not all schoolwork could be done outside of the school, given the student has a computer and an internet connection. This situation frees the young to become less segregated in the schoolhouse, and more integrated in the adult world of work, where they could learn firsthand how to do many useful things, rather than specializing in only literacy-based tasks. We could even foresee a future in which digital communication technology facilitates the renewal of an age integrated culture, in which the young learn experientially through work, adults are encouraged to continue learning in order to broaden their work lives as generalists rather than specialists, and the elderly can remain integrated in the broader society by continuing their roles as workers, learners, and educators to the young. Thus, in the new virtual environment of the digital arena, people will not be segregated and pigeon-holed into rigid roles and vocations based on specialist skills and arbitrary age brackets, they will be integrated into ongoing communities of lifelong learners—as lifelong-learning workers will engage in an ever-widening variety of skills in many different areas. Ultimately, the distinctions between learning, work, and leisure will be blurred and dissolved, as learning how to do useful things for work could be fun as well.

Another issue raised by living in an age segregated culture is the end-oriented or goal-oriented mindset evoked by functioning in age segregated institutions. If learning is something done by the young in school, and not a lifelong process, then one can easily believe that the goal of going to elementary school is to graduate and go to middle school, where the goal is to graduate and go to high school, where the goal is to graduate and go to college, where the goal is to graduate and go to grad school, where the goal is to graduate and get a job, where the goal is to move up the corporate ladder rung by rung, with the eventual goal of retiring from work altogether. Each phase of life offers another goal to focus on. Schools in particular indoctrinate the goal-oriented mindset, as its structure is set through the many quarters, semesters, grades, and schools, each with their many assessment-based goals and objectives. Being goal-oriented has its benefits (financial success being the most obvious), but ultimately, a goal-oriented life will be unfulfilling, because anything that's really worthwhile is a process, not a goal.

I love others because the process of loving and being loved in return is joyful and fulfilling. Applying an external goal to love would cheapen the experience itself, while not adding anything of true value to the experience. Life itself must be process-oriented—we must live for the sake of living—and enjoy that process. If life is conceived of as goal-oriented or end-oriented, then the goal of life would be the end of life, which is death. Many people believe that the purpose of life is to gain good life-credit or karma so they can go to heaven or be reincarnated favorably after they die, but I don't advocate that point of view. I don't want to live for death, I prefer to live for life. And finally, if learning is conceived of as goal-oriented or end-oriented, then when school is over and the final diploma received, learning is over too.

However, if we move beyond the rigid segregation and specialization fostered by both our education industry as well as our vocational industries in general, we can create a process-oriented system of lifelong learning, in which learning is engaged in for love of the process itself. As a result, the work we learn to do would become less end-oriented—focusing on the paycheck and the retirement date—and more process-oriented, engaged in for love of the process itself. Ultimately, we could one day see a world in which most people learn what they love in order to work at what they love, so that leisure as a concept is somewhat obsolesced, as both learning and working will be process-oriented, enjoyable, leisurely endeavors.

Manufacturing Anxiety in Schools

> It is in our IQ testing that we have produced the greatest flood of misbegotten standards... [22]
> ... [O]ur intelligence tests exist only for measuring left-hemisphere achievement, and take no cognizance of the existence of the (qualitative) right hemisphere.[23]
>
> —Marshall McLuhan

If Education is perceived as an industry with student learning as its product, then it seems that the primary byproduct of this industry is anxiety. I discussed the issue of generalized anxiety in a previous chapter, but the more specific anxiety that is manufactured in schools—"school anxiety"[24]—needs to be discussed here, as yet another "disorder" created in and by the classroom.

The issue of standardization is the culprit. If all student learning is to be standardized in order for the industrialized system of mass education to work seamlessly, then standards not only need to be met in the student body, but standards have to be ever-increasing, in order for the American education industry to remain competitive with the education industries of foreign nations with whom we're competing for market share. Johnny not only has to learn how to read, but he must learn how to read quicker, better, and earlier than Yuki, as the Japanese students are apparently learning earlier, better, and quicker than we are. The anxiety that we as a nation feel as we compare our economy and workforce to other countries such as Japan is passed down to our children in the form of ever-increasing standards, which take the form of ever-increasing assessments, which in the mind of the child is experienced as ever-increasing school anxiety.

Of course, this system is self-perpetuating and self-escalating. If standards are ever-rising, then we'll never reach a point of satisfaction, a point where anxiety can be reduced. If we hold a "standard of excellence" for all students, that literally means that every student must be excellent, or that simply being average or satisfactory is never acceptable for anyone. Thus, the drive for universal excellence is always raising the average bar, like a pool constantly being filled, so that the people in the system must keep treading water at higher and higher levels just to survive. Some people will excel, most will struggle, some will drown. If that's not a system designed specifically to produce anxiety as a motivation for performance, what is?

The self-perpetuating and ever-escalating system of assessment, driven by anxiety and fear, is quite out of control, because nobody with power over the system is completely outside of the system. It's become a runaway train, rushing our children in a headlong race to nowhere. We teach our children that they must race against the rival "other"—the Japanese, the Russians, the Europeans—while in fact, they're merely racing the phantoms of the machine that they've been thrust into. There are a variety of tragic results from this self-perpetuating cycle of ever-escalating standards for performance. One is the issue of "extrinsic" versus "intrinsic" motivation for learning. When we're intrinsically motivated to learn something because we like it, we'll freely engage ourselves in that subject without the need for pressure, assessment, or anxiety. I could learn new songs on the piano and guitar all day because I love it. I need no pressure to do so, no outside motivation is needed, nor do I need or want to be assessed in any way. I feel no anxiety when I learn and play music. In fact, playing music reduces anxiety for me.

However, when there's no intrinsic motivation to learn, and if learning in a specialized mode of instruction is mandated by the state, then schoolchildren must be forced to learn via extrinsic motivation, such as the consequence of failing an exam or a class. Assessments, therefore, are only required in a system in which intrinsic motivation is lacking, and extrinsic motivation is the norm. And if assessments work by creating fear and anxiety in those being assessed, then we have a system of education in which both teachers and students are motivated primarily by a fear of failing assessments, and not, ironically, by a desire to learn or a desire to teach.

When a system is confident in what it's doing, the system administrators don't feel the need to constantly assess themselves. Assessment is only needed when we doubt the work we're doing, and we fear that we're doing it wrong or ineffectively. The more doubt, the more fear, the more we assess. The assessment-driven culture of academia can therefore be seen as a process driven by doubt and fear: Doubt as to the legitimacy of what we're doing to our kids in schools, and fear that what we're doing isn't working. Assessment, in this way, is both the product and the cause of school anxiety. We assess because we're afraid that we don't know what we're doing, but the process of assessment itself simply creates more doubt and more fear, which we allay by—one can easily guess—even more assessment. The assessment process is a positive feedback loop of self-perpetuating and ever-escalating assessments. Students assessed by teachers, teachers assessed by students and by principals, principals and schools assessed by superintendents, superintendents assessed by the district board of education, the districts are assessed by the county, the county by the state, the state by the federal Board of Education... In the end, everybody—including the children—is motivated solely by fear of the extrinsic motivator, the external assessment.

Teachers may bemoan the fact that school kids seem to care only about the grade and the diploma, and not about learning or appreciating the curriculum, but the kids are merely responding normally to the abnormal environment they've been forced to endure. From a media ecology perspective, the teachers are media providers, the students media consumers, and the media content itself—the information used to develop mastery in literacy in verbal and mathematical language systems—is the product. In most situations, a consumer wants the product provided by the provider.

In the case of education, the whole system is backwards. Students, in general, don't really want the product (the facts and figures they're required to memorize and regurgitate via assessments), they want the pieces of paper that show they've acquired the product satisfactorily (report cards and diplomas). They want those pieces of paper because they've been told by parents and teachers their whole lives that they're exceedingly important.

So now the teacher is in the dubious position of providing a product that their students don't really want, so they're forced to rely ever more on the threat of the assessment, the threat that the students won't receive that all-important piece of paper unless they do well on the assessments. As such, the teacher is not so much a provider using assessments as learning tools but a "servo-mechanism" to the assessments, teaching to and for the tests—but they're not to blame—because just like their students, they're functioning within the same system of assessment, in which their jobs depend not so much on how well they facilitate learning, but on how well they prepare their students for assessments.

Assessment is a learning tool, not an end-in-and-of itself. However, because the education industry is providing a product that the consumers don't really want, it's forced to put the cart before the horse, as it were, by giving assessment precedence over everything else. In essence, that means that students are forced to learn due to fear of failing assessments. Fear, however, is not a very good motivator for learning. If I'm afraid of failing, I'll study, but once the test is over, I won't study anymore. When the external motivator passes, the learning does too. Fear only creates temporary motivation to study, it cannot inspire a love of learning. To the contrary, forcing someone to study is invariably the best way to instill an abiding hatred for learning. Fear is also a bad motivator because it creates anxiety, which is unconducive to learning, and actually hampers the quality of learning for most people. Moreover, the external motivator, the standard assessment, is not a very good evaluator of learning.

Standardized testing in particular is notoriously bad at assessing knowledge and cognitive skills in populations of diverse students. In particular, nobody has figured out how to accurately assess really important things, like creativity, originality, and critical thinking. Standardized tests actually penalize students who think creatively and originally, because standardized tests work by establishing normative solutions to problems, so that any solution that isn't normative—any solution that's original, creative, or divergent from the norm in any way—is graded as being wrong. For the most part, standardized tests are only good at assessing types of learning that have become obsolete in the Digital Age, such as the ability to memorize and regurgitate specific facts and details. Possibly the worst aspect of an assessment driven education system, aside from the anxiety it manufactures, is that it leads to poor teaching, because teachers who are afraid of losing their jobs if their students fail the standardized tests have no recourse but to "teach to the test," relying on obsolete teaching methods that we all know discourage creative and original thinking.

In the race to meet ever-escalating standards, we feel we must drop things that are slowing us down, things that are deemed unessential because they aren't assessed directly on the all-important standardized tests, and also because they don't produce the product that modern industry requires, which is a workforce that specializes and excels in "STEM" subjects (science, technology, engineering, and math). So music, art, drama, dance, and all the other creative fields are bit-by-bit cut back and dropped by the school system. The ultimate irony is that the fields that students want to engage in because they're intrinsically motivating, are the fields that are being dropped by the education system in favor of fields that need to be extrinsically motivated by testing. Thus, the tests created to assess learning become the determinants of what is to be taught and learned, as teaching an untestable subject has become pointless and futile in a world where only assessments—rather than actual knowledge and skills—matter.

Parents stress their kids out when they're young so they can stress themselves out when they're older, fretting about exams and papers so they can get into a good college, where they can stress out about exams and papers so they can get into a good grad school, where they can stress out about exams and papers so they can get a good job. This is all so everyone can earn a good living and live a good life—but ultimately, it's all the stress and anxiety that kills us.

Dyslexia

Returning to the topic of brain lateralization, there's a great deal of evidence to support the hypothesis that dyslexia is a condition associated with either hemispheric symmetry in the ways that we attend to information or right hemispheric dominance.

> In nondyslexics, the left hemisphere of the brain, where language processing takes place, is somewhat larger than the right hemisphere. In dyslexics, the two hemispheres are the same size. Researchers theorize that dyslexics have equal-size brain hemispheres because the language processing centers in their left hemispheres are not as well developed as the left hemispheres of nondyslexics.[25]

Put simply, most or even all dyslexics probably have brains that attend in ways that do not reflect the normative pattern of left-hemispheric lateralization. Left handedness and ambidexterity are strong indicators of right hemispheric dominance for functions such as language, that are usually lateralized in the left hemisphere. Nonright-handedness is un-proportionally present in people with learning disabilities such as dyslexia, and also among biological relatives of people with learning disorders.[26] Studies have repeatedly found a "markedly higher rate of dyslexia ... among strong lefthanders than among strong righthanders."[27]

In one particularly influential study, researchers found the "rate of dyslexia was fifteen times as high in strong lefthanders as in the strong righthanders."[28] There's also a fair amount of evidence to show that, while dyslexics tend to be below average in the left-hemispheric specialization of literacy, they also tend to have exceptional talents in areas that depend on right-hemispheric specializations, such as music and the visual arts.[29] These divergences in brain anatomy and functioning have a genetic foundation, as twin studies demonstrate a concordance rate of 85 percent for dyslexia among identical twins, which breaks down to a heritability factor of 60 percent, with similar concordance rates between dyslexia and other learning disabilities as well.[30]

Oftentimes, we can get a hint to the underlying cause of a problem by looking at its functional opposite. If dyslexia is marked by extremely late or slow reading acquisition, then its opposite is a condition called "hyperlexia," in which children begin reading at an unusually early age (as early as two years old), and read "too much"—that is—they read all the time and have no desire to play games or socialize or engage in any other form of media, such as watching TV or playing videogames. Children who are hyperlexic are very fast and accurate readers, but they often don't grasp the overall meaning of what they're reading, and they also tend to be delayed in oral language, as well as in the development of social skills. If you're thinking that these symptoms seem rather "autistic," you're right. Hyperlexia is a symptom of autism, and it's rarely if ever seen in someone who isn't "on the spectrum."

So, if hyperlexia is a symptom of autism, and autism is a condition related to over-dominance of the left hemisphere, then it would make sense for the functional opposite of hyperlexia—dyslexia—to be a condition related to reduced dominance of the left hemisphere. If hyperlexia and dyslexia represent opposite sides of the same coin, then the coin in question is, once again, hemispheric lateralization for attending to stimuli.

Returning to my spectrum model of hemispheric lateralization, it seems highly probable that hyperlexia may occur if dominance is too far to the left, and dyslexia may occur if dominance is too far to the right. This give and take function between the hemispheres would also explain why hyperlexics display deficits in socialization and strengths in detail-oriented tasks such as reading, while dyslexics display diametrically opposite tendencies.

> The way we each balance the work of these two hemispheres (our *hemisphericity*) has a great deal to do with how we learn. For example, reading researcher Guinevere Eden describes an area in the right rear cortex called the *fusiform face area* that is specialized to recognize faces. The same area in the left hemisphere becomes specialized for recognizing words.[31]

The work of scholars such as Noam Chomsky and Eric Lenneberg in the field of cognitive linguistics has demonstrated that human brains are "hardwired" for language acquisition. The fact that any normal human toddler can acquire a fully functional use of any given language without any deliberate education or training, but merely by being exposed to that language, is proof enough that our brains are hardwired for language; but if you want more proof, I encourage you to read the work of Chomsky and Lenneberg. Literacy, however, is not hardwired, which is why children must attend school for years and experience years of deliberate training and education in order to acquire an even rudimentary level of mastery in literacy. Because literacy is not hardwired, modern brains must adapt themselves to this relatively new medium. Nonstandard adaptations for literacy—i.e., "dyslexia"—reward their hosts with certain cognitive advantages that offset the advantages for standard adaptations. Put more simply, thinking differently than most people can be advantageous, which reduces the tendency for the brain at the population level to harbor just one-and-only-one way for brains to adapt to literacy.

Complications also arise because literacy is not the only game in town. Competing media may favor and support nonstandard adaptations, such as media that convey music, the visual arts, the performing arts, etc. The evolutionary pressure for the brain to conform to one standard adaptation for literacy is offset by simultaneous pressures to adapt to nonliteracy based media. In the past century especially, nonliterary media such as photography, film, radio, television, video games, and many of the other different forms of electronic and digital media, have all entered the fold as active competitors for the brain's attention, making them competitors for the brain's adaptation to media in general, and to literacy in particular.

Because the development from oral language to written language represents an extremely recent adaptation in the brain (an adaptation that shifts the focus from auditory to visual processing of language), it's no wonder than an estimated 10–15 percent of children in schools are diagnosed with a reading disorder such as dyslexia.[32] It also makes sense that the most effective method of instruction for these children, "phonics," aims to refocus their attention on the auditory element, the original seat of language processing, even though they're struggling to comprehend language in a new and confusing visual format. Phonics is somewhat effective because it aids the auditory mode of language reception—oral language—which is the primary and only linguistic mode in both early childhood and in preliterate oral societies.

There's a strong correlation between stuttering and dyslexia. Many dyslexics stutter as young children. Studies show that the rate of stuttering as a child is five times greater among dyslexics.[33] This correlation suggests a common issue between the two conditions that has to do with phonological processing of word sounds. To be clear, the issue is not hearing—neither dyslexics nor stutterers are hard of hearing—the issue is the neurological processing of the specific sounds that the brain perceives and interprets as words. This very specific task, "lexical phonological processing," is carried out by the left hemisphere in most people. Studies have shown that for most people, our right ear (corresponding to the left hemisphere), hears speech sounds far better than our left ear (right hemisphere); while the left ear has superior hearing for nonspeech sounds, especially music.[34]

Geschwind and Galaburda (1987) argued that the processing of phonemes (the most basic unit of speech sound, such as the sound of a single letter), is ever-so-slightly slower in dyslexics and stutterers, because they have a "nonstandard" pattern of lateralization, in which language is not being processed completely by the left hemisphere, but is shared to varying degrees by the right hemisphere.[35] The result of this disinhibition of right hemispheric input for the processing of speech sounds for stutterers might be a slightly slower processing time for their own speech sounds. Since speech happens fast, and since we need to process our own speech sounds instantaneously in order to self-monitor our own pronunciation and articulation, even a tiny delay in phonological processing of phonemes could cause noticeable problems, such as stuttering.

While oral language is a strength for most dyslexics, the commonness of stuttering in their early language development is a clue to the neurological root of their condition. Reading is a phonological task. When learning to read, we read aloud, associating the sight of each letter and word with their correct sound. As we progress in our reading career, we cease reading aloud, but we still move our lips. We also unconsciously move our larynx as if we were speaking, and we still hear the word sounds we are reading in our heads. Eventually, with practice, our lips stop moving, but the word sounds are still there, "silently speaking" out the written words in our mind. "Silent reading," however, speeds up the reading process, as the words spoken silently in our heads while reading go faster than the words we speak aloud.

Our ability to read faster than we can listen or speak is related to our brain's ability to process visual stimuli significantly faster than we can process auditory stimuli.[36] One reason for this variance in processing time is that visual stimuli come to us at the speed of light, while auditory stimuli come to us at the speed of sound, which is much slower. Once reading becomes a primarily visual as opposed to auditory neurological task, it speeds up considerably. "Speed reading" is accomplished by intentionally curtailing our "subvocalization" of the words so that our lips and larynx remain perfectly still, and only our eyes move, making the task almost entirely visual rather than auditory.

In dyslexia, phonemic processing is apparently slightly slower than "normal." This slight delay is probably the cause of stuttering in early language development, a problem that the vast majority of children outgrow (that is to say, their brains adapt to the delay). However, since visual information is processed much faster than auditory information, the same delay is not as easily adapted to by the brain for reading, because the brain needs to decode the visual alphabetic symbols into phonemes at a miraculously fast rate of processing, and then translate and combine those phonemes into meaningful words, all in a matter of milliseconds per word. Even an infinitesimal delay, when multiplied by the thousands of phonetic symbols on a single page, will add up to a major delay in reading. Dyslexic children unconsciously try to compensate for their neurological weakness in phonological decoding by falling back on their neurological strength in visual-spatial pattern recognition, but this, unfortunately, is not a good strategy, as reading expert Dr. Jane Healy explains in her book, *Different Learners* (2002):

> The best readers seem to "listen" to print as if they were hearing it in their heads, while poorer readers are trying to do it all with their eyes.[37]
> There's both anecdotal evidence, from the way dyslexic children try to read, and empirical evidence, from fMRI studies of the functioning of the brains of dyslexic children as they try to read, that the right hemisphere of the brain in dyslexic children is trying to do the job that the left hemisphere usually does, which is the phonological decoding of written letters into heard sounds... "The right hemisphere, however, is not very well suited for this task.... The "style" of the right hemisphere would tend to look at whole words and guess from the shape, length, first letter, or some other *visual* feature instead of *analyzing the sounds in order....* This kid is reading with the wrong part of her brain!"[38]

Dyscalculia

> *What is a number that Man may know it?*
> *And what is Man that he may know number?*
>
> —Warren McCulloch

What is math? From our traditional educational experiences, most of us relate math to numbers and calculations. However, numbers and mathematical operators such as + and - are just the abstract symbols that express mathematical ideas, just like the letters and punctuations on this page are abstract symbols that express linguistic ideas. If we say that mathematical thought is about numbers and logical symbols, we've made the mistake of defining a medium by the symbols that represent it, just like if we said that the letters and sentences on this page are "language," when they're actually the representations of language. Letters and sentences represent an expressive mode for the medium of language, while numbers and logical symbols represent an expressive mode for the medium of mathematical thought. Saying that math is all about numbers and operators is tantamount to saying that language is all about letters and punctuation. In both cases, we're mistaking the symbols for a medium of thought with thought itself. But what is mathematical thought?

Mathematics, in its broadest, most inclusive, and, therefore, most *correct* definition, is the study of *patterns* in quantity, structure, and in space. Numbers are merely abstract representations of quantity. But why does this matter?

If we separate numbers from mathematics, we can get a clearer picture of what math is as a medium of thought, and thereby get a clearer picture of what dyscalculia is, and how it affects the medium of mathematical thought in people who are dyscalculic. Mathematicians generally distinguish between the specific discipline of "arithmetic" and the broader field of mathematics. Arithmetic is the area of math that deals with the manipulation of numbers using logical operators or functions (e.g., +, −, ÷, × etc.). In this sense, arithmetic is to math as literacy is to language. Arithmetic deals with the written representation of mathematical thought using abstract logical symbols, just as literacy deals with the written representation of linguistic thought using abstract phonetic symbols. As it turns out, just as dyslexic people have severe problems with the written representation of linguistic thought (i.e., literacy), and not necessarily with language in-and-of-itself—dyscalculics have severe problems with the written representation of mathematical thought (i.e. arithmetic)—and not necessarily with math in-and-of-itself. The problem, it seems, in both cases, is difficulty in automatically translating abstract visual symbols, whether they be numbers or letters, into meaningful bits of mathematical or linguistic thought. This is why, I suspect, the comorbidity rate for dyslexia and dyscalculia is so very high (well over 50 percent, by some estimates): "Dyslexia can occur in association with dyscalculia. **Co-occurrence of learning disorders appears to be the rule rather than the exception** and is believed to be a consequence of risk factors that are shared between disorders...."[39]

If dyslexia and dyscalculia share a common etiology—difficulty automatically translating abstract visual symbols into meaningful thoughts—then they also share a common obstacle to learning. Dyslexics are not intellectually or linguistically impaired, they have fine mastery of oral language (often superior to the average), and can think perfectly well. The problem is that their brains have difficulty translating the abstract visual symbols into contextualized phonetic sounds (words), so that for them, the medium of literacy is not efficiently providing the content of literacy (language), as the meaning gets lost in translation in their brains. Difficulty in reading—difficulty mastering the written representation of thought—is a huge obstacle to learning, because our traditional academic system places such a huge emphasis on literacy. If a dyslexic student cannot read, he cannot proceed to advanced subjects of thought, because reading must come first.

"Reading is fundamental" has been the creed of academia since its inception in the Middle Ages. Indeed, the entire purpose of school to begin with was to teach children their "letters and numbers." So, a very bright student with a good head for scientific ideas cannot move ahead in academia and study higher scientific thought unless he's thoroughly mastered the media of literacy and arithmetic, making all areas of higher thought practically inaccessible to most severe dyslexics and dyscalculics. As of yet, no shortcut or bridge around or above literacy and arithmetic is offered to any student, even if that student is profoundly dyslexic and/or dyscalculic, and even though we have the digital tools to allow these students to temporarily bypass literacy and arithmetic, in the form of voice-to-text and text-to-voice software, calculators, and other digital tools that we all have on our smartphones.

For these dyslexic and dyscalculic students, school is typically a long and grueling hazing process in which they cannot proceed to what they're good at until they've mastered what they're bad at, even if their brains are neurologically indisposed towards mastering what they're bad at. In other words, it's a game where certain students are put on a path straight to failure, even while other paths are wide open, but are forbidden to tread.

While the "alphabet" of numbers and the "grammar" of logical arithmetical functions provide an entryway into the field of mathematical thought, arithmetic is not the only way to think of mathematical patterns. It's just the only way taught to schoolchildren. Other methods of teaching mathematical thought rely more on visual-spatial pattern recognition and less on abstract symbols. It's clear that dyscalculics have difficulty with arithmetic—calculations, computations, and equations of abstract symbols—but it's equally clear that many dyscalculics and dyslexics are extraordinarily adept at recognizing and manipulating visual-spatial patterns. Indeed, once mathematical problems get complicated due to lots of data, visually creating, recognizing, and manipulating computer-generated graphical displays of patterns becomes the only way to comprehend the data set. "Faced with information overload, we have no alternative but pattern recognition," writes Marshall McLuhan.[40]

For the average schoolchild (not just dyscalculics), mathematics as approached via arithmetic is too much information. When patterns of quantity, structure, and shape are decontextualized and coded into abstract symbols, they become long strings of meaningless information that contain all the details but provide absolutely no sense of the whole. Those decontextualized lines of detailed logico-mathematical code are comprehendible by people who have left-hemispheric dominant brains that decode abstract symbols automatically. To people with right-hemispheric dominant or nonlateralized brain functions for decoding abstract symbols, the information is incomprehensible. Those who can "get their heads straight" in school—those whose brains can adapt to the left-hemispheric dominant approach required by the curriculum—will do fine in math, though the shift towards left-hemispheric dominance may impede or stunt their ability to recognize and manipulate visual patterns, as that function is a right hemisphere specialty. Those who cannot "get their heads straight" will be labeled dyslexic, dyscalculic, and most probably dysgraphic, and ADHD as well. With incredible feats of hard work, patience, determination, and resilience, these kids will make it through school. If they're lucky, the same students will find that their somewhat unusual neurological dispositions will allow them to build skillsets that pave the way to extremely successful careers in virtually every field of human endeavor, as linguistic and mathematical thought go way beyond the basic arithmetic and basic literacy learned in grammar school, and these students found ways of getting around or through these barriers. But the burning question is, why can't these kids learn to master the skills they need to succeed *in* school, rather than learning these skills *despite* school.

Literacy and arithmetic are the written symbolic expressions of language and math. As such, they are media. When a specific medium is serving as a barrier rather than a bridge to the content that it contains, it should be adapted or changed. A medium that is a barrier rather than a bridge is a dysfunctional medium. What's happened in academia is that the significance of the *media* for linguistic and mathematical thought—literacy and arithmetic—have taken such precedence over the actual *content* of linguistic and mathematical thought, that we've completely lost sight of the forest for the trees. We only care that the child masters the media, while the content of the media remains curiously irrelevant. If a child cannot understand a written passage, the focus and concern of the school is to force the child to read better, rather than enabling the child to understand the same information using a different medium. Similarly, if a child cannot figure out how to do a calculation or equation, the focus and concern of the school is to force the child to calculate better, rather than enabling the child to understand the patterns of quantity using a different medium, such as a computer generated graphic display.

To be clear, I'm not saying that we shouldn't be focused on teaching children how to read, write, and do arithmetic. What I'm saying is that the media of literacy and arithmetic are so engrained within the institution of academia that we've forgotten that the point of school is to learn how to think, not just to learn how to master a couple of specific media for thought. This distinction is extremely important when we consider the fate of millions of schoolchildren whose brains don't decode alphabetic and numerical symbols in a streamlined way, because when we deny these children access to linguistic and mathematical thought via alternative media, then we deny them access to thought itself.

On a broader level, we may also be concerned with the fate of every schoolchild. The brain is a mirror of our environment; its functioning directly reflects the demands of its surroundings. If we teach children to think in only one way, they're likely to develop brains that think in only one way. If our schools are teaching children to think of math only in numbers, then we're doing them a disservice, because math is much, much more than numbers. Mathematics is inherently fun and engaging in the visual-spatial realm of thought—recognizing and manipulating patterns—as in puzzles and videogames. But for most of us, math is not particularly fun or engaging, because we're exposed to it only through the code of logico-mathematical symbols, a mode of mathematical thought that, for most of us, is dry, abstract, and decontextualized from our senses.

Similarly, our schools are teaching children to think of ideas only in words. In this case, we're doing them a disservice as well, because there are many media for ideas, and words are only one of them. It's quite possible that our current schooling system is limiting rather than broadening the minds of our schoolchildren, by limiting the media in which they're trained to think. J. Robert Oppenheimer, the "father of the atomic bomb," said, "There are children playing in the street who could solve some of my top problems in physics, because they have modes of sensory perception that I lost long ago."[41]

When we open only one door of perception to a mode of thought, people will only perceive through that one door. But there are many doors. When they remain shut, we not only limit the thought of the individual, we limit the thought of society. The ones who defy the system, either by dropping out, scraping by, or muscling through, often become quite successful—not *despite* of their different ways of thinking but *because* of it. In his book, Thomas West recounts the struggles and eventual successes of creative thinkers who displayed clear symptoms of learning disorders, people such as: Albert Einstein, Leonardo da Vinci, Winston Churchill, Thomas Edison, W.B. Yeats, and Michael Faraday. All of these men had great difficulty with mastering either basic literacy or basic arithmetic or both, yet in time, they all eventually found their own ways of understanding linguistic and mathematical thought, and they all found brilliant, original, unique, and highly creative ways of expressing their divergent thoughts.

Schools are in "crisis" because test scores of reading, writing, and arithmetic seem to be going down. Many blame electronic and digital media for taking away schoolchildren's time and focus from reading and other literary or academic tasks. The basic principle of media displacement—time spent engaging in one medium will subtract from time spent engaging in another—would substantiate those claims. The schools approach to decreasing test scores are invariably to double-down on the only media they know how to teach—literacy and arithmetic—which by the same principle of displacement, draws time and attention away from other media. Hence, schools are cutting music, art, drama, dance and other media of expression, in favor of adding remedial and supplementary instruction in literacy and arithmetic.

Perhaps the time has come for Education as an institution to take a good look at itself and its five-century-old curriculum and wonder if an update is needed? Perhaps the reason students choose to engage in media other than literacy and arithmetic is because for many or even most students, the alternative media are more engaging? Perhaps if schools used more engaging media to teach ideas, students will be more engaged? McLuhan's adage, *the medium is the message,* could be no more apt than it is right now, when applied to the field of education. When a medium such as literacy or arithmetic is taught in a way that limits understanding of concepts in most students, and is obstructive to the understanding of the same concepts in a large minority of students, then the instruction of that medium should be changed and supplemented with other media that are less limiting and un-obstructive. This cannot happen in an institution that perceives literacy and arithmetic as the fundamental and thus exclusive paths to knowledge. In terms of understanding what media are, how they can be taught interactively rather than just passively, and how they can both form and limit our knowledge and skills, the field of education is in the Dark Ages.

The Gift of Dyslexia?

> *We must consider another apparently paradoxical possibility: that minor malformations may often be associated, not with abnormal function, but with distinctly superior capacities in certain areas.*
>
> —Geschwind & Galaburda[42]

"Dyslexia" and other labels for students whose brains aren't predisposed to the literacy-focused curriculum of academia have posed an ironic issue for the academic world. If the function of school is to prepare students for vocational success, then why do certain students who do not succeed in school wind up succeeding greatly in their vocations—oftentimes finding much greater success than their nondyslexic peers who did perfectly well in school. For example, a 2002 cover story in *Fortune* magazine entitled "The Dyslexic CEO" cited a British study done by the London School of Business, which found that nearly half of a group of successful U.S. entrepreneurs in their study met the diagnostic criteria for dyslexia.[43] Geschwind & Galaburda, pioneers in the neurological study of hemispheric lateralization, explain the phenomenon of vocational success among dyslexics—despite struggles and failures in school—as a byproduct of atypical right-hemispheric dominance for representational thought:

> The idea that a "pathological" disorder could manifest itself primarily by superior abilities is alien to standard modes of thinking about neurological disease.... If the growth of one portion of the hemisphere is delayed, then other regions will be larger than they normally would have been. When this increase in size is marked, superior or even remarkable talents may develop.... The superior right hemisphere talents of dyslexics ... illustrate the same point.... The occurrence of high talents though this mechanism may also help to explain the high frequency of such disorders as childhood dyslexia. The high spatial talents of many of the affected individuals may counteract the evolutionary disadvantage of their disabilities. This would, of course, be even more conspicuously the case in nonliterate societies, in which failure to learn to read would not be a problem. Even in a literate society the manifest disability may be overcome through great effort and good teaching, so that only the superior talents may be evident. The fact that family members may manifest the high talents without obvious disabilities raises the possibility serious difficulties may occur in only a fraction of those in whom left hemisphere development is slowed to a greater degree than in most people. These considerations raise the possibility that the mechanisms that delay left hemisphere growth have been selected in the course of evolution because they often produce individuals of elevated talent. The advantage to these individuals presumably outweighs the disadvantage of the learning disabilities, which probably appear in a small number in whom the slowing on the left is excessive. Again, a disability such as dyslexia would have been of minor importance in nonliterate societies.[44]

As we move hopefully move towards a more neurologically tolerant society, we'll be obliged to construct new names for various conditions, not just as a function of nominal political correctness, but as true expressions of the notion that neurodiversity is an accepted fact in the educational and psychological communities, and hence neurodiversity is not only tolerated, but encouraged. We'll have to come up with names for types of attending that aren't based on negative functionality, as in "attention deficit," "dis-order," "dys-function," "dis-ability," and "dys-lexia." Perhaps the new names could note the functionality of the individual's manner of attending, rather than its dysfunctionality?

At a neurological level, the theory that ADHD, dyslexia, dyscalculia, and dysgraphia are byproducts of a nonleft-hemispheric dominant mindset is supported by much evidence. The dyslexic's and dyscalculic's relative strength in visual-spatial pattern recognition, and relative weakness in phonetic and logico-mathematical symbol decoding, point to a strength in a right hemispheric specialty and a corresponding weakness in a left hemispheric specialty. "Children who are virtuosos at building and fixing things—the ones who can visualize three-dimensional space—often have trouble in school, where abstract symbolic learning is favored."[45]

Ellen Winner, a renowned researcher in the psychology of art, found that children with delayed speech development displayed superior visual-spatial skills, and "most had relatives working in professions that require strong spatial skills."[46] Winner also found that the "association between verbal deficits and spatial gifts seems particularly strong among visual artists."[47]

The right hemisphere seems to specialize in primary cognitive processes, basic thoughts and behaviors that don't require a lot of special training or education, such as remembering what something looks like, or imagining what something might look like. These facilities are strong in both the preliterate societies outside of the Western world (what sociologists used to call "primitive" cultures), as well as the preliterate societies within the Western world (little children). When we were little children, we had a primary way of attending based on visual pattern recognition, imagination, intuition, visual memory, etc. As we learned more about the world, and especially as we began to read, write, and think in words, our right hemispheric primary processes were gradually displaced and supplanted by our left hemispheric secondary processes, which attend to the world by representing stimuli symbolically in words.

Our prehistoric preliterate ancestors navigated the glacial landscapes without the aid of maps or compasses, just an excellent visual memory and an intuitive sense of direction. The Truk Islanders, a contemporary preliterate society in the South Pacific, routinely sail hundreds of miles within a crisscrossing maze of tiny coral islands, finding their way using the same time-tested faculties.[48] Small children sometimes display "eidetic memory," also known as "photographic memory," an ability to recall in exact detail a visual memory of things they've seen. This ability is usually lost soon after the child starts school, obsolesced by the more practical medium of linguistic memory. Other media, such as written diaries, photograph albums, and social media sites and apps, have also come along to displace our innate visual memory, by recording memories extra-somatically, eliminating the need for long term visual memory altogether.

Autistic savants who do not completely master language sometimes retain their eidetic memory, allowing them to perform seemingly miraculous feats of visual memory. Stephen Wiltshire, for example, is a British savant artist who can recall an entire landscape after seeing it just once, reproducing the landscape from memory in detailed drawings. On an episode of *60 Minutes,* Wiltshire took a helicopter ride around Manhattan, and based on a single observation, made dozens of detailed drawings of the entire Manhattan skyline from a variety of different perspectives that were extremely vivid and precisely detailed—he even remembered which specific windows in which particular apartment buildings were either open or shut.[49]

In short, though the benefits of school and literacy are quite obvious, it's also useful to remember what we give up as well, for in the zero-sum game of neural networking, nothing in the brain is gained unless something else is lost. In school, the extremely vivid and detailed visual memory that most people are born with and experience in early childhood, is displaced by the highly organized verbal system of memory that we learn by reading, writing, and thinking in words. Though it may seem the natural order of things for a primary process to be displaced by a secondary process, we should note that for some people, the secondary process does not come naturally at all, and when that happens, it behooves us to recognize it and understand it. There's nothing natural about forcing someone to think in a medium that his brain is indisposed to.

Furthermore, as the world of digital media technology continues to evolve, it may come to pass that the primary processes that we're born with will become more useful and expedient than the secondary processes we learn in school. At a certain point, we may even come full circle, and start focusing on developing primary processes in school, while the secondary processes ("three R's") will become extra-curricular. This particular re-ordering of the natural order would be particularly useful in art schools, and in schools designed for people whose minds very evidently attend in the primary rather than the secondary way.

Researchers in dyslexia often mention the case of Albert Einstein—the man whose name has become synonymous with the term "genius"—whose speech development was severely delayed in childhood. Einstein's genius arose from his unusually vivid visual imagination, which allowed him to do thought experiments with three-dimensional representations of time-space, and which aided him in his mathematical reconceptualization of the physical universe, which was based more on visual patterns of time-space matrices than on arithmetical numbers. Einstein's mathematical thought experiments were entirely visual-spatial. He saw it all in his head. The numeric calculations came afterwards, which he supplied in his papers only as empirical proofs of the visual patterns he already saw fully formed in his mind.

His calculations, by the way, were notorious for being full of minor arithmetical errors that most high school students who were reasonably good in math would've spotted, clearly indicating that in Einstein's math, visual space and pattern both preceded and superseded the significance of numerical calculation. It's also been noted that Einstein had lifelong issues with written language, especially in the areas of word memory and spelling. This well-documented pattern of "great strengths and surprising weaknesses"[50] has led "some researchers to theorize that Albert Einstein had a lifelong difficulty with language because he was more in touch with the right hemisphere of his brain."[51]

Literacy in the Digital Age

> *The right hemisphere, with its greater integrative power, is constantly searching for patterns in things. In fact its understanding is based on complex pattern recognition.*
>
> —Iain McGilchrist[52]

The different forms of digital media are vast and divergent. Most of these media are more appealing to the right hemisphere's manner of attending than the left's. With its scrolling procedure, digital screens present information in a vertical fashion, as opposed to print, in which text is laid out horizontally. Thus, at a purely ocular level, screens of words and images foster right hemispheric attending, while pages of print foster left hemispheric attending: "The right hemisphere prefers vertical lines, but the left hemisphere prefers horizontal lines," writes Iain McGilchrist.[53]

Furthermore, the focus on images in digital media recalls a media that preceded literacy based on the phonetic alphabet, media found in ancient writing forms such as pictographs, ideograms, and hieroglyphics. To a large extent, digital media—with their emphasis on audio and video—is pushing the species away from print literacy and towards means of communication that are much more similar to the nonspecialist media of the preliterate ages; that is, media based in images, music, and the spoken word. It's entirely likely that digital media are actually turning the pendulum of hemispheric lateralization away from the literate left hemisphere, moving communication and perception more towards the holistic right hemisphere, which prefers the spoken word over the written word, images over letters, and interactive movement over isolated, static, fixed positions.

Literacy, obviously, will not become obsolete. To the contrary, it will continue to spread throughout the world. However, there's a distinction that must be made between basic literacy and advanced literacy. The former refers to reading and writing at the basic literal level, in which words are read and written in terms of their literal meaning, and no secondary or deeper analysis is required in order to understand the subtext, the underlying meaning, the symbolism, or the implications of the words that go beyond the text. Advanced literacy is required for this deeper level of reading and writing. Advanced literacy is needed for the critical analysis that's required for reading Heidegger or Proust or Joyce, or if one intends to write poetry or profound exposition. It's this latter level of literacy that may be destined to become a "specialist" skill—just as the ability of a professional musician to fluently read and write music is a specialist skill—or the ability of a computer programmer to read and write binary code. While everyone can appreciate and even create music on the basic level, and while everyone can use computers on a basic level, the more advanced use of these technologies is mastered only by the specialists in their respective fields.

Many of the children being labeled as "learning disabled" now in the current literacy-centric education system, may ironically be better suited than their "normal" peers on a cognitive level, for the age of digital media that they're entering. The tables are being turned. Those considered blind will be the visionaries of the future. Those who cannot see the future ahead of them will be left behind.

The Future of Literacy

> It is now obvious that all languages are mass media, so the new media are new languages. To unscramble our Babel we must teach these languages and their grammars on their own terms. This is something quite different from the educational use of audio-visual aids or of closed circuit TV.
>
> —Marshall McLuhan[54]

There's a long history behind the argument that "photography is not an art, it's a technology." The argument goes back to the birth of photographic technology in the 19th century, a time when artists spent many years of toil and trouble perfecting their abilities to create extremely realistic visual representations of subjects in the form of paintings, portraits, drawings, sculptures, etc. The argument, of course, is hollow, because all art forms are also technologies, thus the two categories are not mutually exclusive; but my point in mentioning the argument is the traditional response to the argument from photographers: That photography is not necessarily the art of *creating* an image, but the art of *framing* an image. Photography is the "art of the frame"—the art of selecting, setting, framing, and capturing images on film (or in digital memory) using the photographic medium.

Because the technology of photography is relatively accessible to anyone, it eventually opened up the media of image-making to nonspecialists, people who are untrained or untalented in the classical media of image-making, such as painting, drawing, sculpting, etc. The technological medium of photography thus created a population of visual media artists who can practice their art without the burdensome necessity of years of training or the need for innate talent.

Applying this metaphor to literacy, we may see the future of writing as a nonspecialist medium, in which expression is more about the "art of the frame" than about creating original written expressions. If I ask you a question—"How is the current president better or worse than the previous president?"—you might sit down with pen and paper and organize your thoughts; or you may google the question and find multiple websites with appropriate answers. In the first instance, critical thinking is applied via reflection on one's own internal thoughts, noting one's own original ideas, organizing the best ideas, researching the ideas of others to compare with and supplements one's own ideas, and then constructing sentences in a linear fashion to build a solid argument. In the latter instance, critical thinking is applied via external searching on the internet of other people's ideas, noting the ones that seem to be the best, or the ones that you agree with the most, organizing these ideas in a lateral fashion (based on their appearance on the internet), and then stringing them together to represent a broad argument (based on the wide variety of opinions on the internet).

Critical thinking is achieved in both instances, but the more traditionally "literate" method is introspective, linear, sequential, and logical. The newer "digital" method is "extrospective"—seeking outwardly, laterally—jumping quickly via hyperlink from one idea to the next, nonsequential, and intuitional. McLuhan would note here that the newer digital method is actually a retrieval of the dialectic thinking of preliterate oral cultures, in which knowledge was formed through discussions and the asking of others' opinions, and a strong argument was based on persuasive rhetoric that gains a large consensus, as opposed to the linear depth or singular logic of one's argument in the literate mode.

When I ask my college students to write a paper on a specific subject, I'm often disappointed. I, with my very traditional background in academic literacy, am expecting a paper in which ideas are built up with original thought and buttressed by research, and then stacked one upon another in logical, sequential, and linear fashion. What I often get are papers that consist of various unoriginal but related ideas collected from the internet and strung together in no particular order. If I were an art teacher, it would be like I asked for a work of art, expecting an original painting, but instead I got a montage composed of clipped photographs. My disappointment is my own fault, both for having predetermined expectations, and also for assuming that my students will have the same affinity for the literate media as I do. But my students grew up in a digital media environment, not a literary media environment. In their minds, why write new words when there are perfectly good words on the internet to gather and put together? Why build when you could collect? Why create new ideas from scratch when you could find ones on the internet that are just as good or even better and then connect and assemble them in record time. The montage is simply much more efficient than the painting. I'm asking my students to *build*, but their media environment encourages them to *connect*.

Similarly, when I complain about plagiarism (the use of other people's words or ideas without proper citation), my students seem rather oblivious, and it's easy to see why. Of what importance is authorship in a world of limitless, free, and infinitely accessible ideas? Worrying about authorship in the digital environment is like worrying about paying for a single apple in the midst of a vast orchard. Just take it. They're everywhere!

My purpose here is not to suggest that one method is better or more proper than the other, but simply to point out that the media themselves—literacy vs. digitality—foster and create different modes of thinking and expression. Each child now enters the classroom already adapted to the digital environment of their homes. In the classroom environment, the child that is used to and adapted to the digital method will find it frustrating to have to readapt to the literate method, which is dull and methodical, slow and burdensome, under-stimulating and downright boring. The digital method of leaping from hyperlink to hyperlink in a fast and furious torrent of ideas is much more engaging, as it's unpredictable in terms of what you may find, self-directed, interactive, and highly stimulating on auditory, visual, and tactile levels. The child who's forced to remold their cognitive operations into the literate mindset will likely show patterns of resistance that are completely unconscious to the child, and will appear to the teacher as resistance to the process and reluctance towards the task. The child will appear distracted as their mind automatically seeks more audio-visual-tactile stimulation. They'll appear impatient as the unbearably slow process of methodically and laboriously building one idea upon another seems like an eternity. They'll appear fidgety and hyperactive as the lack of physical movement combined with the anxiety of the task itself are released in "hyperactive" jaunts away from their desk. In short, many of the symptoms of ADHD will appear and are likely to be perceived as internal deficits within the child's brain, rather than as a maladjustment of the child's mind to a media environment that is unconducive to the child's own method of information processing. At this point, it seems like the brain of the modern child (molded in large part by the digital media environment of the modern world), is at odds with—and in certain ways is at war against—the medieval media environment of the traditional classroom...

> There is a rather tenuous division between war as education and education as war.... It is simple information technology being used by one community to reshape another one. It is this type of aggression that we exert on our own youngsters in what we call "education." We simply impose upon them the patterns that we find convenient to ourselves and consistent with the available technologies. Such customs and usages, of course, are always past-oriented and the new technologies are necessarily excluded from the education establishment until the elders have relinquished power. This, of course, leave the new technologies entirely in the sphere of entertainment and games.—Marshall McLuhan[55]

So what's to be done? The fact that all children will have to be forced to read and forced to write over many years of schooling with often excruciating levels of anxiety and pressure brought to bear on each child, has been communally accepted as the price we pay for mass literacy. To realize that some children, no matter how much pressure or psychosocial damage is inflicted upon them, will never master literacy to the standards of modern academia, has only been grudgingly accepted. However, when we reach the point in our society when about a third of the population of school children are labeled as "disordered" because of their struggle with the medium of literacy, and when we've reached the point where we've deemed it necessary to drug millions of these children with powerful psychoactive substances in order to subsume the behaviors that are evoked by the media environment being forced upon them, isn't that the point when we should question the system itself and ask: What is "disordered," the brains of these children, or the system that refuses to accept their brains?

I'm certainly not advocating the removal of literacy as a universal standard for academics. Even the digital medium requires a certain level of literacy, though these requirements seem to be diminishing each day. For instance, young people are increasingly using emoji in favor of words in their text messages, and using digital images and voice recordings in their personal expressions on social media in favor of written words. Among the young, email is obsolete, and written posts and texts have given way to the emoji, pic, selfie, image, or audio-visual clip. In his book, West notes that some dyslexics create a shorthand for themselves, in which letters and words are replaced by nonphonetic symbols: "If one has special difficulty with conventional written language, one may devise one's own written language. Often it takes a form based on pictures (like Chinese ideographs or ancient Egyptian hieroglyphs) or on forms that can be written quickly and read as wholes (like stenographic shorthand)."[56]

West provides Leonardo da Vinci and Woodrow Wilson as examples of famously successful men who displayed clear signs of dyslexia, and who utilized their own personal shorthands when writing in their notebooks.[57] Using a symbolic shorthand based on visual patterns that represent whole concepts would sidestep the need for the brain to decode phonetic symbols into phonemes (the sounds of the alphabet), thus shifting neural processing away from a dyslexic's weakness (phonological decoding), and towards a dyslexic's strength (recognition of visual patterns and whole concepts).

This is somewhat similar to the way that small children rely on the use of "sight words" when first learning to read. Sight words aren't read phonetically—children recognize the visual pattern of the words—and relate the patterns to the meaning of the words as a whole. Eventually, as reading speeds up, children adopt the standard method of reading by decoding each letter into a phoneme and then combining all the phonemes together to create a word. It's well known that dyslexic children rely on the use of sight words for a much longer time than nondyslexic children, which causes problems, as this strategy works ok for a few dozen very small and easy words, but it becomes a hindrance when the child is expected to read countless words of all sizes and difficulty levels, as even the best visual memory can never hope to recall all the written words in a language system that is constantly generating new words.

So, while the phonetic system is really the only practical way to read using the phonetic alphabet, there are other ways of reading and writing that are nonphonetic. The ideographic, pictographic, and hieroglyphic writing systems of both ancient cultures and contemporary non–Western societies predate phonetic literacy by thousands of years, and may obsolesce phonetic literacy in the near future, as digital media foster the use of nonphonetic visual communication, by offering users the option of replacing words with emojis, pictures, streaming video, and other visual symbols and images that rely on the eye rather than the ear for interpretation.

We may see later in this century that emerging populations in the Third World will simply leapfrog over literacy straight to digitality, in which written words are replaced completely by digital images and sounds. In post-industrial nations, we may soon begin to realize that digitality provides a nonspecialist medium of communication and information processing that is easily accessible to virtually all children, including the millions labeled as ADHD and learning disordered. Just as the camera simultaneously invented the art of photography and changed (but did not eliminate) the role of the traditional artist, digital media is inventing a new mode of communication, while it simultaneously changes (but does not eliminate) the traditional role of literacy. As this process occurs, will we still find it necessary to drug children into submission in order to master literacy, or will we allow them the option of adopting digitality as their primary medium for nonoral communication?

The concerned educator and parent may ask: By allowing some children to "opt out" of literacy, aren't we embarking on a slippery slope that declines precipitously towards mass illiteracy? I don't think so.

Basic literacy—being able to read or write at the elementary school level—will continue to be of vital use to just about everyone in modern society for a very long time. However, the masters of literacy, the writers of novels and stories and poems and articles, and the critics and deconstructors of those works, will be the members of the specialist craft of literate masters, just as the scribes and scholars were members of the specialist craft of literate masters in the days before Gutenberg's press, when relatively few people could read or write. On a broader level, we could imagine that in the primordial era of archaic hominids, when our ape-like ancestors could build fire and tools but not speak, the average human was probably quite adept at communicating mimetically with hand gestures. When spoken words became the dominant medium of communication, average people were not nearly as fluent in mimetic communication as they used to be, because the medium had changed and they didn't have to be.

Nevertheless, the ability to "speak" fluently using only mimes and gestures remains part of the human neurological legacy, as demonstrated by deaf people who, when given the opportunity, can communicate fluently using only sign language. Similarly, when all communication in ancient societies was oral, the bards and sages committed entire epics and mythologies to memory, that they recited at will with the aid of only a harp or a lyre. These astounding and eloquent feats of memory and oratory became quite rare when the medium for long stories changed to the written word. There are few bards left in the world now, as the script and then the book have replaced them. Nevertheless, there are still people who can recite entire epics by heart—such as the zealous scholars who memorize the Torah and the Koran—and there are still bards who can sing entire canons of lyrics relying only on their memory (Bob Dylan comes to mind here).

No, literacy will not die, but it will not remain the same.

For children who are truly suffering by being forced to adapt to a medium that is not a good fit for their ways of attending, I truly hope that literacy will not be forced upon them the way it's being forced upon them now, with drugs and stress and anxiety, and then more drugs for the anxiety. For those children who struggle, I foresee an eventual slackening of the standards required for literacy, especially once it's established that communication and information processing could be achieved digitally with only a basic level of literacy required. Also, as Thomas West points out in his book, dyslexics and other children with learning disabilities are *notoriously slow learners* when it comes to literacy. In other words, all but the most profoundly dyslexic will eventually learn at least basic literacy skills in due time, and possibly proceed to very advanced literacy skills if they want or need to. The current academic standards are based on age-based norms for literacy skills. Hence, it's not necessarily the academic expectations for literacy that are the issue for dyslexics, but the rigid timeline for meeting the age-based standards in academia. If the age-based standards were loosened, we'd see much less storm and stress over literacy acquisition in schoolchildren.

So, in the future, there will certainly be the literary specialists whose mastery of the medium will allow them to write at increasingly higher levels of sophistication, for an increasingly sophisticated but dwindling audience of literary specialists, who will still be able to read and critique these literary creations. But for the rest of us, I think most people will be able to read and write, but they will not be writers, and they will read very little. (Come to think of it, rather than describing the future, I may be describing the present.)

What will school be like in the post-literate digital age? Writing for many will become the art of the montage, the mastery of the link rather than the mastery of the written word. Voice recognition software that translates the spoken word seamlessly into digital text will switch the focus of mastery from the medium of writing to the content of writing: the thoughts themselves. Teachers will accept the fact that writing is merely a medium for thought, not thought itself, and that digital technology can help students struggling with the mastery of the written word to express their thoughts just as clearly, if not more so, than if they wrote the words by hand rather than speaking the words into a device that prints out the words for them. Dysgraphia as a construct will no longer exist.

Reading will remain fundamental, but it may not be required for all students to go beyond the fundamentals, if they prefer to focus on images or sounds or other post-literate elements of communication. Dyslexia as a construct will no longer exist. Artists in the post-photographic world changed their focus from representational art to nonrepresentational art, because cameras are better than people at capturing exact visual representations. Artists' work became more nonrepresentational—expressing impressions, concepts, and moods—rather than realistically representing actual subjects.

Similarly, digital media fosters nonliterate and "post-symbolic communication."[58] If I want to message you about my dog's appearance, I could send you a text message with words describing my dog, or I could send you an emoji or clip-art or some other form of ideogram representing the concept of my dog, or I could simply take a photo of my dog and send you that. The latter mode is nonliterate and nonsymbolic, and it's now the easiest, simplest, and most decipherable way of communicating this simple message. A digital media environment fosters nonliterate communication to the extent that literate communication becomes increasingly unnecessary. It may seem odd to create "text" by just speaking, rather than writing; and to absorb text just by listening, rather than reading; but it won't seem odd to a generation that grows up with it. The future of communication seemed so obvious to the creators of science-fiction media environments that the point wasn't even worth mentioning. The characters in *Star Trek* and *Star Wars* generally speak to their computers and robots. Captain Kirk (William Shatner) always spoke out his "captain's log" to his computer, he never actually "wrote" his log. Keyboards are rarely if ever used in science fiction.

In the future, children who are struggling with attention and distraction will be allowed to reconstruct their media environments to a point of proximal adjustment—a point at which both student and teacher agree that the student is communicating and integrating information at the rate and in the mode that is most comfortable for his neurological disposition. As a construct, ADHD will no longer exist. Children will no longer be drugged in order to function in the classroom without distracting others or frustrating the teacher. The media environment will be physically adjusted, rather than the neurochemicals in the child's brains. The square peg will no longer be pounded into the round hole, but rather the holes will be made flexible in order to accommodate a diverse and limitless variety of pegs.

The Musical Literacy Metaphor

"Back to basics" is the last bugle call of the diehards.

—McLuhan & Powers[59]

For many thousands of years, humans have been both musical and linguistic. Music is intuitive and spontaneous, everyone can both enjoy it and participate in it, even if just by humming, singing, or playing a simple instrument, like a drum. Oral language is acquired by young children via simple exposure. In both cases, language and music are not taught, they are simply acquired and eventually mastered merely by practice. As such, we can say that oral language and music are nonspecialist media, as in their traditional forms, they require no training, study, or exceptional talent. Within the past few millennia, and especially within the past few centuries, both forms of media have been adapted into new modalities: the written format. In both cases, the written format for music and literature are specialist media. Without a good deal of training and study, one cannot read, write, or play sheet music. Similarly, without extensive schooling, one cannot read or write literature. The creation of specialist modalities for both forms of media created elite classes of specialists: scribes and classical musicians.

Only some people can read or write music, just as only some people can read or write words. This does not exclude anyone from the pre-literate, nonspecialist forms of the media. One can enjoy listening to as well as both playing and singing music without having to know how to read or write music. Similarly, one can speak and listen to words, without having to know how to read or write. One can imagine a society in which musical literacy (being able to read and write music fluently) was required of all people. (Indeed, there probably were and are some schools and households that did and do require children to be musically literate.) However, one need not imagine a society in which all people are required to be able to read and write words fluently, because we live in such a society. But media and society are changing...

If I was the principal of a school and you a parent, and I told you that your child was "failing" because he or she is required to be musically literate at a proficient level of fluency, you might ask: "Why? My child can appreciate listening to music, and can enjoy singing and playing music, without having to go through the trouble of learning how to read and write music."

I, the principal, may reply: "But if your child doesn't learn to be musically literate, how will he ever be able to express his musical ideas in the written form" (i.e., compose), "and how will he be able to understand and perform musical ideas in the written form?"

You, the parent, may reply: "Look, if my child wants to become a composer or a professional musician or a music teacher" (i.e., a musical specialist), "then by all means, let her spend countless hours learning how to read and write sheet music fluently. But if she doesn't want to be one of those things, then why force her to learn how to read and write sheet music, especially if she doesn't enjoy it, isn't naturally good at it, and has no desire to learn it? After all, she can still listen to both live and recorded music, and can still sing and play and even write songs without having to learn how to read and write music."

This conversation seems to make sense self-evidently in the case of music, but when it's applied to linguistic literacy, it gets more complicated.

"Mr. Johnson, I called you into my office today because Johnny, your nine-year-old son, cannot read or write."

"So, Mr. Principal. What's the problem?"

"Well ... don't you see ... if Johnny cannot read or write, he cannot go to middle school."

"Why not? He understands ideas perfectly well when they're spoken to him. Why can't the teachers explain the information he needs to know orally?"

"Well, they can, but then how will he take the tests?"

"If the questions are read to him, he can give the answers orally."

"But the teacher doesn't have the time to sit down with each child in order to read out the questions and listen to the answers."

"Well, just digitalize the test and have a computer ask the questions and dictate his answers."

"Yes, ok, that's all well and good, but what about outside of school?"

"Perhaps you haven't noticed, Mr. Principal, but the world outside of school has changed...." Our digital devices can read and write for us. Cars can drive themselves, and can be controlled by our voices, so we don't even need to know how to read directions or how to read a map. Stories can be watched as moving images on screens, or narrated to us by our devices. Business can be done in face-to-face real-time meetings using Skype, Zoom, or FaceTime. In short, anything that needs to be read can be read to us by our computers, and anything that needs to be written can be dictated to computers. As Dylan sang, "The times they are a changin'"; and as McLuhan foretold, only the "diehards" are interested in conserving obsolete learning structures...

... Western (visual and sequential) man now discovers himself habitually relating to information structures which are simultaneous, discontinuous, and dynamic. He has been plunged into a new form of knowing, far from his customary experience tied to the printed page.... As such, by the next century it will destroy all existing forms of school structures. "Back to basics" is the last bugle call of the diehards.—McLuhan & Powers[60]

The world of the very near future is a world in which literacy is becoming a specialist skill, just like the ability to read and write sheet music. There will always be books, and there will even be new books published in paperback and hardcover for quite awhile, as there's a tactile as well as textual allure to the paper book that's as satisfying as old records and record players to vinyl album lovers. Who knows how long these nostalgic attachments to obsolete media will survive? But regardless of the means of delivery, there will always be music, there will always be music lovers and music makers. Similarly, there will always be writers and readers. I suspect that over a large period of time, the effects of digitality on literacy will mirror the effects of musical literacy on music. That is, pretty much everyone will use language and enjoy music in both the expressive and receptive forms (playing and listening), but the literate forms of language and music—the written modalities—will be the domain of specialists. People will still be able to read at a basic level, but text messages and tweets will be the standard length of the typical written expression, though even these very brief agrammatical missives will be increasingly corroded by ideographic emojis and digital imagery.

In time, as the digital medium becomes universal, the preliterate masses of what used to be called the Third World will learn to read with cheap used smartphones exported by developed countries. Most will learn only enough to read and create brief digitalized messages, but functional illiteracy will to all extents and purposes become a thing of the past. At the same time, advanced literacy will also decrease, as the proportion of people in the population who choose to read and write long and ever more sophisticated literary works will decrease in ratio to the people who can get along just fine with reading and writing only brief messages annotated with cartoon emojis and video clips.

The Teacher as Artist

At present our system of education seems almost a guarantee that while we teach them how to use words and concepts, we wipe out this other world of beauty and higher reality which so many children live in.

—Aldous Huxley

Painting is like teaching. When the focus is on the individual figures within the painter's field of vision, such as the subject of the portrait or the mountains in a landscape, we call this type of painting "Art." When the focus is on the ground within the painter's field of vision, such as a wall or the side of a house, we call this type of painting "house painting." The goal of the artist is clarity, to make the figures within the frame seem distinct, to stand out as individuals. The goal of the housepainter is congruity, to make the ground of the wall appear smooth and homogeneous, an even and flawless continuum of sameness. The goal of the teacher is unclear in relation to this metaphor. If the teacher is an artist, her goal is to see her classroom as a frame, and to view the figures in the classroom as individuals, who need to become distinct from each other, and distinct from the ground of their environment. The teacher as artist must use tools that favor distinctiveness and individuality—small brushes that bring out the details and idiosyncrasies that come from within the student. The teacher as artist must use a small brush.

Standardized tests and standardized curricula are big brushes—paint rollers and spray cans—whose primary function is to roll or spray over all of the details and idiosyncrasies within the field of vision. The goal of the big brush is to make everything look the same. The teacher as house painter uses her brushes to grade and score each student on the basis of how closely their expression resembles the sameness of the general standard. The individual student is perceived as an embedded figure within the ground of the classroom, who must remain congruent with the other embedded figures in the ground. Their performance is only meaningful in relation to the class, and the class' performance as a whole is only meaningful in relation to the standardized measures for all classes. The ultimate goal, therefore, is to promote conformity to the standards, a smooth and even coat of paint. Individuality, idiosyncrasy, and divergence are graded negatively in this system of standardization, whose aim is to brush over everything in order to achieve perfect homogeneity.

What the big brushes cannot do effectively is evoke intrinsic motivation. A child, given paper and crayons, will naturally make art, with no external motivation needed. Children, given music, will naturally sing and dance. But it is the rare child indeed who will study for a standardized test, or practice his spelling in a workbook, or memorize multiplication tables, in the absence of an external motivator, such as a teacher wielding a red marker and a big brush. Standards and standardization are outside forces inflicted upon the child from without, for the purpose of comparing the child to everyone else. The teacher as artist must recognize the individuality within each student, and encourage the children to think and express themselves like nobody else. When teachers see their students as distinctive works of art rather than uniform blank slates, they're bound to encourage modes of learning that favor intrinsic motivation and individuality, rather than extrinsic motivation in the form of standardized tests, that penalize cognitive divergence and reward conformity.

The Classroom of the Future

> *No one has a perfect brain. Most of us have some sort of "learning disability" or weakness, for which we learn to compensate by using our strong points. Whether or not a difference becomes a disability depends on the environment—what it encourages, what it expects. Rigid or punitive schools can turn a difference into a disability. As a society, we need to preserve a variety of mental skills, which may become very important in an unknown future.*
>
> —Jane Healy[61]

In order to accommodate the reality of neurological diversity, the education industry will have to abandon its current model of standardized education for everyone. When will this happen? As always, one must follow the money. Currently, there are millions of children who receive federally mandated special education services for all sorts of psychological issues. Special education services are exceedingly expensive, requiring specially trained teachers, individualized education plans (IEPs), specially developed resources, and—probably the most expensive factor—lots and lots of lawyers to handle all of the inevitable lawsuits brought by parents who realize that, despite the existence of special education, their children are still not being served in the classroom with the dignity they deserve, because their neurodiversity is treated as a deficit rather than as a divergence.

When the number of students requiring special education hits a critical mass—let's say 50 percent of the student population—the industry itself will either collapse under its own weight of inefficiency, or it will realize that "special education" is just too expensive and, also, it just doesn't work. Then and only then will the industry be forced to totally revamp its service model, and create a new classroom that is tolerant of all expressions of neurodiversity, a classroom that accepts each student as an individual with a unique brain, rather than as a lump of clay or "tabula rasa," to be shaped into a standardized mold. Digital media will be the key technology that can be used to accommodate neurological diversity in the classroom, by individualizing educational products and assessments, making the standard "one-size-fits-all" model obsolete.

For nearly all of the human experience, the hundreds of thousands of years leading up to the modern age, children learned by seeing and doing, with hands-on experience. Children learned to hunt and fish by hunting and fishing, they learned to farm and ranch by farming and ranching, they learned to cook and sew by cooking and sewing. So, one reason why classroom learning is so inefficient and so inaccessible to so many students is because classroom learning is anathema to the natural way that children learn and have been learning for eons. Classroom learning, book learning, is abstract and decontextualized because the knowledge acquired in the classroom from books is divorced from any real life experience.

If "learning disordered" children in general are not left-hemisphere dominant in the way that they attend to stimuli, then it would follow that the abstract, decontextualized, academic approach to learning that the left-hemispheric brain specializes in would be anathema to these children's minds. It would then follow that learning which is holistic, contextualized, and practice-based would be more conducive to a mind that is not left-hemisphere dominant, and therefore learns better in an environment where knowledge is attained through interaction with the material, rather than the passive and distanced academic approach of studying decontextualized knowledge by decoding abstract symbols in books that re-present the knowledge. The right hemisphere's gestalt approach would favor learning that's experiential rather than academic, hands-on rather than abstract, and contextual rather than decontextualized.

If this sounds eerily familiar, it should, because educators and psychologists have known for decades that children who struggle with classroom learning, whether due to behavioral issues such as ADHD or due to a learning disorder such as dyslexia, usually thrive in settings where the approach is experiential. If this is so, then why hasn't the classroom evolved to better engage students with learning difficulties? The answer, in short, is because these children have, for most of the history of education, been incorrectly considered to be a small minority of the student population. However, anywhere from 80 to 90 percent of children receiving special education services in America are there because of reading failure, which is just a drop in the bucket, as the U.S. Department of Education has estimated that only 20 percent of students who need special services for reading actually get a diagnosis in order to receive them; and while there are many success stories to relate about "learning disabled" children who go on to rule the world, like Richard

Branson and Anderson Cooper, there are also the grim statistics. Such as, up to 85 percent of U.S. prison inmates meet the criteria for having a "learning disorder" and 75 percent of school dropouts experienced reading failure.[62]

Now that improved awareness and detection have revealed that the students who are not well equipped neurologically for typical classroom learning constitute such a substantial proportion of the student population that they can't be considered a minority at all, there's been a concerted effort at every level of education, from preschool through graduate school, to incorporate more experiential learning in the curriculum. Children go to the zoo to study animals, the museum to study art, and the theater to study Shakespeare. Undergraduates are required to complete internships, externships, fieldwork, practicums, etc. This is a move in the right direction, but it's certainly too little and too late and moving too slowly for the millions of children who will suffer anxiety, depression, academic and social failure, and the stigma of clinical diagnoses such as ADHD and dyslexia, that may hobble their self-esteem, simply because they're being forced to learn in a manner and in an environment that is antithetical to the way their brains naturally process information.

If education is to become truly tolerant of neurological diversity, it will need to prove it by providing diverse learning experiences, rather than paying lip-service to the notion of diversity, while simultaneously stuffing all children in the same basic classroom environment, where they're measured using the same standard assessments, and taught the same standard curricula. Prior to Gutenberg's invention and the revolutions of information and industrialization that followed, virtually all learning was contextual, hands-on, experiential learning. Hunting and gathering societies and agricultural societies did not need schools, as everything one needed to learn was learned directly from others while on the job. In the case of crafts, young apprentices learned directly from their masters, also on the job.

It was only after the Industrial Revolution that the effects of the revolution of information that preceded it—the Print Revolution—came full circle. The rise of literacy, the first mass media, and the "Enlightenment" that came in its wake, paved the way for the application of new knowledge in the form of rampant industrialization. The new world created by industrialization in turn created a need for mass literacy, creating the need for mass education, which led to the current system of decontextualized learning. School, a quiet place removed from the adult work environment where children could learn to master the medium of abstract decontextualized knowledge, was a place created by and for the book.

The new information revolution, the Digital Revolution, is now creating effects that are similar to that of the Print Revolution, but in the time frame of years and decades, rather than centuries. As digital information fosters post-literate and post-symbolic communication, we will see a reversal from academic learning to experiential learning. Why learn about the rainforest in a classroom using a textbook, when you can take an educational virtual tour via the internet using virtual reality technology? Why study about marine life in a classroom with a textbook, if you can swim with the virtual dolphins? Learning will exit the classroom via the digital door leading to the infinite. Learning will be remarried to experience. Young people will no longer be sequestered in school—away from the "real world"—in order to academically prepare for the "real world." In the future, the world itself will be one big school, integrated and interconnected via digital technology.

The new information technology will herald new ways of communicating information—new media environments—in which new ways of teaching and new ways of learning will be inducted. When the primacy of learning-through-doing is re-established, the current academic system, based on specialism in any of the myriad fields of abstract learning, will obsolesce. It's likely that the age-old system of apprenticeship will be revived, as many trades are better learned via one-to-one hands-on instruction with a "master," rather than decontextualized classroom learning, in which a credentialed "master" pontificates abstractly to scores or even hundreds of students in a vast lecture hall. Digital conferencing technology can foster this one-to-one pedagogy, thus eliminating the obstacles of time and space that made the traditional school structure the only viable way that society could educate the masses. The teachers of the future will be everyone.

In this scenario, it's quite likely that every teacher will be a student as well. As learning is and should be considered a lifelong process that doesn't end with a degree, we will see less age segregation in the various fields of learning, with adults spending more time engaged in learning, and children spending less time in the traditional classroom, and more time engaged in practical vocational-educational experiences within "real world" settings. In the new media environment, there will be fewer distinctions between teacher and student, author and reader, master and apprentice, as those roles will become increasingly fluid and interchangeable. There will be less focus on granting and earning specialized degrees to prove qualification, less concern about the assessment of decontextualized knowledge, less focus on people needing to prove what they know; and a renewed focus on what people can actually do and show to others in the "real world."

The classroom of the future will be the world.

SEVEN

Social Media

NARCISSUS LOST IN THE HALL OF MIRRORS

*I call this peculiar form of self-hypnosis "**Narcissus narcosis**," a syndrome whereby man remains as unaware of the psychic and social effects of his new technology as a fish of the water it swims in ... .*

—Marshall McLuhan (1969)[1]

... What if the left hemisphere were able to externalize and make concrete its own workings—so that the realm of actually existing things apart from the mind consisted to a large extent of its own projections?

*... It would make it hard, and perhaps in time impossible, for the right hemisphere to escape from the **hall of mirrors**, to reach out to something that truly was "Other" than, beyond, the human mind.*

—Iain McGilchrist, (2009)[2]

Have you ever used your phone as a mirror?

Ironically, the super-intelligent smartphone is in its purest form when it's turned off and its screen darkened, for only then do we see that the screen is *truly* a mirror. Once the phone is turned on and the device's digital media activated, the images floating by on the screen deceive us into believing that the phone is a window to the outside world. Like Narcissus gazing into his pond, we're oblivious to the underlying nature of the medium in front of us, and therefore oblivious to the fact that, when gazing at our phones, we're not looking outwardly at the world, but inwardly at ourselves. What we mistake for the images of others are merely our own reflections in the mirror, the mirror that both creates and allays the unbearable anxiety of being.

The words we hear in our heads, the voice of consciousness, are ruminations about our own existence. But even when thinking about others, our words cannot truly reflect the true nature of other people's existences. Our thoughts can only reflect *our own impressions* of other people, and those impressions in turn could only be understood by comparing them to our own experiences. I can never truly know how you think or feel, because I have no direct experience of your thoughts and feelings. I have only my impressions of you, garnered primarily from my interpretations of your words, which are merely metaphors for your thoughts and feelings, not your actual thoughts and feelings. The only way I could understand you or your experience is to compare my subjective impression of you to myself and my own experience. That comparison, however, does not mean that I understand *you.* It only means that I understand the *reflection* of me that I compare with my *impression* of you. Hence, all my thoughts about others are merely personal reflections on my own experiences and impressions, projected outwardly onto other people and then reflected back onto me. Since I cannot understand anything unless it's in relation to myself, I can never truly understand anything without first filtering it through the interpretive mirror of myself.

The purpose of this brief diatribe on subjectivism is merely to illustrate that all media, from the most basic—oral language—to the most technologically complex—streaming videos on an iPhone—are experienced cognitively as *mirrors* of our own thoughts and reflections about our own experiences and our own selves.

McLuhan used Narcissus as an extended metaphor for our relationship with our media devices, which is, in essence, a technologized relationship with ourselves: "It is this continuous embrace of our own technology in daily use that puts us in the Narcissus role of subliminal awareness and numbness in relation to these images of ourselves. By continuously embracing technologies, we relate ourselves to them as servomechanisms."[3] The Narcissus role is one in which we're aware of what we're doing, but unaware of the motivation, nor of the consequences. More specifically, it's a role in which we use technology for our own purposes, while remaining unaware that the technology, in turn, is using *us* for its own purposes.

Consider social media in general, and a medium such as Facebook in particular. The media world lures us in with images and information about infinite people. Its promise is that of connection and relatedness with others. As a digital representation of our own identities, Facebook becomes an "extension" of ourselves. People can discover and explore our identities online, and we can do the same to others. Yet the process itself is entirely self-referential. When exploring another person's Facebook identity, we're either consciously or unconsciously comparing them to ourselves. Are his pics prettier than mine? Is his house nicer than mine? Is he on a better vacation than me? With better kids?

A better car? A better wife? A better life? Though the "purpose" of Facebook and other social media is to relate to others, in practice its function is as a medium for *social comparison*, a way for us to compare our lives with other people's lives. In other words, it's a mirror, but a fancy mirror, because rather than providing a direct reflection of ourselves, it provides a projection of ourselves based on comparisons with the digital reflections of others.

And while the medium functions as a hidden mirror, it also functions as a hidden camera, funneling our personal expressions, our preferences and desires, back to Facebook Corp., Inc., who then commoditizes our personal information into advertisement and solicitation revenue for companies who want to sell us toothpaste and kitty litter. Every time we respond to a notification from Facebook regarding someone else's post or comment, we're being used by a corporation that promises connection but offers only reflection. In responding to the "Echo" call of Facebook, we become the "servomechanism" to our own media device, dutifully logging in to demonstrate how engaged we are with others, as we anxiously obsess over our self-comparisons with them, even as our identities are mined by corporations seeking a new angle through which to sell us what we don't even know we need.

Social media, like the fortune-telling mediums of old, provide us with a mirror, and then in capturing our images and identity, sell them back to us through ads and targeted marketing.

> The Greek myth of Narcissus is directly concerned with a fact of human experience, as the word *Narcissus* indicates. It is from the Greek word *narcosis*, or numbness. The youth Narcissus mistook his own reflection in the water for another person. This extension of himself by mirror numbed his perceptions until he became the servomechanism of his own extended or repeated image. The nymph Echo tried to win his love with fragments of his own speech, but in vain. He was numb. He had adapted to his extension of himself and had become a closed system.[4]

The "numbness" or "narcosis" that McLuhan refers to above is the essence of narcissistic self-indulgence.

Have you ever googled yourself? It can easily become a never ending process of reflecting upon images and information of yourself reflected by Google, clicking on link after link to discover more and more images and information about yourself, as well as images and information about past friends, acquaintances, and paramours, whose connection with you cast them in the mirror as comparison reflections, a means of looking at yourself through the silhouettes of others. The process of digital self-reflection, whether mediated through Google or Facebook or Instagram or some other form of digital or social media, is a "narcotic" process. The narcosis or numbness that we feel after the umpteenth hour of digital self-reflection arises from the addictive desire to continue gazing at these mysteriously engaging images. We can't stop gazing because we've unwittingly fallen desperately in love with those uncannily engaging and familiar images. The mystery behind their narcotic attraction is at the heart of the numbing effect. The attraction, the obsession, is with *ourselves*. The addictive quality of the obsession stems from our unawareness of our own narcissism, as the magic mirror of social media offers images of others. Only in our unconscious minds do these images flip back into socio-comparative reflections upon ourselves. "[The] wisdom of the Narcissus myth does not convey any idea that Narcissus fell in love with anything he regarded as himself."[5]

In olden days (and modern ones too), there were mediums who, for a nominal fee, could read your fortune and reveal your future. The classic method was to use a crystal ball—a wonderfully symbolic object—for as we gaze into the crystal ball, we see nothing but ourselves. What the medium reveals is merely what she can guess from the things you've already said, and the images that are manifest in the mirror image of the crystal ball. In short, the crystal ball was and is just a mirror, and the medium was and is just a woman who fools you into believing that your own reflected image is more than just a simple reflection.

The modern mediums—digital social media—perform similar functions. For a hidden fee, they provide delusory reflections of ourselves that we believe are something other than ourselves. The significant difference between the old mediums and the new media is that, in the old days, you had to go to a gypsy tent or a witch's hut to hear your fortune. That is, you had to enter a mysterious and eerie environment in order to experience the peculiar sensation of connection with the invisible spirit world. In the digital age, we live entirely within the mystical environment of infinite connection. The ether surrounding us is filled with invisible electromagnetic signals that transmit infinite images and information directly into the phones in our hands. And it's precisely the *invisibility* of this new media environment that imbues it with the power to lure us into it, to envelope and embed us within it, to blind us to its hidden costs and unseen agendas, to dazzle us with its infiniteness while keeping us completely unaware of its true nature.

> As a result, precisely at the point where a new media-induced environment becomes all pervasive and transmogrifies our sensory balance, it also becomes invisible. This problem is doubly acute today because man must, as a simple survival strategy, become aware of what is happening to him, despite the attendant pain of such comprehension.[6]

McLuhan's warnings, now over a half-century old, about invisible media environments, seem to strike a more urgent tone in the digital age. Our relationships with our media devices—our phones, tablets, laptops, consoles, etc.—have become so tightly embedded in our daily lives, that we may not only safely say that these devices are now extensions of our selves, but that to a significant extent, we have become "servomechanisms" to our own devices, witlessly responding to each beck and call with dutiful servility. While McLuhan was able to see with oracular vision the changing media landscape around him and predict their effects, his understanding of the inner media landscape was limited.[7] For the internal media environment—the way that information is perceived and processed in the brain—I return to psychiatrist and neurologist, Iain McGilchrist.

In *The Master and His Emissary*, McGilchrist warns us of another narcissistic trend fostered by technology:

> … the right hemisphere delivers "the Other"—experience of whatever it is that exists apart from ourselves…. But what if the left hemisphere were able to externalize and make concrete its own workings—so that the realm of actually existing things apart from the mind consisted to a large extent of its own projections? Then the ontological primacy of right hemisphere experience would be outflanked, since it would be delivering—not "the Other," but what was already *the world as processed by the left hemisphere.* It would make it hard, and perhaps in time impossible, for the right hemisphere to escape from the hall of mirrors, to reach out to something that truly was "Other" than, beyond, the human mind.[8]

The digital age provides us with a virtual world that is, without exaggeration, created by the left hemisphere of the brain. Digitality—a communication system based on sequential and linear strings of abstract logico-mathematical code—is a medium that epitomizes left hemispheric attention. The digital medium is ubiquitous and all-inclusive, subsuming all other media in its wake. A webpage, for instance, is able and likely to include print media in the form of written words, oral language in the form of podcasts, mimetic representations of people or animals in video clips, images in both static and moving format, music, art, theater, etc. As the digital medium can literally deconstruct any content into the most basic code imaginable (binary code), there is no media content that cannot be digitalized … a fact that portends manifold overarching consequences.

Though nondigital media frame their content, thus framing our perception and comprehension of that content, they're limited in the type of content they can purvey. Print is a medium for only one type of content, the written word. The same is true for oral language and the spoken word. Radio is a medium only for auditory stimuli such as music and talk, television and film are media only for audio/visual stimuli such as sitcoms and films, theater is a medium only for human movement, music, and voice, and so on. The limitations of these non-digital media is also their saving grace, because they're fundamentally limited to only bits and pieces of our mental lives. Digital media, however, are all-encompassing, allowing them to subsume all other forms of media, thereby giving them the potential to consume our entire mental lives. While this potentiality is a grave matter of concern, it would be both impossible and impractical to discuss the effect of digital media on *everything.* The discussion in this chapter, therefore, focuses on just one form of digital media—social media—selected because the psychosocial effects of this form of digital media are particularly insidious, invasive, and entirely invisible.

If digital media are all-encompassing and all-subsuming, if they have the potential to take over our mental lives entirely, and if they are the products of a typically left-hemispheric manner of attending, then the danger invoked in McGilchrist's thesis is embodied most fully in the form of social media. For if, in McGilchrist's words, "the right hemisphere delivers 'the Other'—experience of whatever it is that exists apart from ourselves"—and that "Other" is now becoming experienced indirectly via digital media, then the right hemisphere is indeed being "outflanked" by the left, because the left is quickly grasping control of the means of discourse and relation for all information. Via the process of digitalization, we can imagine a near future in which the left hemisphere has reshaped the world, in the way that we conceive and perceive it, in its own image—*"the world as processed by the left hemisphere."*

While there is danger in this idea in toto, the greatest danger by far arises when the thing that must never by any means be deconstructed into atoms and reprocessed analytically, is deconstructed and digitalized. This thing is human relations with other humans; and it's this thing in particular that's being digitized and deconstructed via social media. When the left hemisphere "outflanks" the right hemisphere by outpacing and replacing the traditional media of social relations (spending real time with real people in the real world), with a virtual reproduction of social relations via social media, then the entire experience of relationship with "the Other" is devitalized ... reprocessed, altered, and made virtual rather than real and alive. To recall Martin Buber's classic distinction, a person that I relate to in real time and in real space is a subject (a "Thou"), while a virtual reproduction of a person that I relate to in unreal time via the unreal dimension of the digital ether, is no longer a subject but an object (an "it").[9]

Social media presents the biggest danger within the invisible hall of mirrors that the left hemisphere is making of the Western world, because it imperceptibly alters our perception and experience of social relationships—downgrading real relationships into unreal digital interactions—and downgrading our experience of real people as subjects into the processing of unreal media profiles as objects. In short, social media does not provide us with a means of relation with real people, but rather, it offers us the left hemisphere's virtualized version of people, which ultimately is merely a projection of ourselves, as we can never truly relate to an object on a screen as if it were a real person. The person on the screen appears to us as the other, but like the facade that appears in the magic mirror or crystal ball, the image is merely our own projection, masking the reflection of our selves in the persona of an other.

As a reminder that virtual relating is not, of course, in any way real, we could note that in the real world, we have real friends that we relate to as real others. In social media, we have virtual "friends" that we may never meet in the real world and never relate to as a real other, making them quite unreal. The effect is such that, while in the real world, we can make friends and relate to friends and even distance ourselves from friends, but only in the virtual world of social media could we "unfriend" someone with a click of a button. The verb "unfriend" exists only in the virtual world of social media, because one can only "unfriend" a virtual object, one cannot "unfriend" a real person. There is no "unfriend" function in the real world.

And so we find ourselves increasingly lost in the virtual hall of mirrors created by and for the left hemisphere. What's worse, the left hemisphere is a narcissist, because only a narcissist prefers gazing at his own projected self to the company of real others, and only a narcissist is so unaware of his own narcissism that he mistakes a mirror for a window, and on object for a person.

The Self as Object

> ... for thousands of years the left hemisphere has suppressed the qualitative judgment of the right, and the human personality has suffered for it.
>
> —McLuhan & Powers[10]

In his paper "On Narcissism" (1914), Freud introduces the concept of narcissism as a form of neurosis, in which the individual redirects the love and adoration usually focused towards an external love object, back onto himself. Because the narcissist loves himself more than anyone else, he tends to shut himself off from others, and tends to ignore the needs of others, while simultaneously expecting that others will always fulfill his own needs. While the term "object" in psychoanalytic theory generally refers to anything that satisfies a psychosexual drive or need, in practice, it usually refers to a person who satisfies a desire, like a mother, father, husband, or wife. The term "object" is significant, because it suggests that we often treat people like objects—as things whose function is to please us—rather than as subjects, who are people just like us. McGilchrist (2009) pointed out that the left hemisphere of the brain specializes in dealing with objects that can be manipulated, as the left hemisphere controls the right hand for physically manipulating objects, and it also controls speech and the written word, for mentally manipulating objects. The right hemisphere, on the other hand, specializes in dealing with subjects, that is, with other people.

When we enter the parallel dimension of social media, we enter a world of subjects who, in projecting their personae into the ether, objectify themselves, turning their mirror images into objects for others to behold, and who in turn relate to other personae as objects as well. Perhaps the greatest danger of social media is the way it erases the line between personal and professional personae, especially on networking sites such as Facebook and LinkedIn, that encourage this incestuous intermingling of personal and professional interests. When someone is trying to get ahead professionally, they need to promote themselves, "package" themselves, to appear appealing to potential employers or clients. Once we begin to package ourselves, we begin treating ourselves like objects—like commodities to be promoted and sold—losing sight of our true selves as subjects.

> Our private and corporate lives have become information processes just because we have put our central nervous systems outside us in electric technology.—McLuhan (1962)[11]

When self-objectification, self-promotion, and self-commoditization get intermingled with our personal personae via the double-sided card of social media, we run the risk of self-exploitation ... selling our souls for a quick profit. We also run the risk of seeing others as mere objects, and treating them as such. The ubiquity of "camming" within the digital generation—dancing nude or masturbating for tips on streaming video sites such as Chaturbate—reveals the ease in which people who grew up on social media are willing to exploit their bodies and identities for a little bit of cash and recognition.

The dramatic rise in the popularity of tattooing, piercing, scarring, cutting, and other forms of self-mutilation and self-injurious behavior, all point to an increasingly objectified attitude towards the body and the self. The need for recognition and the need to stand out in the predominantly visual world of social media is a primary motivation for the digital generation in making permanent and damaging alterations to their bodies. These alterations do provide visual uniqueness—a commodity that comes at a premium on social media—and a commodity that young people are all too eager and willing to adopt, even at the extremely high cost of permanently mutilating their bodies.

Personal identity in pre-digital generations was a personal thing we kept inside of us, expressed outwardly in our words and deeds. The digital generation, however, is pressured both by peers and by multi-conglomerate social media corporations to express their identity on the outside, via social media. This puts all of the focus on outward appearance and none on inward character, because inner character doesn't pop off the screen in social media, the way that a naked teenaged body covered in tattoos and piercings pops off the screen. On social media, identity must be externalized in order for it to be shown, and the only way this is accomplished is through altering and projecting the surface of the physical body.

Identity on social media must be visual—but this can be expressed in less permanent and damaging ways than mutilating the body. The permanent and damaging aspect of the digital generation's unprecedented obsession with body alterations has to do, I believe, with the way the experience of the "word" has changed in the digital generation. In previous generations, the word was invariably experienced as marks on paper that were physical, material, and permanent. In the digital generation, the word is primarily experienced as transitory little images scrolling down the screen of a digital device. The digital word is entirely impermanent, and therefore less impactful, making words in general less important. So, if one wishes to make a significant statement of identity on social media, words are simply insufficient. The statement needs to be permanent in the way words used to be but no longer are; and it also needs to be dramatic, in order to capture the attention of a generation of people who, by pre-adolescence, have already seen everything. Only the tattoo, or other permanent skin or body damaging signs of identity, meet those criteria.

When we permanently damage our own bodies as a show for others, we turn our bodies into show things, objects, billboards for the commodities we're promoting, which is our selves. Now, the individual doing the damage to their body doesn't see it that way. They see the damage as an adornment that expresses their identity, and that's exactly the point. It's precisely because they have turned their own body into a *medium* for their identity, that the individual engaged in damaging self-mutilation is blind to their own self-exploitation; for as McLuhan taught us, the user is generally unaware of the psychological impact of the medium their using. The digital youth is like Narcissus, who sees only the figure within his visual field, which is the same as the content of his medium, which are both, of course, himself. The ground of the visual field, the effects of the medium of communication—social media, in this case—remain invisible.

The naked, tattooed, pierced, and scarred teen—gyrating on a cam for virtual penny tips—is completely unaware that he's being used by a corporation, and that he's engaging in self-exploitation. No one, obviously, would knowingly exploit himself. It's the complete invisibility of the effects of the medium that conceals the attention economy behind the scenes, in which each second of a user's attention is mined by media corporations selling advertisements and subscriptions. Only in this virtual realm of invisibility could media corporations use their users so conspicuously, luring the gullible children into the digital den of iniquity, enslaving them in a sinister half-world of sexual self-exploitation, and selling their images to voyeurs for pennies on the dollar. The beauty of it all, from the corporate point of view, is that the children exploit themselves, with hardly any encouragement necessary.

In *The Master and His Emissary,* McGilchrist notes that "the body was never so much on display, here or in cyberspace. The body has become a thing ... an object in the world like other objects....The left hemisphere's world is ultimately narcissistic, in the sense that it sees the world "out there" as no more than a reflection of itself: the body becomes just the first thing we see out there, and we feel impelled to shape it to our sense of how it 'should' be."

When we regard ourselves habitually from the third person perspective of the social media mirror—from the point of view of someone else viewing us—our inward focus is externalized, until we only care about the surface of our bodies, for that's all that's perceived. We begin to regard our selves quite objectively and entirely visually, like an image on a photographic plate, so that we could imagine "exposing" ourselves to others in a certain light, and we can even consider the risk of "overexposure," in which the virtual image we share on a certain social media outlet leaks into the actual real image we share with our family and friends.[12]

The digital monolith casts an enormous shadow. The common existence of dual identities, shadowy personae with fake usernames and secondary internet identities—the dark web—"oh what a tangled web we weave...."[13]

Kohut's Mirror Model of Narcissism

In his monograph, *The Analysis of the Self: A Systematic Approach to the Psychoanalytic Treatment of Narcissistic Personality Disorders* (1971), Heinz Kohut provided a psychodynamic model of narcissism that (like my model), relied on the mirror as an extended metaphor. Kohut argued that parents provide a psychosocial "mirror" for their child, reflecting his or her own behavior and personality in the way that they respond to the child's needs. The mirror that the parents provide can be flawed in a variety of ways, with each different flaw resulting in a corresponding personality issue developed by the child. Kohut believed that the need to be mirrored is a normal "primary" form of narcissism. Secondary forms of narcissism emerge as a result of the different mirrors that our developing personae reflect in as we grow up. These "selves" evolve into different types of personality traits, each one echoing a different narcissistic need.

Unlike my model, Kohut was interested in how narcissistic personality traits formed in childhood reemerge later in life during psychoanalysis, revealing themselves as different forms of "transference" with their therapist.[14] However, if, for a moment, we replace the "mirror role" of the parent/analyst with the "mirror role" of social media, Kohut's model becomes instructive and elucidating for the current model being discussed.

When parents provide too small of a mirror, they're providing a lack of stimulating responsiveness to their children. As a result, the children experience themselves and their lives as boring and uninteresting. The "mirror hungry personality" develops from this "understimulated self"—a personality that's continually searching for love objects who will admire and nurture him or her—recalling the narcissistic need of the infant to be mirrored by its mother. Mirror hungry personalities may be showoffs, exhibitionists, provocateurs, etc., as they're constantly seeking external responses and reflection from others to ward off feelings of lethargy, depression, and emotional numbness. Certainly, when perceived through the lens of social media, we see a lot of mirror hungry personalities out there. To a large extent, the world of social media seems to be tailor made for the mirror hungry personality, who needs daily affirmation and responsiveness from others, no matter how distant, in order to feel stimulated, appreciated, and whole.

When parents provide a cracked mirror, they're only offering responsiveness to select parts of the child's self. For instance, parents may only be responsive to their children when they get good grades, remaining indifferent to other aspects of the children's lives. As a result, the children experience themselves as healthy in only one aspect of life, and unhealthy in others. The "fragmenting self" reveals itself as a "contact-shunning personality," as the fragmented ego is so fragile and its fear of rejection or abandonment so acute, that the individual is afraid of close emotional contact with others. Contact-shunning behavior obviously leads to isolation and loneliness. Of course, social media are ironically filled with people who shun contact with others in the real world.

Social media give us an inordinate amount of control over social interactions, so that the user—sitting safely in solitude on his sofa—may pick and choose his virtual interactions, and bail out of any one at any time. He also picks and chooses what he responds to, and what he ignores. For example, if my friend posts something about a joint project we're doing, I'm likely to post a comment about that project and that project only, while ignoring completely everything else on my friend's profile. This is a fragmented response to a fragmented page of web content, facilitated by a medium that engenders fragmentation by its very nature. (Everything on social media is digitized, i.e., fragmented into bits of digital information, as a function of being uploaded onto the internet.) Thus, the fragmented self on social media fragments its own interpersonal relationships, responding only to bits of other people's profile personae that the self selects, and in turn, being responded to by other personae in the same fragmented manner. Social media does not provide real interaction with real people, only fragments of interactions with fragments of virtual people. When this type of fragmented interaction becomes the norm, we will have created an entire society of contact shunning personalities, who can interact only when their fear of rejection and close emotional contact is completely allayed by a technology that promises connection, but in reality, offers only reflection, fragmented interaction, and disconnection.

When parents provide an enlarging mirror, it has a magnifying effect on the child's ego, resulting in an "alter ego hungry personality," who seeks relationships with others who are perceived as being just like them, as their inflated ego craves to be mirrored. Real interpersonal relationships typically end relatively soon for the alter ego hungry personality, because they eventually realize that the other person is somewhat different from themselves, and they cannot accept the other for who he or she truly is.

Virtual relationships on social media, however, would seem to be, once again, tailor-made for alter ego hungry narcissists, who only appreciate people exactly like themselves (betraying in their preferences the self-love embodied in narcissism). In exchanging relationship quality for relationship quantity, social media creates a world where one can find limitless fragments of people that reflect the same ideals, preferences, and lifestyle choices as your own. If one profile turns out to reflect ideas that are not exactly the same as yours, another profile can be found with a simple swipe of the finger. The ease in finding people with similar personae on social media leads to yet even more irony about the medium itself. We use social media, theoretically, to connect and communicate with others, yet we often tend to use social media only to relate to virtual others who think like us—hence we're not so much relating to others, but relating to reflections of ourselves. When the virtual other's reflection becomes less than identical, we move on to another virtual other.

Similarly, while social media have a plethora of information and opinions, rather than using the medium to broaden our own ideas and our own concerns, we tend to use the medium to seek out profiles of only those who reinforce and reflect our own positions, making us even more entrenched in our own solipsistic reference points, and even less open or tolerant to the ideas of others. Social media thus have the paradoxical effect of narrowing rather than broadening people's viewpoints, and radicalizing rather than moderating political positions.

Social media and online gaming operate via the user's creation of a "profile" or "avatar," which is, in essence, an "alter ego" that reflects not only the user's personality, but also their penchant for fragmenting their own personality into an alternative identity. The online alter ego interacts with other online alter egos in a virtual hall of mirrors where infinite reflected images give the semblance of lots of "friends," until we look close enough to discover that the myriad images are all just projections of the user's need to be reflected.

And finally, when the parents provide a broken mirror, they've abandoned, abused, or neglected the child, in which case the child will perceive the world as a hostile and dangerous place, preconditioning them to overreact with hostility, aggression, and anger to even minor frustrations or fears, as they're unable to rationalize the threat to their ego. The "overburdened self" reveals itself in the "merger-hungry personality." In relationships, "merger-hungry" types continually merge their own selves with figures that they idealize, losing their own individuality as they seek refuge within the ego of someone they perceive as being greater than themselves.

Kohut also referred to the same basic type as "ideal-hungry personalities," who continually search for others, typically parental figures, whom they could admire. They may often cast a blind eye towards the defects in the people they idealize. Contrastingly, they may become hostile or distressed when the reality of the actual person doesn't live up to the ideals that have been projected onto them, in which case the projector is quickly disillusioned, immediately un-merging and re-merging again with another object of idealization.

The "borderline" behavior of users on social media bear witness to this "merger-hungry" and "ideal-hungry" type of narcissistic personality. By "borderline," I'm referring to behavior similar to that of someone with Borderline Personality Disorder, which is marked by a desperate need for attachment. Borderline personalities rush much too quickly into relationships, which they falsely believe to be more intimate than they truly are. Then, just as quickly, they become disillusioned with the relationship when it fails to live up to their need for support, typically ending with hostility, as the borderline personality promptly moves on to another doomed relationship. This unstable cycle of idealization, merger, disillusionment, disconnection, and re-merging, is so common on social media that it's practically the norm.

"The Age of Narcissism"

The notion that we're living in an age of unprecedented narcissism is not new. In his book *The Cry for Myth* (1991), Rollo May, the renowned existential psychologist, dubbed the latter half of the 20th century, "The Age of Narcissism." May argued that the decline of traditional values in the West—religiosity, nationalism, patriotism, as well as "family values"—has had the effect of "hollowing" out the human spirit, what Sartre famously referred to as the *"God-shaped hole in the heart of man where the divine used to be."* In efforts to fill that existential hole, the disenchanted (that is, the *de-spiritualized*), modern American turned to materialistic rather than spiritual fulfillment. Seeking subjective meaning by elevating his own ego to the level of deity, modern Americans began worshipping themselves, expressing their self-devotion with expensive pretty objects, lavish self-adornments, ultra-luxurious homes and cars, hedonistic lifestyles, and endless self-obsessions.

Somewhat similar arguments were made over a decade before by Christopher Lasch in his National Book Award–winning *The Culture of Narcissism: American Life in an Age of Diminishing Expectations* (1979). More recently, psychologists Jean Twenge and Keith Campbell approached narcissism from a psychological disease model of study. Their book *The Narcissism Epidemic: Living in the Age of Entitlement* (2009) points the finger at over-indulgent parenting, a culture of excessive self-admiration and bloated self-esteem, unrealistic economic mindsets towards credit and debt, and, of course, new media. Obviously, the focus in this chapter is specifically on media's contribution to the apparently accepted notion that narcissism is the psychosocial plague of the modern world. My focus on media, however, is not just because I'm a media psychologist, but because the new media that has entered our world in the past two centuries has created entirely new environments of information and perception that have extremely significant effects on the way that we think about ourselves. If every medium is, indeed, a mirror, then the explosive level of magnification and multiplication of our media mirrors, will undoubtedly be reflected in our mirror-bound perceptions of ourselves.

The English word "mirror" is derived from the Latin word mīrus, "to wonder" or "to marvel at," a derivation which seems to recapture the initial wonder and marvel of a new technology, composed of polished metal and glass, that lures us in and hypnotizes us with an otherworldly charm. It wasn't just Lewis Carroll who saw magic in the looking glass, and wondered if the parallel dimension it reflected was real or just a dream. The secret of the mirror's spell, however, is not in the technology, nor in the image it reflects, but in the space between the mirror reflection and the user, the space where the user wonders at the mysteries of his own identity, and marvels at the apparent duality of his own being.

The Soul Photograph

> *When everything happens at once, when everybody becomes totally involved in everybody, how is one to establish identity?*
>
> —McLuhan (1962)

Prior to the advent of the new medium of photography in the 19th century, any representation of a person had to be created by hand, with ink, pencil, paint, clay, or some other means of artistic impression. A photograph, however, is a completely different medium than a painting, drawing, or sculpture. A portrait is an *impression* of the model, representing a combination of the model's actual appearance, transposed and interpreted through the hand and eye of the artist, and transformed via the physical aspects of the medium itself. A photograph, on the other hand, is not an impression of the model, but rather, it's a direct *representation* of the model. That is, a re-presentation—a means of taking what is presented to our eyes in the real world—and then re-presenting it to the eye afterwards in a medium that captures the physical reality of the model, without distortion at the hands of the impressionable and impression- izing artist. (For this discussion, photography is considered a means of creating direct representations. Photography as an art form, in which photographers are indeed trying to create impressions rather than rep- resentations, is relevant, but not the point here.) Photography presents us with a medium that is much more mirror-like than any medium that came before it.

Consider, for instance, the famous painting by surrealist painter René Magritte, entitled *The Treachery of Images* (1929), which is just a painting of a tobacco pipe, with the subtitle *"Ceci n'est pas une pipe"* (This is not a pipe). Magritte's point, made at a time when the modern media of photography and film were quickly displacing the traditional arts as media of mass attention, is that the painting of a pipe is actually not a pipe at all, but a depiction or impression of a pipe. "Could you stuff my pipe?" Magritte asked. "No, it's just an image of a pipe, is it not?"[15]

Magritte's intention was to show us how we often mistake the rep- resentation of something for the thing itself. (Just like we often mis- take the symbols of numbers and logical operators for the entire field of mathematics.) Magritte's point, however, would've been entirely lost if he'd used photography as his medium, rather than paint. A photograph of a pipe with the subtitle "This is not a pipe" would've elicited mass confusion rather than enlightenment. That's because when we look at a photograph, we think of it as a veritable reflection of reality, in a manner that can never be evoked by handmade media.

There are apocryphal stories about the Lakota chief Crazy Horse (1840–1877) refusing to be photographed, because he believed that the camera would steal his soul and imprison it on film or photographic paper. These legends, whether true or untrue, persisted and were pop- ularized, because we truly do sense the difference between the reality- capturing nature of a photograph, and the impressionistic depictions of earlier media. In capturing our actual physical likeness without human impression or distortion, photography does indeed seem to partake of our own personal identity in ways that paintings and drawings cannot.

Furthermore, if our personal identity is in some way related to our "soul," than Crazy Horse was more correct than anyone could've con- ceived at the time. For if we fast forward through the decades in which photography was democratized and put into the hands of the people, so that everybody could take a snapshot of themselves or their friends; and if we proceed into the Digital Age of photography, when every- one carries around a camera in the form of a smartphone, and is fre- quently engaged in taking snapshots, mainly of themselves, in the form of "selfies"; and if we note that most if not all of these selfies are posted on the internet for the world to see—then is it not correct to suggest that our sense of personal identity (our soul), has indeed been captured in the form of digital photographic images—and that our souls, in the digital age, are no longer inside of us (as Rollo May suggested) but exteriorized into the ether, as public re-presentations of whatever it is about us that we cherish and wish to display to others. The image that somehow captures the essence of our soul?

The power of a medium lies in the invisibility of its effect on its users. When we watch a movie, for instance, we're drawn into the story and imagery as if it were a dream or flight of fantasy. The technological equipment of the medium itself—the cameras, microphones, lights, even the physical screen and physical film running through the projector—must all remain invisible in order for the illusion to work. The medium of digital photography has, quite invisibly, created a means for us to capture our own personal image, manipulate it and "photoshop" it, and then re-present it to the world, so that we could bask in the reflected glow of our own imagery. The invisibility of the technology behind digital photography, the fact that we can take a snap in a matter of seconds and then post it instantly onto the web for millions to see, without once having to think about communication satellites or silicon micro-transmitters, endows us with a tremendous amount of technological power.

The gods of old were revered for their "temporal duality," their ability to be in two places at once. Zeus, for example, could be sitting on his throne above the clouds, yet at the same time, he could project his image earthward, where he could be perceived by a mortal in the guise of a bull or a swan. Temporal duality has always been a "condition of the gods,"[16] but not anymore. The internet allows our online personae to be everywhere at once. In this way, we get to experience the condition of the gods firsthand, a condition that may predispose us towards feeling godly about ourselves. This godly feeling is, by definition, narcissistic, for what was Narcissus' great crime, for which he was punished so famously for by the gods? Was it not the hubristic sacrilege of believing himself to be grander than mortal—putting himself at the same level as the gods—displayed in his obliviousness to Echo, and the other nymphs who adored him?

The Old Gods and the New

In my previous book, *The Digital God* (2015), I argued a line of thought (following Carl Jung) that humans seem to be predisposed towards a "spiritual drive," which, in essence, is a need to connect or commune with something larger than ourselves. Existential psychologists such as Erich Fromm and Rollo May have referred to the same drive as an existential need to transcend one's own ego. Fromm, in particular, suggested that people need an "object of devotion," something outside of ourselves that we could devote ourselves to and worship. Historically, the object of devotion has been a communal spiritual figure that connected members of the community together through their collective worship and devotion to a common deity. The deity is entirely symbolic. It could be a totem animal, a fallen hero or king, or an entirely spiritual entity, such as the almighty "God" of the Judeo-Christian tradition. The key facet of the deity is that it exists simultaneously in two dimensions of being (temporal duality). The deity is outside of us, so that in reaching out to commune with it, we are transcending ourselves. More importantly, the deity is simultaneously *inside* of us. "God" is in our soul, in our spirit, in our innermost self. Thus, we've been told time and again by the prophets and sages of every religious tradition, that the path to "God" is inside of us, or as Jesus said, "The Kingdom of God is within."

> Whoever worships another divinity than his self, thinking, "He is one, I am another," knows not.—*Brihadaranyaka Upanishad*

The object of devotion is both inside and outside of us. This is the key to its spiritual power. It is "I," and it is also, "not-I."

In a similar manner, I can compose a digital image of myself and project it into the ether as my "avatar." (Significantly, the ancient Sanskrit term "avatar" is derived from the Hindu tradition, referring to the mortal form taken on by the gods when they descend to Earth.) My avatar embodies all of the conditions of the gods. It has temporal duality—it can be seen in millions of places simultaneously by millions of people. My avatar has the Protean power of the shapeshifting Greek water god, in that it can change its form at will. Also, as it exists in the ethereal mist of the internet, my disembodied soul, in the form of my avatar, is immortal, like the gods of old in their abode above the clouds. With its instant access to infinite information via its own medium, the internet, the avatar, in its own way, is not only omnipresent, but omniscient as well.

Most importantly, my avatar is both "I" and "not-I." By splitting my ego in two (as in the ego/alter-ego duality of comic book heroes), I create a mirror-image doppelganger that combines a reflection of my real self with a projection of my idealized self.[17] It is this split in the self, this dissociative doubling of my own self-concept, that sets the stage for the avatar aspect of myself to step forward into the spotlight as the dei-fied version of myself, while the mortal aspect of myself, which remains mired in the real world, humbly steps back into the role of worshipper and devotee.

Like the titular character in *The Wizard of Oz* (1939), we've become both the mystical Wizard projected outwardly, as well as the mortal shapeshifting trickster behind the curtain. The only difference is, Professor Marvel was quite aware of the illusion he was project-ing, while modern users—blind to the invisible psychological effects of our own media—are apt to become lost in the delusion of our own divinity. Again, Narcissus was quite unaware that he had unwittingly displaced the position of the gods in worshipping himself, thus his curse of eternal genuflection to his own mirror image was fittingly ironic, both for the ancient mythical Narcissus, and his modern digi-tal counterpart.

Celebrity Worship and the Social Media Mirror

Everyone, in the back of his mind, wants to be a star.
—Chad Hurley (co-founder of YouTube)[18]

Returning to the existentialists, the need for an object of devotion puts us in the position of spiritual seeker, though we may not be aware that what we're seeking is spiritual in nature, and we may not even be aware that we're seeking at all. When we use the internet, we inter-face with a "search engine" such as Google's. By default, then, an inter-net user is a "searcher," seeking information, even if they're unaware that they've taken on this role. McLuhan mused that the internet/user interface retrieves the hunter-gatherer role of Homo sapiens, replac-ing the natural wilderness with the virtual badlands of the world wide web, and replacing physical prey and quarry with metaphysical information...

> What seems to have happened is that after many years centuries, in fact, after many thousands of years, we have left this Neolithic time and have leapfrogged into a period of the hunter once more; only we live in a an age of information, and the hunter now seeks information.—McLuhan (1967)[19]

In order to transcend our own egos, we require the object of devo-tion as a focus point for our need to worship something that connects us to something larger than ourselves. Historically, the focal point of our devotion has been the gods, or the mortal heroes who embodied our desire to partake of the divine by communing with the gods and becoming semi-divine themselves. Kings of old partook of the divine via the "divine right of kings," which not only affirmed their claim to absolute power, but also their worthiness to be worshipped. Hence, the tendency for old myths, folktales, and legends to feature as their primary characters semi-divine heroes, aristocrats, and gods. This tendency was begun with scriptural media in the form of sacred texts that told the stories of the characters mentioned above, and was propagated further by the theater, which told the same stories in theatrical format, as did much of the print media, especially in the early days of print.

Following the Enlightenment, all of the popular media formats began to be secularized, broadening the cast of characters in the stories being told, while not necessarily changing the message, or its meaning. The Industrial Revolution brought with it a concentration of humanity living in the cities, who now had commodities that were rare for the average farmer or rancher of those times—money and leisure time— both of which were capitalized upon by entrepreneurs, creating amusement parks and vaudeville theaters to bring a level of entertainment to the masses that was previously enjoyed only by the wealthy. The explosive growth of the theater industry gave birth to a new order of heroes and gods—celebrities—whose shrine was the theater, whose sacrament was entertainment, and whose worshippers were not just the audience at their shows, but a new type of devotee that was invented by the new age of theater, the fanatic admirer, or "fan" for short.

When the Electronic Revolution of the 19th and 20th centuries took hold, the theater was democratized once again in electronic format, with the moving picture replacing live theater as a mode of popular entertainment that was cheaper to provide to the masses. It was then (the early 20th century) that all of the new media technology came together as one machine to create a new pantheon of gods and goddesses. The ancients projected the image of their gods onto the dark night sky, and beheld them in the stars of the constellations. The moderns saw their gods projected by electronic machines onto the silver screen, and worshipped those images as "stars," with comparable reverence. Newspapers and fan magazines in the modern age, full of photographs of Adonis-like stars and Aphrodite-like starlets, brought the sacred images of the celebrity gods into the hands and homes of their legions of fans.

The movie theater displaced the church as the house of worship, for the gods on the big screen were more present, more vital, more real than the faceless gods worshipped in church. The matinee replaced the mass.

The "matinee idol" replaced the holy icon. The gods and divine heroes of old, who were worshipped for their power and wisdom, were replaced by the pantheon of celebrity gods, worshipped for their beauty and talent. As the Electronic Revolution ensued, the godly condition of temporal duality was achieved when the sacred presence of celebrities was broadcast directly into our homes, first aurally via radio, then visually via television.

With the Digital Revolution came the technological ability to close the circuit between our inner need for something to worship, and our drive to project that need outwardly onto an external object of devotion. Television and radio brought with them the television and radio "personality," the person who was not necessarily beautiful or talented to any great degree, but who somehow got to be on radio or TV anyway. Television personalities like Paris Hilton and Kate Gosselin had no discernible talent, they were just famous for being famous. This new kind of celebrity partook of the divine by consorting with the divine in the sacred realm of broadcast news and entertainment, which exists neither in the studio where the broadcast is made, nor in the home where it's heard or viewed, but in the vast space of electromagnetic-signal-filled ether between them.

This new ability for an ordinary person to become extraordinarily famous despite the lack of any extraordinary talent or beauty, gave rise to a new possibility for all mortal beings. If fame in-and-of-itself is the new sacrament, and if being famous is to be a celebrity, and to be a celebrity is to be divine, then digital media provides the means of sanctification. If I can create my own virtual space online, fill it with photographs, videos, blogs, and all of my personal music, images, and other preferences that reflect me, and if I can get "fans" to tune into this space, then, in effect, I have deified myself.

In creating this virtual alternate identity—this avatar—I project myself outwardly into the sacred ethereal realm of the gods. I experience a doubling of my self-concept, a temporal duality of my soul. I achieve a certain level of immortality in projecting my virtual self into the ether, and I gain the adoration of my devotees, even if my principal devotee is myself.

This narcissistic onanism of being at once one's own god and one's own worshipper is not a problem in the digital age. In fact, it's precisely my point. When we get into the practice of creating a virtual self to sell, promote, and exploit online, we double ourselves, creating both a self that is to be worshipped, and a self that worships that same self. In short, when we put ourselves into the Narcissus role of self-adoration in the digital realm, we close the circuit of our need to worship something outside of ourselves (the object of devotion), with our complementary desire to be worshipped and adored by others (narcissism). This doubling of roles is quite efficient, satiating one neurotic need with another; but it's also quite dangerous, for Narcissus was quite unaware of the fact that he was, indeed, worshipping himself, and he was therefore oblivious to the "narcotic" dangers of this role.

Ouroboros and Erysichton

> In the age-old image of the Ouroboros lies the thought of devouring oneself and turning oneself into a circulatory process … this "feedback" process is at the same time a symbol of immortality, since it is said of the Ouroboros that he slays himself and brings himself to life, fertilizes himself and gives birth to himself.
>
> —Carl Jung[20]

There's a symbol that precedes by millennia the Greek myths, yet the symbol remains as potent today, if not more so, than it was in ancient times. It is Ouroboros, the serpent swallowing its own tail … a ripe symbol, as it can mean many things—fertility, infinity, totality, unity—but the interpretation I'm conjuring is expressed by Carl Jung in the quotation above. Narcissus is indeed an example of a "circulatory process," a man who, by feeding upon himself, closed the circuit of his own existence, by becoming both the object of devotion and the worshipper of himself. The danger of the Narcissus role is that once we close the circuit of our own existential loop, we no longer need or care about others, because we satisfy our own needs ourselves. In closing the loop between devotee and object of devotion, we close ourselves off psychosocially to others, just as Narcissus closed himself off to Echo and the other nymphs.

In *Metamorphoses*, Ovid told us that Narcissus wilted away in his spot by the reflecting pool, his body eventually morphing into the form of a flower, a reminder to us mortals that all beauty is fleeting, that self-adoration is a hunger that can never be sated, and when pursued, is ultimately self-devouring. Ovid told of another man with a similar affliction. There was once a king of old Thessaly named Erysichton, who offended the nature goddess Demeter by felling her sacred grove of oaks. Demeter punished Erysichton for his hubris by casting Limos—the demon of insatiable hunger—into his belly. Each bite Erysichton took only fed Limos more, quickening Erysichton's appetite rather than sating it. The king spent his treasury on food, but still he hungered. He sold his lands, his possessions, his throne, his crown ... but still he hungered. Erysichton even prostituted his own daughter, Mestra, to feed his demon, but he hungered still. In short, no amount of food could satisfy him, until he finally ate himself.

The myth of Erysichton teaches us some powerful lessons about our own media. First, Erysichton's hubris was his total disregard for the sanctity of Nature—he was destructive towards it. Similarly, any new form of media will bring disruption to a prior state of being, and this disruption can be destructive when the usage makes the user estranged to himself, or estranged to the natural condition of a mortal being, which is within Nature. Digital media, in particular, seems to drive a wedge between the user and his context within Nature, driving our bodies indoors and our minds upwards into the unnatural ether of electromagnetic signals. While we might say that it was the savage materialism of industrial humanity that caused global warming and the assault on Nature, it's the current narcissism of digital humanity, with its inherent self-centeredness and obliviousness to Nature or anything outside of ourselves, that perpetuates it.

Second, Erysichton was punished for his hubris with insatiable appetite. So too does the modern media user fall too easily into the bottomless pit of self-indulgent binging, such as watching endless hours of media content on streaming services such as Netflix and Hulu. Each binge draws us down the hole of self-indulgence, and the end of each binge is followed by the inevitable "show-hole"—the sad, empty, lonely feeling a viewer has after watching the last episode of a beloved TV series—which invariably empties out into the next binge. In the throes of his gluttony, Erysichton gives up everything that has any meaning to him, retaining only his appetite. So too does the addicted media user give up meaningful interactions and relationships in favor of the virtual bottomless feedbag of infinite media content. Like Erysichton, the media consumer is ultimately self-consuming. In trying to sate a hunger that's insatiable, we're consumed by our own appetites, and devour ourselves.

The symbols of Ouroboros and Erysichton combine to teach a lesson about media itself. Media as a phenomenon has always been self-perpetuating and self-consuming. In academia especially, books and articles tend to be about other books and articles. Newspapers and magazines report on films and TV shows. Broadcast news nowadays is preoccupied with reporting the tweets and Instagram selfies of celebrities and politicos. Meta-media—media about media—closes the media circuit, as the medium generates its own content by constantly re-generating itself: devouring, excreting, and then re-devouring its own content. The lesson to be learned is that media consumers are propelled by their own appetites, and that the greatest danger for consumers is not in the content media provides, but in the appetites that media arouse (once again, "the medium is the message"). Unlike other appetites, media appetites are never fully sated, and since they're self-generating, the supply of media content is never-ending, putting us all into the Erysichton role of the self-devouring consumer who is never full, and therefore never stops consuming, even when his consumption eats away at his very soul. When the Erysichton role of self-consuming consumer is paired with the Narcissus role of self-admiring admirer, we can imagine an Ouroboros who swallows its tail so completely that it is swallowed entirely, just as Erysichton swallowed himself.

Wounded Narcissism and the Many-Faced God in the Magic Mirror

Numerous correlational studies have demonstrated that social media use is positively related to both anxiety and depression.[21] (In keeping with the construct developed in Chapter Five, I refer to both anxiety and depression collectively, using the label "anxious-depression.") The studies do not implicate social media use as the cause of anxious-depression ("correlation does not imply causation") but the researchers in general see social media collectively as a mediator for other feelings that do cause anxious-depression. In particular, because social media foster *social comparisons* between the users and their perception of other users' profiles, social media foster feelings of jealousy, envy, and even self-loathing, which are experienced cognitively as anxious-depression.[22] Social media users themselves often note the feeling of "fomo"—fear of missing out—as a reaction they get when viewing the profile of somebody doing better stuff than they are, and that the anxiety of fomo leads to depressing self-deprecatory feelings about themselves.[23]

Particularly virulent among young women on social media is "appearance comparison," a type of social comparison focusing specifically on body image and attractiveness. Appearance comparison on social media is strongly related to body dysmorphia, a condition in which someone is anxiously depressed in an obsessive way about flaws in their body that only they can see.[24] (In this sense, body dysmorphia seems to partake of psychosis, at least a little bit, as perceiving things that are not objectively there would technically be considered delusional or even hallucinatory.)

When we view a photo of someone on social media, our brain immediately judges the attractiveness of that person.[25] This is an instinctive reaction to other people's bodies and faces that we have no control over, and it's certainly related directly to the evolutionary drive for us to find suitable mates for reproduction.[26] Attractiveness is directly related to physical health and fertility, as all of the general markers of attractiveness—clear smooth skin, straight posture, colorful full-bodied hair, symmetrical undisfigured faces and bodies—are also indicators of youth, health, and prosperity.

Studies have found that participants making judgments about the attractiveness of bodies and faces flashed before them rapidly on a monitor, make extremely accurate judgments that correspond highly with the judgments of others, in just microseconds per image.[27] The "microseconds" part of these findings is crucial, because it indicates that we make judgments about attractiveness so fast that we couldn't possibly be consciously thinking about them, our brains just do it instantly and instinctively. This means that we're all inherently judgmental about other people's looks, and that's not a choice, but a biological precondition of our species (and of many other species too). That also means that our inherently judgmental disposition is likely to reflect judgmentally upon ourselves, especially when we objectify our own bodies and faces by digitally capturing our own images and posting them on social media for the world to see, and judge.

When I look in the mirror, I see myself objectively, as if from a third person perspective. However, the regular mirror made of glass and metal is not completely objective, because I still inhabit the image I see in the mirror. I can smile, frown, change my hair, and do any number of things to subjectively change my appearance in real time, and therefore change my self-judgment about my own appearance. More importantly, since gazing into the regular mirror is a private experience, I can subjectively qualify what I see by applying things that only I know about myself: "I usually look better," "My eyes are baggy because I didn't sleep well last night," "I'm having a bad hair day," etc. Therefore, the regular mirror experience offers both an objective third person perspective, as well as a subjective first person perspective, on my appearance and attractiveness.

However, when I post a selfie on social media and then view it, the first person perspective is degraded, because I'm all too well aware that others will be viewing that image, and that others will not cut me any slack for a bad hair day, or for baggy eyes due to lack of sleep, or for any other reason. As the posted pic is a static image, it's no longer inhabited by me in the way my reflection in the mirror is inhabited by me. The social media mirror, made of silicon and digital code, unlike the regular mirror, forces me to view myself as I view others—and I intuitively know the way that I view others—objectively, judgmentally, unforgivingly, and more often than not, disparagingly. The whole phenomenon reminds me very much of the "Magic Mirror" from Disney's *Snow White* (1937)...

In the opening scene of the movie, the vain and narcissistic queen consults her Magic Mirror to compare her attractiveness with the attractiveness of others: "Magic Mirror on the Wall, Who is the fairest one of all?" Her anxious depression about her own appearance is temporarily allayed when the mirror tells her that she's "the fairest one of all." But when it doesn't, her narcissism is wounded. Her "cruel jealousy" is aroused and directed to the one that the Magic Mirror judges to be fairer than she.... Snow White.

Social media provides us with a Magic Mirror that allows us to view the images of infinite users, and of course, our instinctive comparison drive is evoked. If our narcissism is wounded when we feel less attractive than others, both jealousy and anxious depression are roused and directed either at the source of the wound—the pretty person in the innocent role of Snow White—or back onto oneself, in the form of self-loathing, which perpetuates our anxious depression. This "wounded narcissism" model would explain the high levels of aggression on social media, with vicious trolls and lurkers posting nasty spiteful posts, typically done anonymously or via a fake profile, to avoid further wounding of their fragile narcissistic egos. The "wounded narcissism" model would also explain the high correlations between social media use and anxious depression, as well as the correlations with issues such as body dysmorphia, eating disorders, and cutting, which are aggressive thoughts and acts made towards one's own body—self-aggressive, self-harming, self-injurious, or self-punitive behavior.

Like the Magic Mirror in *Snow White*, the social media magic mirror is quite objective, and it also holds an impossibly high bar for attractiveness, for the user—whether she be the Queen or Snow White—can never be "the fairest one of all," because "all" is quite a lot of people. Thus, the magic mirror will always find someone fairer than you, and so the entire process of gazing into the magic mirror is predetermined to elicit feelings of jealousy, envy, self-loathing, anxious-depression, and possibly even anger and resentment towards others whom the magic mirror determines is more fair. The social media mirror, unlike the magic one in *Snow White*, has many faces, and it often speaks an unwelcome truth about ourselves. The media mirror casts a hypnotic spell on us, a "Narcissus narcosis" that fixes us in front of it like a zombie in a trance, all the while dragging us down unwittingly into a bottomless pit of self-pity and negative self-regard.

Locked in to the Double Bind

At this point, one may ponder the notion that social media, like tic-tac-toe—or global thermonuclear war in the movie *War Games* (1983)—is a game that can't be won, so that "the only winning move is not to play." This sentiment works fine for me. I don't engage in social media, not because I don't recognize its benefits, but because I'm all too aware of its hazards. However, the same solution isn't as viable to younger generations who've grown up in the digital arena, and have never experienced life without social media. For my children's generation, socialization has largely moved from the playground and schoolyard to the virtual arena of online interactive gaming and social media.

In a very real sense, though my children and I live in the same house, we're members of two very different media environments. My media environment is dominated by books and emails that I read and write, music that I listen to and play on my piano and guitar, and movies that I watch on TV and occasionally on my laptop. Their media environment is dominated by online games and social media. So, while it's quite easy for me to opt out of social media use, it's not easy at all for my children, especially for my daughter, because opting out of social media altogether would mean, by default, opting out of the majority of socialization within her own peer group. In this sense, while I'm still relatively free to roam in and out of the digital hall of mirrors, my children are "locked in" by force of their generational pressure to conform to the usage of a common communication portal. If they don't stay locked in, they run the risk of getting locked out. (Once again, "fomo" arises as an invisible force, in this case asserting internal pressure in the minds of users to participate on social media.)

Gregory Bateson was an anthropologist whose work bridged many disciplines, including the study of cybernetics (how people and computers communicate with each other). In the 1950s, Bateson developed a theory of psychosis based on his construct of a "double bind," which is sort of like a no-win situation. Bateson theorized that when somebody is locked in to a no-win situation that they can't get out of, their adaptation to that faulty situation is likely to be faulty in-and-of-itself, "psychotic" or "schizophrenic."[28] R.D. Laing, the infamous founder of the anti-psychiatry movement in the 1960s, referred to the double bind adaptation as a "sane response to an insane situation."[29]

An example of a double bind situation would be a small child's relationship with an emotionally needy mother. First of all, the small child is not free to leave the situation, he's "locked in," which is a primary condition of the double bind. Secondly, the child in this situation may be confronted with a pair of "contradictory injunctions" (Laing referred to these as "paradoxical orders"). The first injunction from the mother may be: "I want you to hug and kiss me and say you love me." The second injunction, which is typically implied rather than explicit, may be: "But I only want you to hug and kiss me and say you love me if you really want to."

So, in this situation, if the child doesn't actually want to express affection towards his mother, he's in a double bind. Mother will be angry at him if he doesn't hug and kiss her, but if he forces himself to do it, Mother will detect that he's doing it because *she* wants him to, and not because *he himself* actually wants to, making his affectionate display disingenuous and, once again, angering his mother. The child is locked in to a double bind situation in which there is no way to avoid a negative outcome, and no way to get out of it. Furthermore, no meta-communication—communicating about the way we communicate—is possible, which is another pre-condition for the double bind. A child is unable to communicate to his mother that what she is communicating to him is utterly absurd, because he doesn't know what "absurd" is, and he himself is unaware of the absurdity of his own situation. This emotional maze with no exit creates a world of absurdity that, Bateson believed, was a breeding ground for psychosis.

Double bind scenarios abound in childhood. If Mommy says, "Comb your hair so you look nice," you may trudge to the bathroom to get a comb, prompting Mommy to say, "Don't act like it's the end of the world, you should comb your hair because you want to look nice for yourself ... don't just do it because I'm telling you to do it." This is a double bind. If I don't comb my hair, Mommy will be angry; but if I force myself to comb my hair, Mommy will see that I'm doing it for her rather than for me, which will also make her angry. Double bind scenarios, however, are certainly not limited to childhood. Jack may express the desire to have marital relations with Jane, his wife. If Jane is uninterested, she might say, "I have a headache" (i.e., "No."). If Jack presses his case, she may concede and say, "Ok, go ahead, but be quick about it." If she says that, however, Jack is likely to say, "Well, I don't want to do it *to* you, I want to do it *with* you. I want you to do it because *you* want to, not because *I* want you to." Once again, a double bind situation. If Jane says "No," Jack will be disappointed and resentful; but if she reluctantly gives in just to satisfy his needs but not hers, then he'll be equally disappointed and resentful. She can't win.

Applying these paradoxical orders and preconditions to social media reveals a clear double bind. A friend might say, "Get on Facebook so you and I can share family photos and such." If I resist, my friend may be resentful, while I get labeled as being "antisocial."[30] If I concede and do it half-heartedly, my friend will sense my insincerity and be equally resentful. I can't win.

Another paradoxical order is related to the implicit injunctions behind the "selfie." We all know that a selfie should be a spontaneous photo of oneself in an unplanned situation. That's what separates a selfie from a posed photo taken by someone else. Taking a planned and posed selfie is, of course, clearly narcissistic. However, in actuality, selfies are rarely spontaneous and un-posed. In fact, people generally take multiple selfies in multiple poses and then laboriously go through them all to select the one that looks the most spontaneous and the most candid. So, if you tell me to take a selfie and post it on social media, then I'm in a double bind. How can I plan to be spontaneous? How can I strike a pose that makes me look candid and un-posed? The selfies we're likely to see on social media are aimed at capturing candid spontaneity, but the process is controverted by the act of aiming itself, making the typical selfie appear to be the opposite of what it was intended to be; it becomes a posed candid capturing planned spontaneity.

The selfie problem exemplifies the double bind situation inherent in all social media usage. The implicit injunction in social media is, "Be genuine, be yourself." However, there can be nothing more disingenuous than creating a profile for "yourself," because you're the only person in the world who doesn't need a profile of you to know who you are. Social media profiles are made for others to see, and for others to judge, just as we see and judge the profiles of others. Hence, a social media environment that forces all members to be insincere and disingenuous is actually an "anti-social" media environment that's likely to produce "antisocial" (i.e., sociopathic) members. The vast number of "trolls" and "lurkers" in social media who do nothing but post hateful, spiteful, and vindictive comments is testament to the ironically anti-social nature of social media.

According to R.D. Laing, paradoxical orders, if correctly executed, are disobeyed. If Laing were alive today, his view on social media would likely be based on his original view of the double bind situation, that the "sane response to an insane situation is to be insane." Translated into the absurd world of social media, that would be: "The social response to anti-social media is to be anti-social."

There's a real psychological difference between socialization in real life and socialization via social media, and that difference lies in the level of control we have over the situation. In real life, a social interaction is governed by the implicit rules of interpersonal behavior—etiquette or politeness—and everyone interacting follows the rules, thus sharing control of the situation. On social media, the traditional rules of etiquette don't apply. I can start and end interactions at will, choosing how, when, why, where, and with whom I'll interact at any moment, giving me a free and easy escape route at all times.

The problem arises when someone uses social media as their primary form of social interaction, as the media dependent user is left in a state of hypersensitivity to real-life social stimuli, which are largely out of his control. Personal social interactions are felt as being "too real," because they differ from the virtual social interactions provided by media. The lack of control of real-life social interactions is disconcerting. Real people cannot be turned off like an iPhone. You can't turn the channel, lower the volume, press pause, or switch to a different profile. Hypersensitive media addicts in a real social situation try to numb themselves by receding into the social mode in which they're more comfortable, and in which they have more control. They take out their cellphone and begin texting and tweeting, even as they sit amidst a group of real-life people. This action, however, which seems incredibly asocial, is perfectly acceptable among this particular group, because they're all addicted to the same media, and engage in the same behaviors. Real life socialization is elbowed out by social media, even in real life situations.

In the end, the need to socialize in person becomes completely negated, as real-life interactions are given up in favor of social media. Even when the user is in a real-life situation, like dinner with friends, they'd much rather take out their phone and text a friend than talk to a friend sitting right in front of them. It's just easier, psychologically, to socialize at home via digital media. Social networking is more convenient, easier, and most importantly, more controllable than real-life socializing. It's much better suited to the digital sensibility. However, once a person is completely "locked-in" to social media as their primary form of socialization, they become victim to all of the aspects of the "double bind" situation explained above. That is, they put themselves into the hypnotic Narcissus role of constant self-reflection, which shields their narcissism from wounding, but also makes them incapable of truly knowing someone else.

"The Global Village"

> The new electronic interdependence recreates the world in the image of a global village.
>
> —McLuhan (1962)[31]

This chapter takes an admittedly negative stance on social media, and I'd be remiss in my duty as author were I to dismiss the fact that social media have positive qualities as well. One of McLuhan's last significant contributions to the media ecology paradigm is his construct of the "tetrad of media effects."[32] The tetrad consists of four interrelated principles of new media: Enhancement, Obsolescence, Retrieval, and Reversal.

Every new medium that is successful, succeeds because it's in some way an "Enhancement" on a prior medium. Social media are unusually successful in terms of usage at the population level, because they provide exponentially substantial enhancements on prior media. A bulletin board, for example, is a way of posting an announcement or notification for others to see. Social media are a huge enhancement on the physical bulletin board, because they are immediate, easy to use, communicate to billions of potential viewers with potentially infinite visibility, facilitate direct communication between posters and viewers, etc. Another example is the address book, which people of my age can still remember as a real thing. Social media have largely replaced the physical address book, because the electronic version is easier to maintain and edit, it facilitates connection with addressees rather than just listing them, and—most importantly—it can't be lost or misplaced. I could go on-and-on with examples, but my point, hopefully, is clear: any new media are only as successful as the enhancements over prior media that they offer. Success, in terms of usage and number of users, is directly proportional to the level of enhancement, indicating that social media—with billions of users—are obviously a huge enhancement on prior media for communicating and connecting with others.

Since new media are only successful as a function of their enhancement, new media that are very successful will tend to make prior media somewhat "obsolete" ("Obsolescence" is the second of the tetrad). Case in point, you don't see many people carrying physical address books around anymore, as this medium has been functionally replaced by social media, email accounts, and the smart phone. In new classrooms, offices, as well as in the corridors of new schools and office buildings, we don't see many traditional bulletin boards, cluttered with all sorts of notices, notifications, and announcements, as the bulletin board has also been functionally replaced by social media and the mass email or text message. Physical bulletin boards and address books have been obsolesced in the new generation by social media and other new digital media. While enhancement is generally a positive thing, obsolescence is both good and bad. While it's awesome to be able to connect with grandma instantly via Facebook, this newfound connectivity obsolesces an older means of connectivity that was less convenient—the physical visit in real time and real space—an experience that was surely more personally meaningful to both grandma, and her progeny.

The Enhancement/Obsolescence dyad of McLuhan's tetrad is merely another way of pointing out that in the zero-sum game of media adoption and media usage, nothing is gained without something else being lost. The implicit warning in the top half of the tetrad is in the danger of giving up something of great and irretrievable value, such as a hug from grandma, in favor of the new option offered by the new media, which may seem wonderful and all shiny and new and full of promise and potential, but the gleam of novelty may obfuscate the true value of the old media that the new ones obsolesce. For instance, when modern culture reaches the tipping point where social media functionally subsumes and replaces all prior modes of communication and connection, so that one must be on social media all the time in order to function in both personal and professional spheres, we might suddenly realize that something of great value—personal privacy and the luxury of being able to socially detach oneself for a period of time—have also been obsolesced.

Because new media generally offer a different sensibility in relation to the information that's being communicated and perceived, new media often "retrieve" a sensibility that's been obsolesced by the prior media. For instance, the ability to write and read written letters or dispatches in some ways obsolesced oral language and the spoken message, because it's easier to send a letter to someone far away, then to travel to that person in order to speak with him directly. The written word offered the first form of direct tele-communication (communicating from a distance). Then, in the 19th century, the telegraph came along as a new medium that in some ways obsolesced the letter, because it was exponentially quicker than "snail mail." But then, in the 20th century, the telephone entered the scene as an even newer medium that obsolesced the telegraph, but in doing so, the telephone retrieved oral language and the spoken message as a primary form of tele-communication.

Now, in the 21st century, people carry their phones everywhere, but ironically, when using our phones to communicate, we tend to prefer written modalities, such as the text message and email—retrieving the written word as a primary form of tele-communication once again. (The irony is that the word "phone" is derived from the Greek word for "voice" or "sound," so it's ironic that we use our "phones" more to look and see, rather than to say and listen.) The point that McLuhan was making is that media environments are ongoing processes that are constantly enhancing and obsolescing each other in a never-ending cycle of media adoption and media displacement, so that obsolesced aspects may get retrieved when the next media enhancement comes along.

As for social media, McLuhan believed that immediate and infinite interconnectivity would foster a "Retrieval" (the third of the tetrad) of collective living, like our ancestors experienced living in small agricultural villages, and like their ancestors experienced living in small tribes of migrating hunter-gatherers. The true village or tribal experience is entirely communal. Everybody knows everything about everyone. There's no space for privacy, and no room for individualistic expression, as any expression that deviates from the collective norm will be shouted down by the group. McLuhan famously referred to this retrieval as "the global village," and he referred to the process of collectivization that the global village evokes as "etherealization," in that the individual voice in the global village gets drowned out by the communal "group voice in the ether."[33]

When the effects of a new medium reach their limit, they often foster a "Reversal" in function or form; this is the last part of the tetrad. The example above of the telephone—invented for speech and listening, but now used more for writing, reading, and watching—shows how a medium can suddenly "flip" or functionally reverse itself. One such phenomenon with social media is the reversal of connectivity into disconnection. The "tipping point" mentioned above, where social media functionally subsumes and replaces all prior modes of communication and connection, could also be a "flipping point," in terms of a reversal.

If everyone uses social media all the time for most or all of their personal and professional correspondence and communication, what happens to people like me, who prefer to opt out of social media for philosophical reasons, and what happens to people like grandpa, when he can't master the new technology? What happens is that those who opt out or never join in to social media, are obsolesced as agents in the communication process. That is, the media designed to engender connectivity, functions as a device that *disconnects* those agents that aren't integrated in the new system of media connection. Grandpa and I are made obsolete, because the new media, in certain cases, has a flipping effect, reversing the media's initial intended purpose, and creating in its wake a sub-culture of social media exiles and ex-pats, who've been made socially invisible by the medium designed to increase social visibility.

McLuhan also recalls the ancient metaphor of the Tower of Babel in relation to social media reversals. The Bible tells us that "the whole earth was of one language and of one speech" (Genesis 11:1), but later in the same passage, it tells us that the heavenly host came down to "confound their language, that they may not understand one another's speech" (Genesis 11:7). Contrary to popular belief, the Bible says nothing about the heavenly host creating *different* languages among the builders of Babel, it merely states that the people—who were all "of one language and of one speech"—were confounded in that one language. That's to say, we were all speaking the same language, yet we could no longer understand one another. This interpretation applies quite beautifully and parsimoniously to the social media predicament, in which we see billions of users communicating, but not much being truly understood, as the medium itself fosters brief posts and comments which are so easily misconstrued that the terrain of social media has become a virtual minefield of people taking offense when no offense was intended, and people spreading misleading ideas based on misquotes and misreadings of content taken out of context. Social media is a modern Tower of Babel, in which modern users are mired in misunderstanding, all divided by a common language.

A final thought on social media comes from McLuhan's esoteric notion that when using the medium, "the sender gets sent."[34] If all media are means of communication, and if communication itself is just a means of getting the ideas in one person's mind into another person's mind, then we may say that all content is, in essence, an aspect of a person, and that the function of all media is to deliver this aspect of the person to someone else. When I interact with you in person, my body, my face, my voice, my thoughts and feelings expressed in speech and in physical gestures, and every other aspect of me brought into the interaction, will be conveyed through the medium of me, the person. When I digitalize the interaction, as in a Tweet or an Instagram, I'm forced by the medium itself to "send" only one aspect of me, a brief comment or image. Thus, me the "sender" is reduced to a very narrow range of information that is "sent."

Since most Tweets and Instagrams are sent to dozens, hundreds, or even thousands of recipients, their only knowledge of me comes from these circumscribed snippets of identity, because in the digital age of information, my digital identity is reduced and limited to the amount of information that can be "sent" as a Tweet or Instagram or Facebook comment. The social media user unknowingly accepts this reduction of identity as a condition of social media use. When my identity is self-reduced to that of a "sender" on social media, the message that's "sent" is not merely a single message, it's interpreted by the recipient as an expression of the entire me, not just as an expression of a tiny bit of me. That is, when I reduce my "self" to "sender," I reduce my identity to a single point of information being "sent," and thus, "the sender gets sent."

Conclusion
Media Mindfulness

The fact that we are more aware of those times when we do think explicitly to ourselves in words—and now conceive of all thought as taking place in words—should not deceive us into believing that language is necessary for thought. It could even be an impediment to it. Most forms of imagination, for example, or of innovation, intuitive problem solving, spiritual thinking or artistic creativity require us to transcend language, at least language in the accepted sense of a referential code. Most thinking, like most communication, goes on without language.

—McGilchrist (2009)[1]

The media that we engage in engages us. The media that we consume consumes us—voraciously eating up our time, energy, and attention with insatiable appetite. Parents and children nowadays are constantly at odds, primarily over the issue of media attention. Parents want children to turn off the games and screens so they can read books and focus on schoolwork. In essence, they're saying: "Turn off your preferred media, which are 'bad,' and turn your attention towards media that you don't prefer, which are 'good.'" (Also: "Never mind that we adults are just as immersed in screens as you are, and that as a population, we adults are reading less and less books in favor of more and more games, shows, and other non–literacy based media.")

As children grow into adolescents and adults, the same issues of engagement and disengagement are expressed in our inability to turn off our preferred media in order to go to sleep, or to engage in productive work, or to interact socially with others in person. Addictive disorders and chronic insomnia related to media use are universally experienced by nearly everyone in modern society at some point of their lives, if not all of their lives. The inability to disengage from media, in this sense, could be considered a fundamental psychological issue that affects

us all. Few people in the modern age are insusceptible to the forbidden fruit of media over-indulgence in the forms of media addiction and
binge media consumption. We're all, to some degree or another, being
consumed by our own media appetites.

In an environment saturated with information at every level—oral
language, literary language, imagistic symbols, streaming videos, digital communications—there's no escape from the onslaught of media.
To remove oneself completely from the media environment via sleep or
a practice of mindfulness meditation is helpful and necessary for survival; but just as one cannot sleep all the time, one cannot cloister oneself in mindfulness meditation all the time. Just like the fish out of water,
the average person cannot sustain ongoing total media deprivation and
remain functional in a modern world. Unless you're a monk in a monas-
tery, a nun in a nunnery, or a yogi seeking nirvana, we all need to engage
in our media environments much of the time in order to be productive
and functional members of our media saturated society. Hence, mindfulness as we currently understand it is extremely useful, but not a solution in and of itself.

What we need is a form of mindfulness not aimed at media deprivation (the fish out of water), but aimed at media understanding (the
fish *aware* of water). An occasional or even daily session of brief total
media deprivation would be a potentially helpful practice, to reacquaint
us with the anti-environment of a media-less environment. However, it's
extremely difficult to silence the most basic and most invasive form of
media, the words spoken to ourselves inside our own minds, the voice of
consciousness. Even the most experienced meditators battle the problem of keeping the inner voice silent for extended periods of time.

In order to really deal with the issues raised by media saturation,
we as a species need to create a form of media mindfulness that could
be practiced all the time; rather than just short 20-minute-a-day bursts
of total meditative dissociation from the media environment. We must
develop 16-hour-a-day stretches of media mindfulness, in which we're
aware of the effects of the media as we're actually using it, so we can
adjust our responses to media and our uses of media in adaptive ways.

Ultimately, the role of all media must be as "servomechanisms" to
people, rather than the other way around.

Chapter Notes

Preface

1. "We simply are not equipped with earlids." McLuhan (1962).
2. "One thing about which fish know exactly nothing is water, since they have no anti-environment which would enable them to perceive the element they live in." McLuhan (1968).
3. Comer, R.J. (2015), p. 115.

Introduction

1. Mcluhan (1965), *American scholar, V. 35* (p. 200).
2. Mcluhan (1966), *Mademoiselle, V. 64* (p. 114).
3. "Media Ecology" is a school of thought founded by media scholars such as Marshall McLuhan, Neil Postman, and Susanne Langer.
4. CDC (2014)
5. *Ibid.*
6. McLuhan (1962).

Chapter One

1. McGilchrist (2009), pp. 461-2.
2. Bergmann & Bergmann (2006), p. 990.
3. Weeks & James (1995), p. 76.
4. Rapin (1982), as quoted by Sacks (1998), p. 219.
5. Sacks (1998), p. 87.
6. McLuhan (1973). From the lecture, "Art as Survival in the Electric Age." Retrieved from *Understanding Me: Lectures and Interviews.* (McLuhan, S. & Staines, D., Eds.). Toronto: MIT Press.
7. McLuhan (1964).

Chapter Two

1. Albert Camus, "The Myth of Sisyphus" (1955).
2. Chomsky (1957).
3. Bradshaw & Rogers (1993), p. 322.
4. Bradshaw & Rogers (1993) summarizing Bradshaw & Netteleton (1981), p. 281.
5. Ringo et al. (1994).
6. *Notes sur la Vie*: "Notes on Life," Alphonse Daudet. Quote taken from James (1902), pp. 164–165.
7. Sperry as quoted in McGilchrist (2009), p. 122.
8. McGilchrist (2009).
9. Ramachandran (2011).
10. McGilchrist (2009).
11. Dobzhansky as quoted in Crow (2006), p. 793.
12. Aeschylus (1914).
13. McGilchrist (2009).
14. American Psychiatric Association (2013), p. 88. (The DSM-5's description of disorganized thinking as displayed in speech as symptomatic of schizophrenia).
15. de Saussure (1916), as quoted in Crow (1997), p. 135.
16. Donald (1991), pp. 272–3.
17. *Ibid.*, pp. 276–7.
18. McGilchrist (2009).
19. *Ibid.*
20. Chomsky (1957).
21. McLuhan (1962).
22. Kaas (2006).
23. McGilchrist (2009), pp. 209–33.
24. Abramson, M. & Goldinger, S.D. (1997).
25. McLuhan (1962), quoting Poe, p. 23.
26. McLuhan (1962), pp. 47 & 50.
27. As quoted by Scribner & Cole (1981), p. 14.

28. Sir Edward Dyer, 16th Century.
29. McLuhan (1962), p. 76.
30. The term "necessary distance" is from McGilchrist (2009).
31. McLuhan (1962), p. 22.
32. *Ibid.*
33. McLuhan (1962), p. 43.
34. *Ibid.*
35. Armstrong (2009), p. 133: "For the monks of medieval Europe, *lectio* reading") was not conducted simply to acquire information but was a spiritual exercise that enabled them to enter their inner world and there confront the truth revealed in scripture ... *lectio divina*, ruminating on the sacred page until it had become an interior reality."
36. McLuhan (1962): "In antiquity and the Middle Ages reading was necessarily reading *aloud*."
37. *Ibid.*, p. 54.
38. *Ibid.*
39. McLuhan (1964).
40. *Ibid.*, p. 252: "...the major trauma of the telegraph on conscious life, noting that it ushers in the Age of Anxiety and of Pervasive Dread."
41. Comer (2015), p. 130.
42. McGilchrist (2009), p. 256.
43. Fitzgerald (2014).
44. Comer (2015), p. 130.
45. McGilchrist (2009), pp. 63–4.
46. *Ibid.*, pp. 406–7.

Chapter Three

1. Panksepp as quoted by McGilchrist (2009), p. 244.
2. *Ibid.*
3. McLuhan (1964), p. 88.
4. Deacon (1997), p. 1.
5. *Ibid.*, p. 207.
6. *Ibid.*, p. 221.
7. *Ibid.*, p. 222.
8. Epidemiological statistics are all from the CDC (2020): https://www.cdc.gov/ncbddd/autism/data.html.
9. Boucher (2017), p. 93.
10. Kanner (1943).
11. Comer (2015), pp. 592–593.
12. Quotes are from Silberman (2015), p. 470, paraphrasing Gaugler et al. (2014).
13. Annett (2006) p. 247, and Rutter (1991).

14. Kanner (1943), as quoted in Silberman (2015), p. 182.
15. Kanner as quoted in Silberman (2015), p. 198.
16. Bauman & Kemper (2006).
17. Rimland (1964) p. 127.
18. Silberman (2015), p. 273, paraphrasing Clarke & Lupton et al. (2016).
19. Frith (2003).
20. Grandin (2013), p. 122.
21. Boucher (2017), p.153.
22. APA (DSM-V) (2013), p. 50.
23. McLuhan (1969), *Counterblast*, p. 132.
24. Langdell (1978), as paraphrased by Grandin (2013), pp. 120–1.
25. Boucher (2017), p. 41.
26. Grandin (2013), p. 145.
27. McGilchrist (2009), p. 47
28. Grandin (1986), pp. 28–9.
29. The lack of "earlids" is a famous McLuhanism.
30. McGilchrist (2009).
31. Tremlin (2006), p. 83–85, summarizing Baron-Cohen's theory.
32. McGilchrist (2009), p. 42.
33. *Ibid.*, p. 45.
34. Saxe et al. (2006), p. 288.
35. Tager-Flusberg (2006), p. 46.
36. *Ibid.*
37. In this instance I'm referring to autistic children who *do not* suffer from any intellectual disability related to organic neurological dysfunction, which may affect language development independently of their autism.
38. Asperger (1943), as quoted by Silberman (2015), p. 98.
39. *Ibid.*
40. *Ibid.*, pp. 98–99.
41. *Ibid.*, p. 299.
42. *Ibid.*, p. 103.
43. Rimland as quoted by Silberman (2015), p. 300.
44. *Ibid.*, p. 333.
45. Boucher (2017), pp. 47–8.
46. Mottron (2011), pp. 33–35.
47. *Ibid.*
48. *Ibid.*
49. Clarke et al. (2016).
50. Sacks (1995), pp. 252–3, quoting and paraphrasing Uta Frith (1989).
51. Silberman (2015), p. 469.
52. *Ibid.*, p. 252.
53. Westfahl (2006).
54. Anorexia is the "deadliest psychiat-

ric disorder" because the 10% fatality rate is the highest among all psychiatric disorders—Comer (2015), p. 351.

55. Silberman (2015), p. 10.
56. Grandin (2013), p. 16.
57. *Ibid.*, pp. 105–6.
58. Buchen (2011), p. 26.
59. Sacks (1995) on Temple Grandin, p. 275.
60. Grandin (2013), p. 17.
61. Grandin (2013), p. 200.
62. Grandin as quoted and paraphrased in Silberman (2015), p. 428.
63. Blume (1998).
64. *Ibid.*
65. Grandin (2013), p. 126.
66. Silberman (2015), p. 442.
67. McGilchrist, 2009), p. 256.

Chapter Four

1. Freud, Sigmund. (1917). "A Difficulty in the Path of Psycho-Analysis."
2. McGilchrist (2009), p. 14.
3. Carl Jung (1935), as quoted in Erdelyi (1978).
4. Jaynes (1976).
5. Crow (1997).
6. Comer (2015).
7. Crow (1997).
8. *Ibid.*
9. *Ibid.*
10. Schneider (1959).
11. Crow (1997), p. 128.
12. *Ibid.*
13. Nasrallah (1985) and Annett (1985).
14. Woods (1938), as quoted in Sass (1992), p. 127.
15. Crow (1999), pp. 122–123.
16. Rosenthal & Bigelow (1972).
17. McGilchrist (2009), pp. 212–3.
18. *Ibid.*
19. *Ibid.*
20. Crow (1996), p. 107.
21. Sommer et al. (2000).
22. Crow (1999), p. 123.
23. Sass (1992), p. 129.
24. *Ibid.*, p. 130.
25. Rapaport et al. (1968) as paraphrased and quoted by Sass (1992), p. 130.
26. Sass (1992), p. 130.
27. *Ibid.*, p. 131.
28. *Ibid.*, p. 136.
29. Goldstein (1964) as paraphrased and quoted by Sass (1992), p. 136.

30. Annett (2006) and Gottesman (1991).
31. Dr. Milton Diamond.
32. Jung (1961).
33. Master Chang Chou, 4th Century BCE.
34. Kurtz et al. (2001).
35. *Ibid.*
36. McGilchrist (2009), pp. 84–84.
37. APA (2013), pp. 87–100.
38. Leonhard & Brugger (1998), p. 180.
39. *Ibid.*
40. Rust et al. (1989).
41. Jaynes (1976), p. 432.
42. To be clear, Laing was referring to "insanity," i.e., schizophrenia, as a "rational adjustment," not just specifically the state of paranoia that is typically symptomatic of schizophrenia.
43. McLuhan (1962), p. 245.
44. Max Weber (1917).
45. McGilchrist (2009), p.92.
46. John Wingfield, *Atheism Closed and Open Anatomized* (1597), as quoted in Armstrong (1993), p. 288.
47. Armstrong (1993), p. 288.
48. The topic of the shift from spirituality to religiosity in the Western world is the central topic of my previous book, *The Digital God* (2015), in which this premise is explained much more thoroughly.
49. McGilchrist (2009), pp. 350–1.
50. "Outering" is another classic McLuhanism.
51. McLuhan (1964), p. 86.
52. McLuhan (1962), p. 18: "The interiorization of the technology of the phonetic alphabet translates man from the magical world of the ear to the neutral visual world."
53. McLuhan (1962), p. 21.
54. "Alienation" from our environment, from others, and from ourselves, was a leitmotif of existential psychologist Rollo May's (1953–1991) work.
55. McGilchrist (2009), p. 244.
56. McGilchrist (2009) uses the term "hyperconscious" often, citing Sass (1992).
57. McGilchrist (2009), p. 232.
58. *Ibid.*
59. *Ibid.*, p. 232.
60. *Ibid.*, p. 262.
61. *Ibid.*, p. 262.
62. *Ibid.*, p. 393.

63. Chris Firth as quoted by McGilchrist (2009), p. 395.
64. Nietzsche as quoted by McGilchrist (2009), p. 418.
65. McLuhan (1962), p. 193.
66. McGilchrist (2009), p. 404.
67. Jablensky (2000).
68. See Sass (1992), pp. 360–361.
69. Carothers (1959), p. 307.
70. Sass (1992), pp. 359–366.
71. *Ibid.*, p. 332.
72. Huxley (1944), p. 19.
73. The "double bind" situation, according to Gregory Bateson, is a situation in which an individual is forced to make a decision between two choices, with both choices resulting in a negative outcome. People who must live in environments filled with the "double bind" situation, in Bateson's theory, are stressed to the point of psychosis. My use of the term, in this instance, is rather broad.
74. van Os (2009), Picchioni (2007), and van Os (2004).
75. I owe the distinction between "specialist" and "nonspecialist" media to McLuhan.
76. Stetka (2015).
77. O'Keeffe, G., & Clarke-Pearson, K. (2011).
78. McGilchrist (2009), [paraphrasing Sass (1992)], p. 395.

Chapter Five

1. Comer (2015), p. 217.
2. *Ibid.*, pp. 130–131.
3. Shorter (2013) & Comer (2015), p. 130.
4. Altemus, M., Sarvaiya, N., & Eppersond, C.N. (2014).
5. Shorter (2013), p. 2.
6. Altemus, M., Sarvaiya, N., & Eppersond, C.N. (2014).
7. Sommer et al. (2008).
8. *Ibid.*
9. Shorter (2013), p. 86. The statement by Hippocrates was documented by Galen. Shorter was quoting Galen (130–210 AD) who was paraphrasing Hippocrates.
10. Shorter (2013), p. 58.
11. *Ibid.*, p. 110.
12. *Ibid.*, p. 118.
13. *Ibid.* (2013), pp. 124, 132–33.

14. APA (2013), p. 189.
15. Jaynes (1976), p. 462.
16. *Ibid.*, p. 124.
17. The line about happiness is quoted from dialogue spoken by Don Draper (Jon Hamm) in the AMC television series, *Madmen* (2007–2015).
18. McGilchrist (2009), p. 45
19. "Rumination theory" is from Comer (2015), p. 238.
20. McGilchrist (2012), p. 154.
21. Kirsch (2010).
22. Delgado et al. (1994).
23. Kirsch (2010), p. 80.
24. Comer (2015), p. 280.
25. Dragioti et al. (2017).
26. *Ibid.*
27. My construct of "media mindfulness" as a means of self-treating anxious depression is discussed briefly in the Conclusion of this book, and is planned to be the subject of a follow-up book.
28. McGilchrist (2009), pp. 84–5.
29. *Ibid.*, p. 84.
30. Comer (2015), p. 232.
31. Raichle, Marcus. (2001).
32. Buckner et al. (2008).
33. *Ibid.*
34. Pollan (2018), p. 304.
35. *Ibid.*
36. *Ibid.*, p. 305.
37. *Ibid.* (2018), p. 317.
38. Carr (2010), pp. 87–8.
39. National Center for Education Statistics (2014), the Program for the International Assessment of Adult Competencies.
40. McLuhan, M. (1960). Quote from the lecture, "Popular/Mass Culture: American Perspectives." Retrieved from *Understanding Me: Lectures and Interviews.* (McLuhan, S. & Staines, D., Eds.). Toronto: MIT Press.
41. McLuhan (1964), p. 5
42. McLuhan (1962), p. 214.

Chapter Six

1. Joseph Chilton Pearce as quoted in Healy (2002), p. 162.
2. Marshall McLuhan (1964), p. 316.
3. https://www.aoa.org/patients-and-public/eye-and-vision-problems/glossary-of-eye-and-vision-conditions/myopia

4. Mathematics in its elementary form (arithmetic), is essentially a form of literacy, i.e., a system of symbols with numbers in place of alphabetic letters, and arithmetical operators providing the syntactic rules or 'grammar' for combining symbols. (Arithmetic as a form of literacy is explained in more depth later on in this chapter.)

5. Healy (2002), p. 15.

6. https://www.cdc.gov/ncbddd/adhd/data.html

7. Friedman (2014).

8. *Ibid.*

9. *Ibid.*

10. Lanier (2010), p. 28.

11. McLuhan (1995), p. 302.

12. *Ibid.*, p. 250.

13. *Ibid.*

14. McLuhan & Powers (1989), pp. 37–8.

15. McLuhan (1967). Quote from the lecture, "Fordham University: First Lecture." Retrieved from *Understanding Me: Lectures and Interviews.* (McLuhan, S. & Staines, D., Eds.). Toronto: MIT Press.

16. McLuhan (1966).

17. UNESCO (2017). Reading the past, writing the future: Fifty years of promoting literacy. Paris: UNESCO. pp. 21–23, 26.

18. McLuahn & Powers (1989) p. 129.

19. West (1997), p. 113.

20. McLuhan (1972). Quote from the lecture, "The End of the Work Ethic." Retrieved from *Understanding Me: Lectures and Interviews.* (McLuhan, S. & Staines, D., Eds.). Toronto: MIT Press.

21. The term "age segregated culture" is commonly used in the field of developmental psychology. I don't know who originally coined the term.

22. McLuhan (1962), p. 17.

23. McLuhan (1995), p. 373. (Quote is from *Essential McLuhan*, taken from an excerpt from McLuhan's book, *Laws of Media: The New Science* (1988).

24. Though I didn't invent the term "school anxiety," the term is used often enough to be recognized as a common condition.

25. Clark (2005), p. 32.

26. Annett (2006), p. 245.

27. Geschwind & Galaburda (1987).

28. Geschwind and Behan (1984) (as cited in Geschwind & Galaburda (1987).

29. Grandin (1986), p. 144: "For example, autopsies of brains from dyslexics indicate that left cortex development is impaired, and neurons have grown in the wrong direction. Impairment on the left side could allow the right side of the brain to develop larger neural circuits. Albert Galaburda from the Harvard Medical School concludes: "Such a system could help explain the anecdotal evidence suggesting that among dyslexics there is a disproportionately large number of individuals with special talents in music, visual-spatial abilities and left handedness.'"

30. Wicks-Nelson & Israel (2015), pp. 266–7.

31. Healy (2002), p. 106.

32. Comer (2015).

33. Geschwind and Galaburda (1987).

34. Pinker (1994), p. 161.

35. Geschwind and Galaburda (1987), pp. 62–3.

36. *Ibid.*, p. 169.

37. Healy (2002), p. 142.

38. *Ibid.*, p. 138.

39. https://www.bdadyslexia.org.uk/dyslexia/neurodiversity-and-co-occurring-differences/dyscalculia-and-maths-difficulties

40. McLuhan (1969), p. 387.

41. Oppenheimer as quoted in McLuhan (1969), p. 345.

42. Geschwind & Galaburda (1987), p. 65.

43. Healy (2002), pp. 9 & 361(n).

44. Geschwind & Galaburda (1987), pp. 65–6.

45. Literacy expert Sylvia Richardson, as quoted in Healy (2002), p. 236.

46. Ellen Winner's research as summarized and quoted by Clark (2005), p. 86.

47. *Ibid.*, p. 87.

48. McCrone (1991), p. 134–7.

49. Indick (2015), pp. 46–7.

50. West (1997), p. 150.

51. Clark (2005), p. 88.

52. McGilchrist (2009), p. 47.

53. *Ibid.*, p. 276.

54. McLuhan (1962).

55. McLuhan (1968), p. 149.

56. West (1997), pp. 68–9.

57. *Ibid.*

58. Lanier (2010), p. 190.

59. McLuhan & Powers (1989), p. 14.

60. *Ibid.*

61. Healy (2002), p. 222.
62. *Ibid.*, p. 16.

Chapter Seven

1. McLuhan, *Playboy* interview (1969).
2. McGilchrist (2009), p. 107.
3. McLuhan (1964), p. 46.
4. *Ibid.*, p. 41.
5. *Ibid.*
6. McLuhan, *Playboy* interview (1969).
7. McLuhan did address the dichotomous roles of the twin hemispheres in our relationship with media. McGilchrist's coverage of the topic, however, is far more systematic and comprehensive.
8. McGilchrist (2009) p. 386.
9. See Martin Buber's seminal essay, *I and Thou* (1923).
10. McLuhan & Powers (1989), p. 4.
11. McLuhan (1964), p. 52.
12. My ideas about 'self-exposure' were in part inspired by McGilchrist's notion of passivity in modern technophilic culture: "They would see themselves as 'exposing' themselves before culture, like a photographic plate to light, or even think of themselves as '*being* exposed' to such things" (McGilchrist [2009], p. 433).
13. "*Oh, what a tangled web we weave / When first we practice to deceive!*" From the poem, *Marmion: A Tale of Flodden Field*, by Sir Walter Scott (1808).
14. "Transference" in psychoanalysis is when the patient unconsciously projects his own issues (typically with one of his parents), onto the psychoanalyst.
15. Torczyner (1977), p. 71.
16. "Temporal duality" as a "condition of the gods" is a point made by Joseph Campbell in his televised discussions with Bill Moyers in the PBS series, "The Power of Myth" (1991).
17. The terms "real self" and "idealized self" are derived from Adlerian personality theory.
18. Hurley, as quoted in Twenge & Campbell (2009), p. 121.
19. McLuhan (1967). Quote from the lecture, "Canada, the Borderline Case." Retrieved from *Understanding Me: Lectures and Interviews*. (McLuhan, S. & Staines, D., Eds.). Toronto: MIT Press.
20. Jung (1964).
21. Facebook use, especially, has been found to correlate with anxiety and depression, because Facebook is so ubiquitous and has been around so long, therefore it's been studied the most.
22. Tandoc et al. (2015), is just one study among many that has found a correlation between social comparison on social media and feelings of anxiety and depression among users.
23. *Ibid.*
24. Fardouly & Vartanian (2016).
25. Thornhill & Gangestad (1999).
26. Buss & Barnes (1986) & Rhodes (2006).
27. Møller & Thornhill (1998).
28. Bateson et al. (1956).
29. Laing (1960).
30. The psychological term "antisocial" actually refers to someone who actively and maliciously hurts others, i.e., a sociopath. For someone who refuses to engage in a communal social activity or gathering, the correct term would be "asocial."
31. McLuhan (1962), p. 36.
32. The entire discussion of McLuhan's tetrad is based on the model put forth in *The Global Village* (1989), by McLuhan and Powers.
33. *Ibid.*, pp. 175–178.
34. *Ibid.*, p, 173.

Conclusion

1. McGilchrist (2009), p. 107.

Bibliography

Abramson, M., & S.D. Goldinger. (1997). "What the reader's eye tells the mind's ear: Silent reading activates inner speech. "Perception and Psychophysics." Vol. 59 *(7)*, pp. 1059–1068.

Aeschylus. (1914). *Prometheus Bound.* Vol. VIII, Part 4. (E. H. Plumptre, translator). Harvard Classics. New York: P.F. Collier & Son.

Altemus, M., N. Sarvaiya, & C.N. Eppersond. (2014). Sex differences in anxiety and depression clinical perspectives. *Frontiers in Neuroendocrinology*, Vol. 35, Issue 3, 320–330.

American Psychiatric Association. (2013). *Diagnostic and Statistical Manual of Mental Disorders*, 5th Ed.: *DSM-5.* Arlington, VA: American Psychiatric Association.

Annett, M. (1985). *Left, Right, Hand and Brain: The Right Shift Theory.* London: Lawrence Erlbaum.

Annett, M. (2006). "The right shift theory of handedness and brain asymmetry in evolution, development, and psychopathology." *Cognition, Brain, Behavior,* Vol. X, No. 2, 235–250.

Armstrong, Karen. (1993). *A History of God: The 4,000-Year Quest of Judaism, Christianity, and Islam.* New York: Ballantine Books.

Bateson, G., D. Jackson, J. Haley, and J. Weakland. (1956). "Toward a Theory of Schizophrenia," *Behavioral Science* 1, 251–254. In Bateson, G. 1972. *Steps to an Ecology of Mind: A Revolutionary Approach to Man's Understanding of Himself.* New York: Ballantine Books.

Bauman, M.L., & T.L. Kemper, Editors. (2006). *The Neurobiology of Autism.* Baltimore: Johns Hopkins University Press.

Bergmann, Maria, & Martin Bergmann. (2006). A Psychoanalytic Study of Rembrandt's Self-Portraits. *The Psychoanalytic Review*, Vol. 93, No. 6.

Bergson, Henri. (1935). *The Two Sources of Morality and Religion.* Oxford: Oxford University Press.

Blume, H. (1998). "Neurodiversity: On the neurological underpinnings of geekdom. *The Atlantic,* September 1998.

Boucher, J. (2017). *Autism Spectrum Disorder: Characteristics, Causes, and Practical Issues,* 2nd ed. Los Angeles: Sage Publications, Inc.

Bradshaw, J.L., & N.C. Nettleton. (1981). "The nature of hemispheric specialization in Man. *Behavioral and Brain Sciences,* 4:51–91.

Bradshaw, J.L., & L.J. Rogers. (1993). *The Evolution of Lateral Asymmetries, Language, Tool Use, and Intellect.* New York: Academic Press, Inc., Harcourt Brace Jovanovich, Pubs.

Buber, Martin. (1923/1970). *I and Thou* (Walter Kaufman, trans.). New York: Charles Scribner's Sons.

Buchen, L. (2011). "Scientists and autism: When geeks meet." *Nature,* Vol. 479, pp. 25–27.

Buckner, R.L., J.R. Andrews-Hanna & D.L. Schacter. (2008). "The Brain's Default Network: Anatomy, Function, and Relevance to Disease." *Ann. N.Y. Acad. Sci.,* 1124, 1.

Buss, D. M., & M. Barnes. (1986). Preferences in human mate selection. *Journal of Personality & Social Psychology, Vol. 50,* pp. 559–570.

Campbell, Joseph, & Bill Moyers. (1991). *The Power of Myth.* New York: Anchor.

Carothers, J.C. (1959). "Culture, Psychiatry and the Written Word." *Psychiatry,* November 1959, 307–320.

Carr, N.C. (2010). *The Shallows: What the Internet Is Doing to Our Brains.* New York: W.W. Norton.

Chomsky, Noam. (1957/2005). *Syntactic Structures.* New York: Martino Fine Books.

Clark, A. D. (2005). *Dyslexia.* New York: Lucent Books.

Clarke, T-K, M. Lupton, A. Fernandez-Pujals and 20 additional coauthors. (2016). Common polygenic risk for autism spectrum disorder (ASD) is associated with cognitive ability in the general population. *Molecular Psychiatry, Vol.* 21, pp. 419–425.

Comer, R.J. (2015). *Abnormal Psychology,* 9th ed. New York: Worth Publishers.

Croen, L.A., J.K. Grether, & S. Selvin. (2002). Descriptive Epidemiology of Autism in a California Population: Who Is at Risk? *Journal of Autism and Developmental Disorders,* Vol. 32, Issue 3, pp. 217–224.

Crow, Timothy J. (1990). "Temporal Lobe Asymmetries as the Key to the Etiology of Schizophrenia." *Schizophrenia Bulletin, 16,* 3, 433–443.

Crow, Timothy J. (1996). "Language and psychosis: Common evolutionary origins." *Endeavour, 20,* 3, 105–109.

Crow, Timothy J. (1997). "Is schizophrenia the price that *Homo sapiens* pays for language?" *Schizophrenia Research, 28,* 127–141.

Crow, Timothy J. (1997). "Schizophrenia as failure of hemispheric dominance for language." *Trends in Neuroscience, 20,* 339–343.

Crow, Timothy J. (1998). "Nuclear schizophrenic as a window on the relationship between thought and speech." *British Journal of Psychiatry, 173,* pp. 103–109.

Crow, Timothy J. (1999). "Schizophrenia as the price that *Homo sapiens* pays for language: A resolution of the central paradox in the origin of the species." *Brain Research Reviews, 31,* 118–129.

Crow, Timothy J. (2006). "March 27, 1827 and what happened later—the impact of psychiatry on evolutionary theory." *Progress in Neuro-Psychopharmacology and Biological Psychiatry, 30,* 785–796.

Deacon, T.W. (1997). *The Symbolic Species: The Co-evolution of Language and the Brain.* New York: W.W. Norton.

Delgado, P., et al. (1994). Serotonin and the Neurobiology of Depression: Effects of Tryptophan Depletion in Drug-Free Depressed Patients. *Arch Gen Psychiatry,* Vol. 51 (11): 865–874.

Donald, Merlin. (1991). *Origins of the Modern Mind: Three Stages in the Evolution of Culture and Cognition.* Cambridge, MA: Harvard University Press.

Dragioti, E., V. Karathanos, B. Gerdle & E. Evangelou. (2017). "Does psychotherapy work? An umbrella review of meta-analyses of randomized controlled trials." *Acta Psychiatrica Scandinavica, Volume 136,* Issue 3.

Ehmke, R., & Child Mind Institute. (2019). How Using Social Media Affects Teenagers. Retrieved from https://childmind.org/article/how-using-social-media-affects-teenagers/

Erdelyi, M.H. (1978). "Dissociationism Revived." *Science, New Series,* Vol. 200, No. 4342, pp. 654–655.

Fardouly, J., & L.R. Vartanian. L. R. (2016). "Social Media and Body Image Concerns: Current Research and Future Directions." *Current Opinion in Psychology, 9 (Social media and applications to health behavior),* 1–5.

Fitzgerald, M. (2014). "Overlap between autism and schizophrenia: History and current status." *Advances in Mental Health and Intellectual Disabilities, 8, 1,* pp. 15–23.

Freud, Sigmund. (1927). *The Future of an Illusion.* New York: W.W. Norton.

Friedman, R.A. (2014). "A Natural Fix for A.D.H.D." *The New York Times,* October 31, 2014.

Frith, U. (2003). *Autism: Explaining the Enigma,* 2nd ed. Oxford: Blackwell.

Gaugler, T., et al. (2014). "Most genetic risk for autism resides with common variation." *Nature Genetics,* 46(8), pp. 881–5.

Geschwind, N., & P. Behan. (1984). "Laterality, hormones, and immunity." In Geschwind & Galaburda, eds. (1987), 211–224.

Geschwind, N. & A.M. Galaburda. (1987). *Cerebral Lateralization: Biological Mechanisms, Associations, and Pathology.* Cambridge, MA: MIT Press.

Goldstein, K. (1964). Methodological approach to the study of schizophrenic thought disorder. J.S. Kasmin, ed., *Language and Thought in Schizophrenia*. New York: W.W. Norton.

Goody, Jack. (1977). *The Domestication of the Savage Mind*. Cambridge, England: Cambridge Universoty Press.

Gottesman, I.I. (1991). *Schizophrenia genesis: The origins of madness*. New York: W.H. Freeman.

Grandin, Temple. (2013). *The Autistic Brain: Helping Different Kinds of Minds Succeed*. New York: Mariner Books. Houghton Mifflin Harcourt.

Grandin, Temple & Richard Panek (1986). *Emergence: Labeled Autistic, A True Story*. New York: Grand Central Publishing.

Haas, M.H., S.A. Chance, D.F. Cram, T.J. Crow, A. Luc, & S. Hage. (2015). "Evidence of Pragmatic Impairments in Speech and Proverb Interpretation in Schizophrenia." *Journal of Psycholinguistic Research, 44*, pp. 469–483.

Healy, J. M. (2002). *Different Learners: Identifying, Preventing, and Treating Your Child's Learning Problems*. New York: Simon & Schuster.

Huxley, Aldous. (1944). *The Perennial Philosophy*. New York: Harper & Brothers.

Huxley, Aldous. (1954). *The Doors of Perception*. New York: Harper & Row.

Indick, W. (2015). *The Digital God: How Technology Will Reshape Spirituality in the Digital Age*. Jefferson, NC: McFarland.

Jablensky, A. (2000). "Epidemiology of schizophrenia: The global burden of disease and disability." *European Archives of Psychiatry and Clinical Neuroscience, 250*, 274–285.

James, William. (1902). *The Varieties of Religious Experience: A Study in Human Nature*. New York: The Modern Library.

Jaspers, Karl. (1949). *The Origin and Goal of History*. London: Routledge & Kegan Paul.

Jaspers, Karl (2003). *The Way to Wisdom: An Introduction to Philosophy*. New Haven, CT: Yale University Press.

Jaynes, J. (1976). *The Origin of Consciousness in the Breakdown of the Bicameral Mind*. New York: Houghton Mifflin.

Jaynes, Julian. (1986). Consciousness and the voices of the mind. *Canadian Psychology*, Vol. 27 (2).

Jung, Carl G. (1961). *Memories, Dreams and Reflections*. New York: Random House.

Jung, Carl G. (1964). *Man and His Symbols*. New York: Doubleday.

Kaas, J.H. (2006). "Evolution of the neocortex." *Current Biology*, Vol. 16, No. 21, pp. 1–5.

Kanner, Leo. (1943). Autistic Disturbances of Affective Contact. *Nervous Child, V 2*, pp. 217–250.

Kanner, Leo. (1971). Follow-up study of eleven autistic children originally reported in 1943. *Journal of Autism and Childhood Schizophrenia, V 1*, pp. 112–145.

Ketteler, D., & S. Ketteler. (2010). "Is schizophrenia "the price that Homo sapiens pays for language"? Subcortical language processing as the missing link between evolution and language disorder in psychosis—A neurolinguistics approach." *Journal of Neurolinguistics, 23*, 342–353.

Kierkegaard, S. (1848). *Christian Discourses*. Copenhagen: Gyldenhal Publishers.

Kierkegaard, S. (1957). *The Concept of Dread*. Princeton, NJ: Princeton University Press.

Killingsworth, M.A., & D.T. Gilbert. (2010). "A Wandering Mind Is an Unhappy Mind." *Science*, Vol. 330.

Kohut, Heinz. (1971). *The Analysis of the Self: A Systematic Approach to the Psychoanalytic Treatment of Narcissistic Personality Disorders*. Chicago: University of Chicago Press.

Kuhn, R., & C.H. Cahn. (2004). "Eugen Bleuler's concepts of psychopathology." *History of Psychiatry, 15*, 361–6.

Kuijsten, Marcel. (2008). *Reflections on the Dawn of Consciousness: Julian Jaynes's Bicameral Mind Theory Revisited*. New York: Julian Jaynes Society.

Kurtz, M.M., P.J. Moberg, R.C. Gur, & R.E. Gur. (2001). "Approaches to cognitive remediation of neuropsychological deficits in schizophrenia: a review and meta-analysis." *Neuropsychology Review, 11* (4), pp. 197–210.

Laing, R.D. (1960). *The Divided Self: An*

Existential Study in Sanity and Madness. Harmondsworth: Penguin.

Laing, R.D. (1967). *The Politics of Experience and the Bird of Paradise.* Harmondsworth: Penguin.

Langdell, T. (1978). "Recognition of faces: An approach to the study of autism." *Journal of Child Psychology and Psychiatry and Applied Disciplines,* 19, no. 3: 255–68.

Lanier, Jaron. (2010). *You Are Not a Gadget: A Manifesto.* New York: Alfred A. Knopf.

Lasch, Christopher. (1979). *The Culture of Narcissism: American Life in an Age of Diminishing Expectations.* New York: W.W. Norton.

Leonhard, D., & P. Brugger. (1998). "Creative, Paranormal, and Delusional Thought: A Consequence of Right Hemisphere Semantic Activation?" *Neuropsychiatry, Neuropsychology, and Behavioral Neurology,* Vol. 11, No 4. pp. 177–183.

Markram, H., T. Rinaldi, & K. Markram. (2007). "The Intense World Syndrome—an alternative hypothesis for autism." *Frontiers of Neuroscience,* https://doi.org/10.3389/neuro.01.1.1. 006. 2007.

May, Rollo. (1953). *Man's Search for Himself.* New York: W.W. Norton.

May, Rollo. (1969). *Love and Will.* New York: W.W. Norton.

May, Rollo. (1975). *The Courage to Create.* New York: W.W. Norton.

May, Rollo. (1977). *The Meaning of Anxiety.* New York: W.W. Norton.

May, Rollo. (1983). *The Discovery of Being.* New York: W.W. Norton.

May, Rollo. (1991). *The Cry for Myth.* New York: W.W. Norton.

McCrone, John. (1991). *The Ape That Spoke.* New York: Avon Books.

McGilchrist, Iain. (2009). *The Master and His Emissary: The Divided brain and the Making of the Western World.* New Haven, CT: Yale University Press.

McGilchrist, Iain. (2012). *The Divided Brain and the Search for Meaning.* New Haven, CT: Yale University Press

McGilchrist, Iain. (2019). *Ways of Attending: How Our Divided Brain Constructs the World.* New York: Routledge.

McGuen, William G. (1988). *The*

Bicameral Brain and Human Behavior. New York: Vantage Press.

McLuhan, M. (1966). Quote from the lecture "The Medium Is the Massage." Retrieved from *Understanding Me: Lectures and Interviews.* (S. McLuhan & D. Staines, eds.). Toronto: MIT Press.

McLuhan, M. (1967). "Canada, the Borderline Case." Retrieved from *Understanding Me: Lectures and Interviews.* (McLuhan, S. & Staines, D., Eds.). Toronto: MIT Press.

McLuhan, Marshall. (1959). Quote from the lecture, "Electronic Revolution." Retrieved from *Understanding Me: Lectures and Interviews.* (S. McLuhan & D. Staines, Eds.). Toronto: MIT Press.

McLuhan, Marshall. (1962). *The Gutenberg Galaxy: The Making of Typographic Man.* Toronto: University of Toronto Press.

McLuhan, Marshall. (1964/2002). *Understanding Media.* New York: McGraw-Hill.

McLuhan, Marshall. (1967). *The Medium is the Massage.* New York: Random House, Inc.

McLuhan, Marshall. (1995). *Essential McLuhan.* (Eric McLuhan & Frank Zingrone, eds.). New York: Basic Books.

McLuhan, Marshall, & Quentin Fiore. (1968). *War and Peace in the Global Village.* New York: Simon & Schuster, Inc.

McLuhan, Marshall, & Bruce Powers. (1989). *The Global Village: Transformations in World Life and Media in the 21st Century.* New York: Oxford University Press.

Møller, A. P., & R. Thornhill. (1998). Bilateral symmetry and sexual selection: a meta-analysis. *American Naturalist. 151,* pp. 174–192.

Mottron, L. (2011) "The power of autism." *Nature,* Vol. 479, pp. 33–35.

Murray, D.B. & S.W. Teare. (1993). "Probability of a tossed coin landing on edge." *Physical Review E. 48 (4),* 2547–2552.

Nasrallah, H.A. (1985). "The unintegrated right cerebra hemispheric consciousness as alien intruder: A possible mechanism for Schneiderian delusions in schizophrenia. *Compr. Psychiatry, 26,* 273–282.

O'Keeffe, G., & K. Clarke-Pearson. (2011). "The Impact of Social Media on

Children, Adolescents, and Families." *Pediatrics, 127* (4): 800–804.

Ong, Walter J. (1982). *Orality and Literacy: The Technologizing of the Word.* New York: Routledge.

Piaget, Jean. (1929). *The Child's Conception of the World.* London: Kegan Paul, Trench, Trubner.

Piaget, Jean. (1952). *The Origins of Intelligence in Children.* New York: International University Press.

Picchioni, M.M., & R.M. Murray. (2007). "Schizophrenia." *British Medical Journal. 335* (7610): 91–5.

Pinker, S. (1994). *The Language Instinct.* New York: William Morrow.

Pollan, M. (2018). *How to Change Your Mind: What the New Science of Psychedelics Teaches Us About Consciousness, Dying, Addiction, Depression, and Transcendence.* New York: Penguin.

Raichle, M. E.; A.M. MacLeod, A.Z. Snyder, W.J. Powers, D.A. Gusnard, G.L. Shulman. (2001). "A default mode of brain function." Proceedings of the National Academy of Sciences of the United States of America. *98 (2):* 676–682.

Ramachandran, V.S. (2011). *The Tell-Tale Brain: A Neuroscientist's Quest for What Makes Us Human.* New York: W.W. Norton.

Rapaport, D., M. Gill, & R. Schafer. (1968). *Diagnostic Psychological Testing.* New York: International Universities Press.

Rapin, I. (1982). *Children with Brain Dysfunction: Neurology, Cognition, Language and Behavior.* New York: Raoen Press

Rhodes, G. (2006). The evolutionary psychology of facial beauty. *Annual Review of Psychology.* Vol. 57, pp. 199–226.

Ringo, J.L., R.W. Doty, D. Demeter, & P.Y. Simard. (1994). "Time is of the essence: A conjecture that hemispheric specialization arises from interhemispheric conduction delay." *Cereb. Cort., 4,* 331–343.

Rosenthal, R., & L.B. Bigelow. (1972). "Quantitative brain measurements in Chronic Schizophrenia." *British Journal of Psychiatry, 121,* 259–264.

Rust, J., S. Golombok, & M. Abram. (1989). "Creativity and schizotypal thinking." *Journal of Genetic Psychology, 150,* 225–227.

Rutter, M. (1991). "Autism as a genetic disorder." In P. McGuffin & R. Murray (Eds.) *The New Genetics of Mental Illness* (pp. 223–244). London: Butterwort-Heineman.

Sacks, Oliver. (1998). *The Man Who Mistook His Wife for a Hat and Other Clinical Tales.* New York: Touchstone.

Sagan, C. (1977). *The Dragons of Eden: Speculations on the Evolution of Human Intelligence.* New York: Ballantine.

Sagan, Carl, & Ann Druyan. (1992). *Shadows of Forgotten Ancestors: A Search for Who We Are.* New York: Random House.

Sass, L.A. (1992). *Madness and Modernism: Insanity in the Light of Modern Art, Literature and Thought.* Cambridge, MA: Harvard University Press.

Saxe, Rebecca, Laura E. Schulz, & Yuhong V. Jiang. (2006). "Reading minds versus following rules: Dissociating theory of mind and executive control in the brain." *Social Neuroscience, 1 (3–4):* 284–98.

Schneider, K. (1959). *Clinical Psychopathology.* New York: Grune and Stratton.

Scribner, S. & Cole, M. (1981). *The Psychology of Literacy.* Cambridge, MA: Harvard University Press.

Seaford, R. (2004). *Money and the Early Greek Mind: Homer, Philosophy, Tragedy.* Cambridge: Cambridge University Press.

Shaywitz, S. (2003). *Overcoming Dyslexia: A New and Complete Science-Based Program for Reading Problems at Any Level.* New York: Alfred A, Knopf.

Shorter, E. (2013). *How Everyone Became Depressed: The Rise and Fall of the Nervous Breakdown.* New York: Oxford University Press.

Silberman, S. (2015). *Neurotribes: The Legacy of Autism and How to Think Smarter about People Who Think Differently.* London: Allen & Unwin.

Sommer, I.E., et al. (April 2008). "Sex differences in handedness, asymmetry of the planum temporale and functional language lateralization." *Brain Research, 1206,* pp. 76–88.

Sommer, I.E.C., N.F. Ramsey, & R.S. Kahn. (2000). "Language lateralization in schizophrenia, an fMRI study." *Schizophrenia Research, 52,* 57–67.

Stetka, B. (2015). "Why Don't Animals Get Schizophrenia (and How Come We Do)? Research suggests an evolutionary link between the disorder and what makes us human." *Scientific American,* March Issue.

Tager-Flusberg, H. (2006). "Language and Communication Disorders in Autism Spectrum Disorders." In Bauman, M.L., & T.L. Kemper, (Editors), *The Neurobiology of Autism.* Baltimore: Johns Hopkins University Press.

Tandoc et al., "Facebook Use, Envy, and Depression Among College Students: Is Facebook Depressing?" *Comp. Human Behavior, 43,* 139–46 (2015).

Thornhill R., Gangestad S. W. 1999. Facial attractiveness. *Trends in Cognitive Science, 3.*

Torczyner, Harry. (1977). *Magritte: Ideas and Images.* New York: H. N. Abrams.

Tremlin, Todd. (2006). *Minds and Gods: The Cognitive Foundations of Religion.* New York: Oxford University Press.

Twenge, J., & K. Campbell. (2009). *The Narcissism Epidemic: Living in the Age of Entitlement.* New York: Free Press.

van Os, J. (2004). "Does the urban environment cause psychosis?" *British Journal of Psychiatry, 184* (4): 287–8.

van Os, J., & S. Kapur. (2009). "Schizophrenia." *Lancet, 374* (9690): 635–45.

Weeks, D., & J. James. (1995). *Eccentrics: A Study of Sanity and Strangeness.* New York: Villard Books.

West, Thomas G. (1997). *In the Mind's Eye: Visual Thinkers, Gifted People with Dyslexia and Other Learning Difficulties, Computer Images and the Ironies of Creativity.* New York: Prometheus.

Westfahl, Gary. (2006). *"Homo Aspergerus:* Evolution Stumbles Forward." *Locus Online.*

Wicks-Nelson, R., & A.C. Israel. (2015). *Abnormal Child and Adolescent Psychology,* 8th ed. New York: Pearson.

Wigan, A.L. (1844, 1985). *The Duality of Mind.* Malibu, CA: Joseph Simon.

Winchester, Simon. (2018). *The Perfectionists: How Precision Engineers Created the Modern World.* New York: HarperCollins.

Woods, W. (1938). "Language study in schizophrenia." *Journal of Nervous and Mental Disease, 87.*

Index

289

www.ingramcontent.com/pod-product-compliance
Lightning Source LLC
LaVergne TN
LVHW042123070326
832902LV00036B/569